PROGRESS IN OBSTETRICS AND GYNAECOLOGY

PROGRESS IN OBSTETRICS AND GYNAECOLOGY

Contents of Volume 4

PROGRESS IN OBSTETRICS AND GYNAECOLOGY
Volume Five

EDITED BY

JOHN STUDD MD MRCOG

Consultant Obstetrician and Gynaecologist
King's College Hospital and Dulwich Hospital, London

CHURCHILL LIVINGSTONE
EDINBURGH LONDON MELBOURNE AND NEW YORK 1985

CHURCHILL LIVINGSTONE
Medical Division of Longman Group UK Limited

Distributed in the United States of America by
Churchill Livingstone Inc., 1560 Broadway, New York,
N.Y. 10036, and by associated companies, branches and
representatives throughout the world.

First published 1985
  Reprinted 1986
  Reprinted 1990

ISBN 0 443 03268 8

ISSN 0261-0140

British Library Cataloguing in Publication Data
Progress in obstetrics and gynaecology.
  1. Gynaecology—Periodicals 2. Obstetrics
  —Periodicals
  618.05   RG1

Library of Congress Cataloging in Publication Data
Progress in obstetrics and gynaecology.
  Includes indexes.
  1. Obstetrics—Collected works. 2. Gynecology—
Collected works. I. Studd, John [DNLM: 1. Gynecology—
Periodicals. 2. Obstetrics—Periodicals. W1 PR675P]
RG39.P73   618   81-21699

Printed in Great Britain by Butler & Tanner Ltd, Frome, Somerset

Preface

I cannot hide the fact that Volume 5 of Progress in Obstetrics and Gynaecology is 'a posy of other men's flowers with nothing but the string that binds them my own'. Looking at the contents it is certainly no worse for that. The alpha to omega has been covered. From the immunology of pregnancy to post-partum problems in obstetrics. From puberty and intersex to the climacteric in gynaecology.

It is hardly possible to express my gratitude to those who have been willing to write for this series during the last five years. Perhaps one should not be surprised at the young lions in training anxious for recognition who produce excellent and punctual chapters. But it is a mystery why senior colleagues invariably accept these invitations for a fee that hardly covers secretarial expenses. It is a tribute to the academic and teaching instincts that heads of departments should be willing to spend so much of their spare time distilling in these reviews their vast experience and enthusiasm into the wisdom of some of the truly marvellous reviews in this volume. The adage that if one wants a job done give it to a busy man is well taken. I and the readers are greatly in their debt.

Of all the variables of training — location of jobs, research, Third World experience, etc — I am of the belief that the most important is to have the good fortune to fall under the influence — the spell — of a great teacher. Some never have that luck. I have had the good fortune to experience this on three occasions with three very different individuals. To the brilliant and eccentric Hugh McLaren I owe almost everything. A man who led by example and no one ever treated his trainees with more concern and decency. To Hugh Phillpott whose ability to pass on his knowledge, skills and commitment to our specialty was quite simply unforgettable. And to Bob Greenblatt's innovative work in so many fields who delighted his many friends and confounded his many critics by being right when the herd was off in the wrong direction. They are all men with the courage and integrity to take unpopular medical, social or political positions. Perhaps the minority is usually right after all! Certainly our profession needs this sort of iconoclastic teacher to question conventional wisdom and keep debate on the boil.

No publisher works fast enough for an unreasonable author or editor. It is only by more experience and comparisons in the publishing world that I can now appreciate the professionalism of Churchill Livingstone's handling of the Progress series. After 5 years I wish publicly to thank Sylvia Hull for her efforts and particularly Mary Lindsay for her prompt and efficient editing.

Contributors

Per B. Bergsjø MD
Professor of Obstetrics and Gynaecology, University of Bergen; Head of Department of Obstetrics and Gynaecology (Kvinne-Klinikken), Haukeland Hospital, Bergen, Norway

Robert C. Cefalo MD PhD
Professor of Obstetrics and Gynaecology; Director, Maternal-Fetal Medicine Department, University of North Carolina School of Medicine, USA

Geoffrey Chamberlain MD FRCS FRCOG
Professor of Obstetrics and Gynaecology, St George's Hospital Medical School, London, UK

Dennis A. Davey PhD FRCOG
Professor of Obstetrics and Gynaecology; Director of Reproductive Medicine Research Unit, University of Cape Town, South Africa

Jacques R. Ducharme MD MSc(Med)
Professor of Paediatrics, Universite de Montreal; Director, The Paediatric Endocrine Research Laboratory Unit of Reproductive and Developmental Biology, Hospital Sainte Justine, Montreal, Canada

Charles C. Egley MD FACS FACOG
Fellow in Maternal and Fetal Medicine and Clinical Instructor, University of North Carolina School of Medicine, USA

H. Gee MD MRCOG
Lecturer, Department of Obstetrics and Gynaecology, University of Birmingham, UK

P. F. H. Giles MSc FRCOG FRACOG
Associate Professor, Department of Obstetrics and Gynaecology, University of Western Australia, Perth, Australia

W. F. Hendry ChM FRCS
Consultant Urologist, Shelsea Hospital for Women and St Bartholomew's and Royal Marsden Hospitals, London, UK

Anthony Kenney FRCS MRCOG
Consultant Obstetrician and Gynaecologist, St Thomas's Hospital, London, UK

R. Kumar MD PhD MPhil(Psychiat) MRCPsych
Senior Lecturer and Honorary Consultant Psychiatrist, Institute of Psychiatry, Bethlem Royal and Maudsley Hospitals, London, UK

F. E. Loeffler FRCS FRCOG
Consultant Gynaecologist and Obstetrician, St Mary's Hospital and Queen Charlotte's Hospital for Women, London, UK

Mary Ann Lumsden MSc MRCOG
Registrar in Obstetrics and Gynaecology, The Royal Infirmary, Edinburgh, UK

John McEwan MA FRCGP
Consultant/Senior Lecturer in Family Planning, King's College Hospital and Medical School; General Practitioner, Southwark, London, UK

I. R. McFadyen FRCOG
Consultant Obstetrician and Gynaecologist, Northwick Park Hospital and Clinical Research Centre, Harrow, UK

Alexander McMillan MD FRCP(Ed)
Consultant Physician, University Department of Genitourinary Medicine, Royal Infirmary, Edinburgh, UK

John M. Monaghan FRCS(Ed) FRCOG
Consultant Surgeon to the Northern Regional Gynaecological Oncology Department, Queen Elizabeth Hospital, Gateshead; Honorary Consultant to the Newcastle upon Tyne Teaching Hospitals, UK

John R. Newton MD FRCOG
Professor of Obstetrics and Gynaecology, University of Birmingham, UK

K. H. Nicolaides BSc MRCOG
Lecturer, Harris Birthright Research Centre for Fetal Medicine, Department of Obstetrics and Gynaecology, King's College Hospital School of Medicine, London, UK

C. H. Rodeck BSc MRCOG
Director, Harris Birthright Research Centre for Fetal Medicine, Department of Obstetrics and Gynaecology, King's College Hospital School of Medicine, London, UK

L. J. Sant-Cassia MD MRCOG
Senior Registrar, Birmingham and Midland Hospital for Women, Birmingham, UK

James S. Scott MD FRCSE FRCOG
Professor of Obstetrics and Gynaecology, University of Leeds; Honorary Consultant Obstetrician and Gynaecologist, Leeds Western Health Authority, Leeds, UK

S. K. Smith MD MRCOG
Lecturer, University Department of Obstetrics and Gynaecology, Jessop Hospital for Women, Sheffield, UK

Gordon M. Stirrat MA MD FRCOG
Professor of Obstetrics and Gynaecology, University of Bristol, UK

M. I. Whitehead MRCOG
Senior Lecturer and Consultant Gynaecologist, Department of Obstetrics and Gynaecology, King's College Hospital Medical School, London, UK

Barry G. Wren MD MHP(Ed) FRACOG FRCOG
Associate Professor of Obstetrics and Gynaecology, University of New South Wales; Visiting Medical Officer, Royal Hospital for Women, Paddington, New South Wales, Australia

Arthur Wynn MA(Camb)
Chief Scientific Officer, Government Scientific Service (retired), UK

Contents

PART TWO: GYNAECOLOGY

PART ONE

Obstetrics

Immunology of pregnancy

To be asked to write about the immunology of pregnancy is akin to a request to discuss the biochemistry of pregnancy. The scope of both is vast. Why then is it impossible to contemplate a comprehensive summary of the latter within the confines of 4–5000 words? The reason is that our knowledge of biochemistry in general and in pregnancy in particular is so much greater than our understanding of immunology. There is, however, no doubt that more progress has been made in general immunology over the past 20 years than in the 100 years from the time of the original discoveries by Jenner and Pasteur which created the new discipline. The immunological implications of pregnancy have only been perceived since Medawar & Sparrow (1956) made their observations in mice. In reproductive immunology it is only within the last decade that a significant body of knowledge has begun to accumulate which can be described as hard scientific fact.

What follows is a distillation of the current understanding of the immunobiology of the feto-maternal relationship as a guide for the bemused clinician. All the data discussed are either referenced specifically or mentioned within referenced overviews.

BASIC IMMUNOLOGY

The presence of a gene system located within a circumscribed chromosomal region which controlled graft rejection was first described 40 years ago. The genes involved were subsequently called the *major histocompatibility complex* (MHC). It was predicted that a similar genetic system would be present in all mammalian species including man. Since no 'in-bred' strains of humans exist, the research into the MHC in man was carried out using the sera from a large number of multiparous women tested against an even greater number of leucocytes taken from unrelated donors. The multiparous sera contained antibodies which had been induced by paternally derived tissue in the fetus. Under appropriate experimental conditions, the extent to which these sera destroyed the donor leucocytes was directly proportional to the genetic differences between them. From statistical analyses of these results, subsequently confirmed by extensive family studies, the presence of an MHC

3

in man was confirmed. Because it was first defined on leucocytes this system was called the human leucocyte system A or HLA. From what has been learned subsequently, we now know that:

1. The MHC is located on chromosome 6.
2. It consists of at least four major subregions or loci now named HLA-A, -B, -C and -D. The D subregion probably contains several loci of which 3 (DR, DC and SB) have so far been recognised.
3. The HLA gene combination on one parental chromosome (called a *haplotype*) is usually passed on as a complete unit. We therefore inherit one haplotype from our mother and one from our father as shown in Fig. 1.1. In general, only four combinations can be passed on from any two parents.

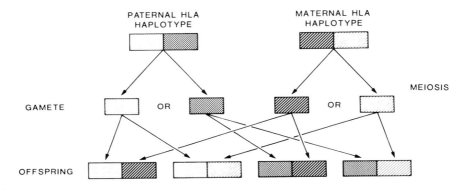

Fig. 1.1 The inheritance of HLA gene combinations (haplotypes)

4. Each haplotype contains genetic contributions from the four main loci. During human development the polypeptide structure of the genes has diversified to the extent that in any one individual each locus contains two of a large number of alternative genes (*alleles*), more of which are constantly being discovered. The end result of this diversity or *polymorphism* is that the number of possible haplotypes is over 1700 with close to 10^6 genotypes. The likelihood of any one unrelated individual being HLA identical to another is, therefore, remote.
5. Each genetic locus codes for the production of glycoproteins which have important functions in the initiation and control of immune mechanisms which are discussed below. The glycoproteins produced by the HLA-A, -B and -C loci are called Class I major histocompatibility antigens: those produced by HLA-D are Class II major histocompatibility antigens. Class I antigens are expressed on the surface of most cells. Class II antigens are only found on certain immunologically active cells. The importance of this difference will become apparent later.

The biochemical structure of these gene products has only begun to become apparent (Peterson et al 1983) and a stylised version of current understanding is shown in Fig. 1.2.

It is becoming increasingly clear that the structure of these antigens is integral to their function which is basic to immunological reactions. It is through the balance of similarities and differences between them that these MHC gene products exert influences which initiate, control, amplify and suppress the immune response at a cellular level.

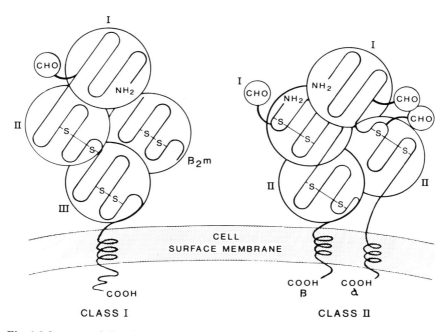

Fig. 1.2 Structure of Class I and II MHC antigens. Class I antigens consist of three convoluted protein chains (or domains), a transmembrane region and a cytoplasmic tail. Another protein β_2 microglobulin is always bound to domain III. Class III antigens have two close but unbound chains (α & β), each of which has two extracellular domains, transmembrane segments and short cytoplasmic tail. The second domain of Class II, and one-third domain of Class I are biochemically similar to one another and do become part of the immunoglobulin molecule

Cells of the immune response (Fig. 1.3)

The most important cells of the immune response are *lymphocytes*. Although lymphocytes look similar, they divide functionally into several different populations. The two major types are:

1. B cells, precursors of the plasma cells which secrete specific antibodies
2. T cells, the orchestrators and drivers of the immune response. Among the most important sub-populations of T cells are those which help B

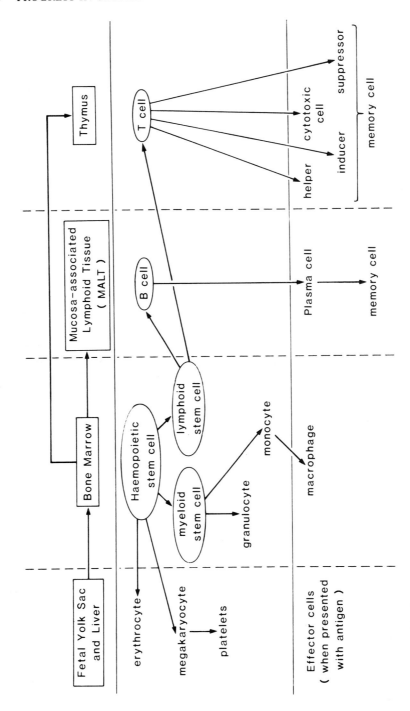

Fig. 1.3 Cells of the immune response

cells to produce antibody (helper T cells), those which kill foreign cells (cytotoxic T cells), those which keep immune reaction within reasonable bounds (suppressor T cells), and those which induce the appropriate reaction in other T cells (inducer T cells).

Macrophages are also important immunologically because they both process antigens for presentation to lymphocytes and act as phagocytes once the battle is over.

Other lymphocyte-like mononuclear cells exist which are also relevant and to these has been given such names as K (for killer) and NK (for natural killer) cells.

Origins of immunologically active cells

Stem cells from which immunologically active cells will arise can be found within the fetal yolk sac within 4 weeks of fertilisation. As can be seen from Fig. 1.3, the bone marrow plays an important part in the maturation of these cells and is their most important source in later life.

A significant proportion of the bone marrow derived stem cells migrate to the thymus where they appear initially in the sub-capsular cortex. Most die within the cortex but about 15% migrate successfully to the medulla where they mature into functionally active T-cells. The amazing thymus is only active during growth and atrophies, with consequent loss of function, when adult stature is achieved. Indeed lymphoid cells processed by the thymus during embryonic and early developmental life may well make up the total T-cell population of the adult. It is while they are within the thymus that the lymphocytes are programmed to discriminate between self and non-self. The exact mechanism by which this is achieved is unknown but the fact that the supporting cells of the cortex and medulla express Class I and II MHC antigens respectively in high-density is probably highly relevant.

About 1% of the total lymphocyte population enters and leaves the thymus daily, moving on to populate the peripheral lymphoid tissue and the lymph-nodes in particular. Mature T-cells probably live as long as the host.

While maturing in the thymic medulla the T-cells develop a receptor for antigens. In those T-cells which are destined to have a cytotoxic or suppressor function, the antigen receptor bears a striking resemblance to Class I MHC antigen. Inducer and helper T-cells carry a receptor resembling Class II MHC antigens. This is integral to the way in which these cells recognise foreign antigens for they can only do so when the antigens are in a cell surface membrane which also contains a MHC molecule which they can recognise. Thus for a T-cell to induce an immune response either by acting on other T-cell populations or by helping B cells produce antibody, it must be able to recognise part of its own Class II MHC antigen make-up in the surface membrane of the foreign antigen. Likewise for an effector response by cytotoxic or suppressor T-cells, part of their own Class I MHC antigen composition must also be present on the foreign cell surface. We will see later how important this mechanism is in the immunology of pregnancy.

IMMUNOLOGICAL ASPECTS OF FERTILITY

The regular insemination of many millions of spermatozoa in a fluid with a high protein content into the vagina will only be relevant immunologically if the sperm and seminal plasma are potentially antigenic and if the female genital tract is capable of mounting an immune response.

Antigenicity of sperm

It is likely that both Class I and II histocompatibility antigens are present on sperm once they have left the epididymis, so, like any other 'graft' between unrelated individuals, they are potentially antigenic. Major blood group antigens have been clearly demonstrated on the surface of spermatozoa. ABO antigens are probably passively acquired from seminal plasma and, to a lesser extent, inclusive components of the sperm membrane. It is, however, somewhat puzzling, but fortunate, that the naturally occurring blood group antibodies in cervical mucus do not agglutinate sperm carrying the relevant A or B antigen. Interestingly, rhesus system antigens do not seem to be expressed. If they were, methods to select out sperm carrying D would have been one way to prevent iso-immunisation in susceptible women. Lesser blood group antigens such as Lewis, MNSs and P, can be found on sperm.

In addition, several sperm-specific antigens have been detected. By their very nature, some of these could cause an auto-immune response if sperm escaped beyond the tubules. They are normally prevented from doing so by the tight junction zones between Sertoli cells.

New evidence using monoclonal antibodies suggests that some sperm-specific antigens are only expressed before capacitation while others only appear afterwards (Menge et al 1983). A sperm-specific lactic dehydrogenase (LDH-C4) has a potential for antigenicity (Goldberg et al 1983) which is being pursued as a potential contraceptive (see p 20).

Antigenicity of seminal plasma

A great deal of information exists but most of it is irrelevant to the question posed here because it involves immunisation of rodents or rabbits with seminal plasma. Up to 15 antigenic components have been described. All but six are also present in human serum and live extracts. Of these one derived from seminal vesicles was designated sperm coating antigen (SCA) before it was found to be a lactoferrin. It is known to be bacteriostatic and this may be one of its physiological functions in seminal plasma.

Immune responses in the female genital tract

There is little doubt on morphological grounds and from experimental evidence that the female genital tract is fully capable of mounting an immune response. Lymphoid cells (including plasma cells) are present in the mucosa of the tract. They are, however, less abundant than in gut or bronchus. It is equally clear that the survival of sperm in the tract is not merely due to its failure to recognise them. Unfortunately little more is known about the immunobiology of the interaction.

The concentration of antibodies in ovarian follicular fluid varies directly with the size of the various immunoglobulins (i.e. relative to blood IgG > IgA > IgM). This suggests passive transfer. The concentration of immunoglobulin in cervical mucus has the same gradation, as shown below:

IgG concentration	up to 6 mg/ml
IgA concentration	up to 1.4 mg/ml
IgM concentration	traces only

Levels are highest during the follicular and luteal phases with a sharp mid-cycle fall. The same fluctuation applies to C_3, one of the important components of complement. These may be no more than dilutional effects consequent on a marked rise in other constituents.

Information on cell-mediated immunity is virtually totally confined to experimental animals. Enlargement of the lymph-nodes draining the uterus as a result of copulation has been noted in rodents and is circumstantial evidence of an immune response. Lack of lymphatics in the endometrium has led to the suggestion that this may prevent induction of an 'immune response'. 'Blocking factors' have also been postulated but none of the evidence provided is firm. For a detailed review of the data up to 1980 the reader is referred to Hogarth (1982). Little new has been added on this issue over the last 4 years.

In summary, therefore, both sperm and semen are potentially antigenic and the female genital tract is immunocompetent. Deleterious immune responses leading to infertility do sometimes occur but they are not common given the population 'at risk'. This is discussed under 'clinical aspects'. Evidence for a facilitating response is circumstantial at best.

IMMUNOLOGY OF IMPLANTATION AND PLACENTATION

The unfertilised ovum poses no immunological problems, being entirely derived from the mother. It is post-fertilisation and particularly in implantation and placentation that the most acute theoretical problems arise.

Pre-implantation

As the zygote traverses the Fallopian tubes its protection may depend on the following:

1. Paternally derived antigens are not expressed from the moment of fertilisation. They have, however, become apparent by the 8 cell stage. The exception to this is the MHC antigens which are thought not to be expressed on the pre-implantation trophectoderm.
2. The immunologically bland zona pellucida may provide some protection at this critical stage.
3. An early pregnancy factor (EPF), the nature of which is unknown, has been described and may have some function in suppressing potentially harmful immune reactions before implantation (for review see Roberts & Smart 1983).

Peri-implantation

By 4 to 5 days after fertilisation the morula has reached the 50–60 cell stage to form the blastocyst. It has already differentiated into the trophoblast which invades the uterine wall and establishes the placenta, and the embryoplant from which the embryonal ectoderm, mesoderm and endoderm develop.

Between day 7 after fertilisation, when implantation begins, and day 14, when it is complete, the most amazing sequence of events takes place which involves the rapid but totally controlled invasion of the maternal tissues by a semi-alien parasite. If this intimate juxtaposition of genetically dissimilar tissues is to be successful, some major deviations from the immunological norm are necessary. The trophoblast is at the forefront of this invasion and it is of it that the most exacting immunological questions are asked. The most vital of these is, does trophoblast express MHC antigens at this stage? Figures 1.4–1.6

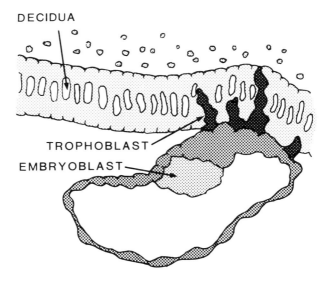

Fig. 1.4 Day 7 — trophoblast begins to invade maternal decidua

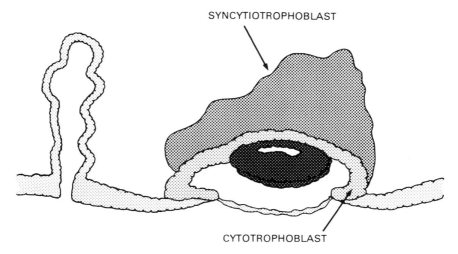

Fig. 1.5 Day 8 — Syncytiotrophoblast (derived from cytotrophoblast) invades into endometrial stroma

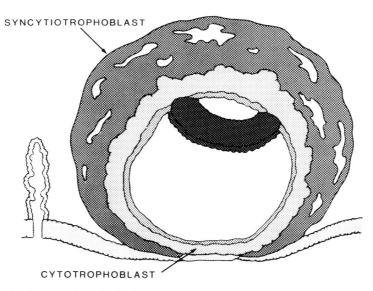

Fig. 1.6 Day 10 — implantation is almost complete

show the sequence of events surrounding implantation with particular reference to trophoblast. As far as can be determined, neither the syncytiotrophoblast nor the cytotrophoblast, closely related to it and from which it is derived, express Class I or II antigens around the time of implantation. An immune response can therefore neither develop nor be effective if it did (see p 7).

It is between days 12 and 14 that the enigma is most acute. Figure 1.7 shows that the cytotrophoblast columns which have formed primary villi within the invading cell columns push through the syncytium to form the cytotrophoblast shell surrounding the whole conceptus. Figure 1.8 is a photomicrograph of one of these cell columns stained with a monoclonal antibody specific for Class I MHC antigens. The dark staining of the column shows that a high percentage of cells — but not the cytotrophoblast from which it sprang — are expressing Class I MHC antigens. Why then does an immune response not develop? The main reason is likely to hinge round the absence of Class II antigens. As we have noted previously, the presence of Class II antigens is required for the induction of an immune response. It also seems likely that the Class I MHC antigens seen here are somehow biochemically different from the HLA-A, -B or -C of the adult (Redman et al 1984).

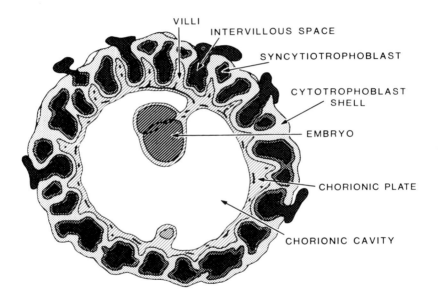

Fig. 1.7 Day 12–14 — The cytotrophoblast shell surrounds the whole conceptus

Post-implantation placentation

All the elements of the haemochorial placenta are developed by day 21–28. In particular feto-maternal interchange has begun. Trophoblast in all its forms remains at the forefront of the feto-maternal interface. Figure 1.9 demonstrates the possible inter-relationships between the various trophoblastic sub-populations. In Figure 1.10 chorionic villi from a term placenta are stained with a monoclonal antibody to Class I MHC antigens and counterstained with haematoxylin. The villous stroma is strongly positive for Class I antigens but the syncytiotrophoblast, of which the counterstained nuclei are all that can be

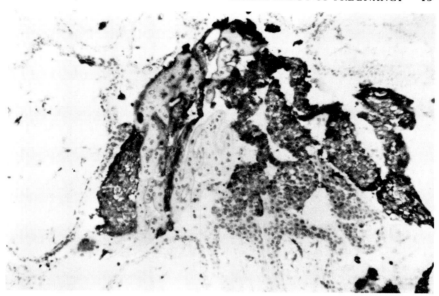

Fig. 1.8 Cytotrophoblast cell column going to make up shell stained for MHC antigens

seen, is entirely negative. In our experience, expression of Class I MHC antigens can be found on all forms of mature trophoblast other than that forming or derived from the chorionic villi (Redman et al 1984). However, the expression is not uniform, amounting to 50% of cells in most sections studied. In Figure 1.11 we see one of the most amazing phenomena of pregnancy — the migration of trophoblast along a maternal spinal arteriole. It can be seen that the trophoblast, which has been positively identified by the appropriate specificity controls, expresses Class I MHC antigens. Its protection too probably depends on the absence of Class II antigens.

Faulk and his colleagues (1978) have proposed the presence of another set of important trophoblast antigens, some of which are shared by lymphocytes.

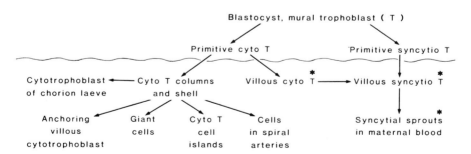

Fig. 1.9 Possible interrelationships between the various trophoblastic sub-populations. All non-primitive trophoblast expresses Class I MHC antigens except those marked*. None express Class II MHC antigens

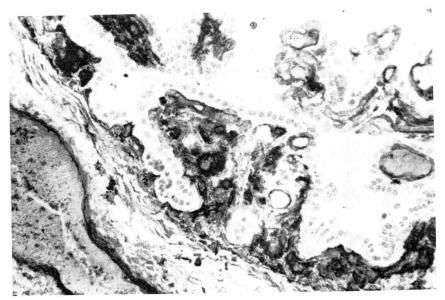

Fig. 1.10 Term placenta stained for MHC antigens. Chorionic villi are negative

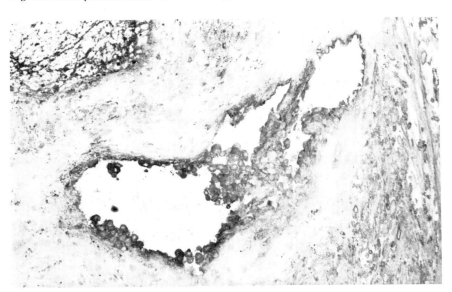

Fig. 1.11 Maternal spiral artery lined by trophoblast which is expressing Class I antigens

They have designated these TLX (for trophoblast-lymphocyte cross reactive) antigens and suggest that their expression on trophoblast might be protective by directly or indirectly modulating lymphocyte functions. Although the presence of antigens shared by trophoblast and lymphocytes has been confirmed (Johnson et al 1981), they have yet to be defined biochemically and no hard evidence exists about any proposed function.

MATERNAL IMMUNE RESPONSES DURING PREGNANCY

This is the most controversial area in reproductive immunology, and anyone trying to review it is faced with a mass of conflicting and confusing data in relation to both cellular and humoral immunity.

Cell-mediated immunity

This term is often used rather loosely in the literature to include general, non-specific aspects of lymphocyte activity. Changes in numbers, non-specific reactivity and the effects of pregnancy-associated proteins and hormones have been used to support rather tenuous hypotheses which explain the success of the fetal allograft in terms of depression of maternal immune reactivity. Non-specific mechanisms are unlikely to be important, particularly in the face of an otherwise normally responsive maternal immune system.

The question remains, 'Does the mother become specifically sensitised to fetal antigens and does she, as a consequence, produce effector lymphocytes against the paternal component of these antigens?' Several techniques have been used over the last 10–15 years to address that question. The details of the methods need not concern us here but the concept behind each of them is the same — specific sensitisation of maternal lymphocytes to fetal or paternal antigens can be detected by their ability to undergo cell division and proliferation as in the mixed lymphocyte reaction (MLR), release detectable quantities of substances called lymphokines such as macrophage migration inhibition factor (MIF), or kill radioactive labelled paternal or fetal cord lymphocytes. The literature (reviewed by Sargent & Redman 1984) contains many reports of positive results in these assays. Unfortunately it is difficult to interpret much of the data from the MLR and MIF assays because the observed effects could have been generated *in vitro*. Time-course studies (which avoid that criticism) using both assays concurrently have failed to find any evidence whatsoever of maternal sensitisation in first or subsequent pregnancies (Sargent et al 1982). Nor has it proved possible to confirm the consistent presence of maternal cells which are cytotoxic to paternal or fetal lymphocytes (Sargent & Redman 1984, Vanderbeecken et al 1984). An effect which can only be demonstrated in some women cannot, by definition, be an intrinsic protective mechanism for pregnancy. On the other hand, the pregnancies in which specific anti-fetal sensitisation occurred suffered no ill effects as a result. Sargent & Redman (1984) conclude, 'There is no evidence that maternal cell-mediated sensitisation to the fetus and production of specific effector cells is a *regular* event in normal pregnancy'. What then prevents it? To explore that question further we must look at humoral immunity.

Humoral immune response

Some pregnant women undoubtedly develop antibodies directed against paternal MHC antigens. There is, however, debate about the proportion who do so in first and subsequent pregnancies. Terasaki et al (1970) found that cytotoxic anti-paternal allo-antibodies (i.e. against HLA) could be found in only 17% of primiparous women and 45% of women who had had four or more pregnancies. Mowbray (personal communication) suggests that in his experience it is the exception for women *not* to develop antibodies against Class I antigens even in a first pregnancy. There is little firm evidence about antibodies directed against Class II MHC antigens.

Several authors propose an important function for these antibodies. Voisin (1983) suggests that these paternal specific antibodies are of the type which will block a harmful immune response, thereby protecting the fetus. There may be evidence for blocking antibody production in some experimental animals but their relevance in human pregnancy is open to question. On the basis of current data it is safest to conclude with Sargent & Redman (1984) 'that the role of blocking antibodies has yet to be defined and it may be that they are merely the consequence and not the cause of a successful pregnancy'. Voisin (1983) and Wegmann (1983) suggest that one important function of the placenta is to act as a sponge or immunoabsorbent for all potentially harmful antibodies.

Two important questions remain. Firstly, against what Class I MHC antigen bearing tissue are these antibodies directed? Although tiny sprouts or buds of syncytiotrophoblast are consistently shed into the maternal circulation we have already noted that this tissue does not express MHC antigens. It is unlikely that fetal leucocytes regularly cross into the maternal circulation (or *vice versa* for that matter) during normal pregnancy. Therefore this is unlikely to be the cause. In fact we do not know for certain the antigenic stimulus. The presence of Class I MHC antigens on the anchoring villi of the placenta intimately related to maternal tissues may be relevant but this is speculative.

The second question is, if these antibodies perform such a basic protective immune function as is proposed, why can they not be found in every pregnancy? According to Billington & Bell (1983) a maternal humoral immune response is not consistent and, indeed, is restricted in relation to the stage of pregnancy, the parity, genotype and immune responsiveness of the mother, and the titre, nature and specificity of the alloantibody produced. They conclude that, on current evidence, 'the high degree of variability in pregnancy-induced alloantibody formation would appear to present serious difficulties in postulating any essential function(s) in the fetal-maternal relationship'.

The hypothesis that the trophoblast and lymphocytes share an important series of antigens called TLX (Faulk et al 1978) has already been noted. These authors have further suggested that a blocking antibody to one set of TLX antigens prevents an immune attack on the trophoblast. Such antibodies have yet to be found in pregnancy sera.

What then is the overall message? It is likely to be that the main protective mechanism in fact of the immunological disparity between mother and fetus is the absence of MHC antigens from the trophoblast. There may be additional and secondary mechanisms but despite many hypotheses and much work, their role in human pregnancy remains unclear.

CLINICAL ASPECTS OF REPRODUCTIVE IMMUNOLOGY

No physiological mechanism functions perfectly at all times and under all circumstances. The clinical problems to which immunological defects have been most frequently attributed and for which immunological remedies have been sought in some cases are male and female infertility, recurrent spontaneous abortion, pre-eclampsia and placental abruption. The main purpose of the following brief overview is to counsel clinical caution. Our immune system is at the very heart of our integrity as individuals and in the vanguard of our fight against hostile forces from without. Potent non-specific suppressors or stimulators of our immune system may in the short-term seem to convey benefit but the long-term price paid by the individual may be high in the fight against infection, neoplasia and auto-immunity.

The basic instinct to reproduce is a powerful one in the human race. Some of those who see themselves as failures in this regard will accept any therapy no matter how speculative or potentially hazardous. Although it is the clinician's role to assist his patients in every way he can, it is equally his responsibility to make as sure as he possibly can that the short or long-term hazards do not outweigh the benefits. In future years we may live to regret some of our current immunological enthusiasms.

Male and female subfertility

Anti-sperm antibodies as a cause for subfertility in the male was first postulated 30 years ago and many subsequent reports have since been published (see Cohen & Hendry 1978). Although anti-sperm antibodies can be found in the sera of approximately 2% of fertile and between 8 and 13% of infertile men, the evaluation of their pathogenic effects is difficult. As Hjort & Hansen (1983) point out, many men with autoantibodies also have semenalyses showing reduced sperm density and motility which contribute to the subfertility, but cannot be assumed to be due to the antibodies. Secondly, pregnancies do occasionally occur in the partners of men with high levels of anti-sperm antibodies.

Sperm from infertile men with significant levels of sperm agglutinating antibodies in the seminal plasma have poor penetrating capacity for cervical mucus. In addition there is reduced penetration by normal sperm of the cervical mucus of women who have developed iso-antibodies to the sperm of their partner. IgA antibodies in semen or mucus are the most potent inhibitors of penetration (Hogarth 1982). It may be that spermatozoa are rendered more antigenic in women by the damage they suffer in the genital tract of the men with auto-immunity. Prolonged use of a condom or abstinence from intercourse are among the therapeutic measures which have been suggested in women with anti-sperm iso-antibodies. There is no convincing evidence that these are of any value whatsoever. Some success has been claimed for the direct insemination of husband's semen into the uterus, thus by-passing the hostile cervix. Not enough data yet exist to assess this approach properly but there is a theoretical increased risk of anaphylatic reactions to antigenic components of seminal plasma with this technique. Corticosteroid therapy has been advocated to suppress antisperm autoimmunity (in the male) and/or iso-immunity (in the female). Unfortunately many of the studies are either badly or totally uncontrolled, vital background information regarding the history of infertility in the patients is often omitted and numbers are usually small. Hendry and his colleagues (1979) report on an uncontrolled series of 47 subfertile men with anti-sperm antibody titres $\geqslant 1/32$ treated with either continuous long-term (up to 1 year) or intermittent high-dose prednisone. The men were treated in three groups divided according to sperm density (>20 and $>20 \times 10^6$/ml) and treatment regimes. Fourteen pregnancies were achieved, five of which occurred in the wives of nine men in whom high dose therapy was prescribed between day 21 and 28 of the menstrual cycle of the wife on alternate months.

The main 'caveats' about this approach are, firstly, the potential for harm which may be produced in otherwise healthy men given short-term high or long-term lower doses of powerful steroids; secondly since 'spontaneous' cures of male infertility are well recognised (Glass & Ericsson 1979), such treatment cannot be generally advocated without much larger properly controlled trials.

Recurrent spontaneous abortion

In 1981, Taylor & Faulk reported successful pregnancies in four women with a history of multiple primary recurrent spontaneous abortion. They had been treated with multiple buffy-coat infusions from donor blood before and during the first two trimesters of pregnancy. In addition the wife and husband of each couple were found to share MHC antigens far more frequently than expected, i.e. their tissues were more compatible with one another than usual. Faulk suggested that this sharing of MHC antigens was not important in itself, but was a marker for sharing of the trophoblast-lymphocyte cross-reactive (TLX) antigens previously described by him (see p. 13). He speculated that, if excessive TLX antigen sharing occurred, protective 'blocking antibodies' would not be produced, laying the trophoblast open to immune attack. This would result in abortion. If, however, an antibody response could be engendered by infusing donor leucocytes, then it was, he reasoned, possible that any subsequent pregnancies might be successful. This uncontrolled study is continuing with seeming success. Also in 1981 Beer and his colleagues reported on the successful treatment of a series of women suffering from recurrent abortion (not all primary) using two intradermal injections of leucocytes from the husband before pregnancy. Not only did they find excessive sharing of Class I and II MHC antigens between husband and wife, but also unresponsiveness by a proportion of the affected women to paternal MHC antigens. They speculated that this interfered with immunoregulation and resulted in abortion. Treatment of 39 women with idiopathic recurrent abortion sharing HLA loci with their husband has now been reported (Beer et al 1983). Four successful and 10 continuing pregnancies have been achieved. In a comparative group of 84 women with a traditionally recognisable cause for recurrent abortion treated appropriately, 17 successful and eight current pregnancies were reported. One of the infants whose mother was treated with paternal leucocytes has been reported as failing to thrive. The nature of the problem is unknown, although a 'graft versus host' reaction is a theoretical possibility.

A third and controlled study is in progress by Professors Mowbray and Beard in St Mary's Hospital, London. They do not confirm HLA sharing between husband and wife in association with recurrent abortion, but do suggest strongly that maternal failure to produce 'blocking' antibody is the missing element in these patients. Treatment is either with lymphocytes taken from the husband or the woman herself (in randomly selected control patients). At the time of writing no definitive results have been reported.

What, then, should the obstetrician's response be to this new approach to a numerically small but therapeutically difficult and emotional subject? The answer can be given in one word — *caution*. The reasons for that advice are as follows:

1. The patients included in the studies are not similar — and 'recurrent abortion' is not always clearly defined.
2. The hypotheses as to aetiology are different and not always compatible.
3. Treatment regimes are very different and yet seemingly equally successful.
4. Similar success has recently been claimed for nothing more than psychological support in recurrent abortion (Stray Pedersen & Stray Pedersen 1984).
5. The women being treated are intrinsically healthy and the use of potent immunotherapy may not be in their long-term interest.

This last point is particularly important. One of the basic tenets of haematology is that one never knowingly immunises an individual (particularly a woman) against antigens present in the partner. Two of the studies do so. In the other protocol women may receive a total of up to 2500 ml of leucocytes — a massive immune stimulus, the long-term consequences of which are unknown. Immune surveillance against neoplasia could be affected and such conditions as SLE may be precipitated in susceptible women. The effect of the accidental transmission of pathogenic viruses is also a possibility. Thus, even although there may be validity in one or other of the approaches, the principle '*primum non nocere*' (first and foremost, cause no harm) means that we must be cautious in our use of such potent non-specific immunological interventions.

Pre-eclampsia and placental abruption

Despite much repeatedly rehearsed circumstantial evidence (see Redman 1980) and a great deal of research effort, there is still very little direct evidence that an immune defect is the primary cause of pre-eclampsia, let alone placental abruption. The suggestion that pre-eclampsia may be caused by an immune reaction to a worm has been withdrawn. It is still most likely that pre-eclampsia is a basic failure of maternal immune adaptation to pregnancy, involving a multiplicity of organs and systems including the immune system.

Immunological contraception

Much time, effort and money have been expended over the last decade in trying to produce safe, effective and reversible immunological methods of male and female contraception. Strategies have included immunisation against:

1. Sperm antigens, e.g. lactate dehydregenase C4 (Goldberg et al 1983). Moderate success has been demonstrated in female baboons but although LDH-C4 remains the most promising antigen for immunocontraception no human studies are in progress.
2. Zona pellucida antigens (Aitken & Richardson 1980) — interest in this seems to be waning.
3. LHRH (Fraser 1980) in male and female — side-effects are likely to be too troublesome.
4. HCG (Stevens & Jones 1983). Inhibition of up to 90% of expected pregnancies has been achieved in baboons. WHO sponsored clinical trials to assess immunogenicity and safety in already sterilised women are due to begin in the near future.

The ultimate place of such approaches on a world-wide scale remains speculative.

REFERENCES

Aitken R J, Richardson D W 1980 Immunisation against zona pellucida antigens. In: Hearns J P (ed) Immunological Aspects of Reproduction and Fertility Control, Ch. 7, pp 173–201. MTP, Lancaster

Beer A E, Quebbeman J F, Ayers J W T, Haines R F 1981 MHC antigens, maternal and paternal immune responses, and chronic habitual abortion in humans. American Journal of Obstetrics and Gynecology 141: 987–999

Beer A E. Quebbeman J F, Semprini A E, Smouse P E, Haines R F 1983 Recurrent abortion: analysis of the roles of parental sharing of histocompatibility antigens and maternal immunological responses to paternal antigens. In: Isojima S, Billington W D (eds) Reproductive Immunology 1983, pp 185–195. Elsevier, Amsterdam

Billington W D, Bell S C 1983 Evidence on the nature and possible function of pregnancy-induced anti-fetal alloantibody. In: Isojima S, Billington W D (eds) Reproductive Immunology 1983, pp 147–155. Elsevier, Amsterdam

Cohen J, Hendry W F (eds) 1978 Spermatozoa, Antibodies and Infertility. Blackwell Scientific Publications, Oxford

Faulk W P, Temple A, Lovins R E, Smith N 1978 Antigens of human trophoblast: a working hypothesis for their role in normal and abnormal pregnancies. Proceeding of the National Academy of Sciences USA, No 75, pp 1947–1951

Fraser H M 1980 Inhibition of reproductive function by antibodies to LHRH. In Hearn J P (ed) Immunological Aspects of Reproduction and Fertility Control, Ch.6, pp 143–172. MTP, Lancaster

Glass R H, Ericsson R T 1979 Spontaneous cure of male infertility. Fertility and Sterility 31: 305–308

Goldberg E, Wheat T E, Shelton J A 1983 Sperm specific LDH and development of a synthetic contraceptive vaccine. In: Isojima S, Billington W D (eds) Reproductive Immunology 1983, pp 215–223. Elsevier, Amsterdam

Hendry W F, Stedronska J, Hughes L, Cameron K M, Pugh R C B 1979 Steroid treatment of male subfertility caused by antisperm antibodies. Lancet i: 498–500

Hjort T, Hansen K B 1983 Autoantibodies to sperm, sperm motility and fertility prognosis. In: Isojima S, Billington W D (eds) Reproductive Immunology 1983, pp 197–206. Elsevier, Amsterdam

Hogarth P J 1982 Immunological Aspects of Mammalian Reproduction. Praeger, New York

Johnson P M, Cheng H M, Molloy C M, Stern C M M, Slade M B 1981 Human trophoblast-specific surface antigens identified using monoclonal antibodies. American Journal of Reproductive Immunology 1: 246–254

Medawar P B, Sparrow E M 1956 The effects of adrenocortical hormones, ACTH and pregnancy on skin transplantation immunity in mice. Journal of Endocrinology 14: 240–256

Menge A C, Richter D E, Naz R K, Lee C-Y G, Wong E 1983 Dissecting the sperm cell by use of monoclonal antibodies. In: Isojima S, Billington W D (eds) Reproductive Immunology 1983, pp 81–90. Elsevier, Amsterdam

Peterson P A et al 1983 Features of Class I and Class II antigens of the MHC at the DNA and protein level. In: Yamamura Y, Tada T (eds) Progress in Immunology V, pp 171–186. Academic Press, London

Redman C W G 1980 Immunological aspects of eclampsia and pre-eclampsia. In: Hearn J P (ed) Immunological Aspect of Reproduction and Fertility Control, pp 83–103. MTP, Lancaster

Redman C W G, McMichael A J, Stirrat G M, Sunderland C A, Ting A 1984 Class I MHC antigens on human extra-villous trophoblast. Immunology 52: 457–468

Roberts T K, Smart Y C 1983 Studies on human early pregnancy factor. In: Isojima S, Billington W D (eds) Reproductive Immunology 1983, pp 157–169. Elsevier, Amsterdam

Sargent I L, Redman C W G 1985 Maternal CMI to the fetus in human pregnancy. Journal of Reproductive Immunology 7: (in press)

Sargent I L, Redman C W G, Stirrat G M 1982 Maternal CMI in normal and pre-eclamptic pregnancy. Clinical and Experimental Immunology 50: 601–609

Stevens V C, Jones W R 1983 Pre-clinical safety studies on an HCG vaccine. In: Isojima S, Billington W D (eds) Reproductive Immunology 1983, pp 233–237. Elsevier, Amsterdam

Stray-Pedersen B, Stray-Pederson S 1984 Ecologic factors and subsequent reproductive performance in 195 couples with a prior history of habitual abortion. American Journal of Obstetrics and Gynecology 148: 140–146

Taylor C, Faulk W P 1981 Prevention of recurrent abortion with leucocyte transfusions. Lancet ii: 68–69

Terasaki P I, Mickey M R, Yamazaki J N, Vredevoe D 1970 Maternal-fetal incompatibility. I. Incidence of HLA antibodies and possible association with congenital abnormalities. Transplantation 9: 538–543

Vanderbeecken Y, Vlieghe M P, Duchateau J, Delespesse G 1984 Suppressor T lymphocytes in pregnancy. American Journal of Reproductive Immunology 5: 20–24

Voisin G A 1983 Enhancing antibodies and suppressor cells in pregnancy: role of the placentation. In: Isojima S, Billington W D (eds) Reproductive Immunology 1983. pp 121–131. Elsevier, Amsterdam

Wegmann T G 1983 The placental immunological barrier. In: Isojima S, Billington W D (eds) Reproductive Immunology 1983, pp 111–117. Elsevier, Amsterdam

Chorionic villus biopsy

Chorionic villus biopsy, unlike amniocentesis and fetoscopy, opens the way to making a prenatal diagnosis of genetic disorder in the first trimester, rather than in the second trimester of pregnancy. In reviewing chorionic villus biopsy, consideration will first be given to genetic information that can be gained from chorionic villi by laboratory procedures. After that, the practical aspects and dangers of chorionic villus biopsy will be discussed and finally, an attempt will be made to define the place of chorionic villus biopsy in current prenatal care.

LABORATORY PROCESSING OF CHORIONIC VILLI

The chorionic villus (Fig. 2.1) contains a wealth of information about the unborn fetus. This information can be obtained by:

Cytogenetic techniques.
Study of enzyme production.
Direct analysis of the DNA within the chromosomes.
Sex chromatin studies.

Cytogenetic techniques

If rapidly dividing cells are exposed to colchicine, cell division becomes arrested in mitotic metaphase. If the nuclei of these cells are 'spread' (or exploded) so that the chromosomes become disentangled and scattered, the karyotype can be determined and numerical or structural chromosome abnormalities can be diagnosed. The identification of individual chromosomes can be aided by special staining techniques which give different chromosomes their characteristic 'banding' patterns. 'Banding' has greatly increased the accuracy of karyotyping.

To date it has been customary to culture cells for 10 days to 3 weeks so as to obtain a sufficient number of dividing cells before adding colchicine. A technique for establishing successful tissue cultures from chorionic villi was described by Niazi et al (1981). However, Simoni et al (1983), using a variant of a method first applied in the mouse embryo by Evans et al (1972), found that

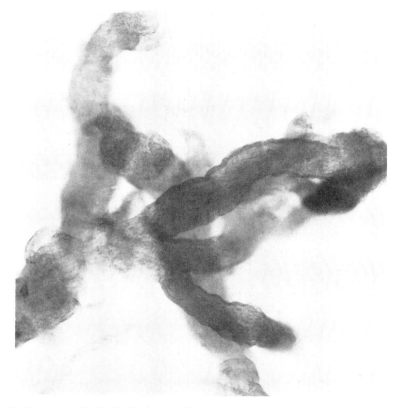

Fig. 2.1 Chorionic villi (× 30). There is sufficient material here for diagnostic purposes

cytogenetic preparations made from uncultured villi exposed to colchicine contained sufficient cells in mitotic metaphase to allow accurate karyotyping and even banding studies. The literature already contains reports of the clinical use of these methods. Thus Lilford et al (1983) and Brambati & Simoni (1983) described cases where fetal sex and trisomy 21 respectively were diagnosed only hours after a successful chorionic villus biopsy. Brambati & Simoni (1983) obtained as many as 58 cells in mitotic metaphase (and therefore suitable for karyotype analysis) from only 15 mg of chorionic villi.

Enzyme studies

Knowledge of inherited metabolic disease has increased enormously over recent years and there are now some 200 disorders characterised by enzyme deficiencies which can be recognised by sensitive biochemical assays on fetal cells. The prenatal diagnosis of affected fetuses has been achieved for some 60 metabolic diseases (Patrick 1983).

Chorionic villi can be used as starting material for tissue cultures on which these enzyme assays are done. Further, a number of workers have reported enzyme assays on homogenates of small amounts of uncultured villi and the enzyme levels that have been measured are listed in Table 2.1 (together with the names of some of the related deficiency diseases). Pergament et al (1983) have reported the exclusion of Tay-Sachs disease by chorionic villus biopsy at $8\frac{1}{2}$ weeks gestation; the pregnancy was in fact terminated because the fetus was found to have trisomy 16 on karyotyping of direct preparations and tissue cultures made from chorionic villi.

Table 2.1 Enzyme levels measured in homogenates of uncultured chorionic villi

Enzyme	Type of disorder	Specific disease
β-D-glucosidase	Lipid	Gaucher
β-D-galactosidase	,,	Krabbe
β-D-hexosaminidase	,,	Tay-Sachs
Arylsulphatase A	,,	Metachromatic leucodystrophy
Sphingomyelinase	,,	Niemann-Pick
β-D-mannosidase	Mucopolysaccharidosis or related disorder	
α-iduronidase	,,	Hurler
β-D-glucuronidase	,,	
α-L-fucosidase	,,	

References: Kazy et al 1982, Simoni et al 1983.

Direct DNA analysis

In the last decade it has become possible for molecular biochemists to make direct analyses of the DNA which goes to make up the chromosomes. Genetic markers for disease have thus been found. These markers involve either direct identification of genes (in which case absence or abnormalities of the gene can be diagnosed with a high degree of certainty) or the detection of associated abnormalities in the structure of neighbouring areas of the chromosome associated with the presence of an abnormal gene (in which case the diagnosis of genetic abnormality becomes a matter of calculating probabilities and is therefore not so accurate as with direct gene identification).

DNA technology has become so refined that only 5 μg of DNA are required for each analysis (Gosden 1983). The cells in 10 ml of amniotic fluid contain this amount of DNA but only a single chorionic villus is needed to give the same yield (Williamson et al 1981).

There are a number of genetic disorders which have been investigated by DNA technology and those for which some form of genetic marker exists are listed in Table 2.2. DNA technology has only really been used on chorionic villi or amniotic fluid cells for the clinical diagnosis of haemoglobinopathy in pregnancies with a fetus at risk of this disorder. It cannot, however, be long before the number of genetic diseases which can be diagnosed prenatally by DNA technology is greatly increased.

Table 2.2 Disorders with genetic markers apparently detectable by DNA technology

Disorder	Reference
α1-antitrypsin deficiency	Kidd et al 1983
Sickle cell trait or disease	Chang & Kan 1982
	Kan et al 1972, 1977
	Orkin et al 1982
	Boehm et al 1983
	Williamson et al 1981
β-thalassaemia	Piratsu et al 1983
	Boehm et al 1983
α-thalassaemia	Kan et al 1976
Antithrombin III deficiency	Prochownick et al 1983
Factor IX deficiency	Gianelli et al 1984
(Christmas disease)	Peake et al 1984
Lethal osteogenesis imperfecta congenita	Pope et al 1984
Becker muscular dystrophy	Kingston et al 1983
Duchenne muscular dystrophy	Murray et al 1982
Lesch-Nyhan syndrome	Nussbaum et al 1983
Myotonic dystrophy	Davies et al 1983
Phenylketonuria	Woo et al 1983
Huntington's chorea	Gusella et al 1983

DNA technology has also been used for the recognition of the Y-chromosome and hence fetal sex (Lau et al 1984). This could be of interest in the direct analysis of amniotic fluid cells; but where chorionic villi are concerned, direct cytogenetic techniques can be employed and because they are simpler and more speedy they would seem to be preferable to DNA analysis for the diagnosis of fetal sex.

For chorionic villus biopsy to be reliable there must be no detectable contamination by maternal DNA. This matter has been investigated by Elles et al (1983) who compared the DNA of chorionic villi obtained at 9–10 weeks gestation from five fetuses with that obtained from the mother's lymphocytes. They concluded that chorionic villi were a reliable and uncontaminated source of fetal DNA.

Sex chromatin

The percentage of cells showing sex chromatin (or Barr bodies) on the nuclear membrane can be used to determine fetal sex. This technique has been used for fetal sexing of chorionic villus samples in China (Department of Obstetrics and Gynecology, Teitung Hospital of Anshan, 1975) but it is unreliable and therefore not to be recommended.

General over-view

Chorionic villi can be analysed by a variety of interesting techniques. What is of particular importance is that it takes only a very few chorionic villi to provide enough cells for enzyme, DNA and cytogenetic analyses without days or weeks spent on preliminary tissue culture. This means that chorionic villus biopsy holds out promise of a very quick genetic diagnosis on samples obtained well before the end of the first trimester of pregnancy and this adds urgency to the need to examine the practical aspects and dangers of this procedure.

TRANSCERVICAL CHORIONIC VILLUS BIOPSY: PRACTICAL CONSIDERATIONS

Techniques

The aim of chorionic villus biopsy is to collect a few villi from the chorion frondosum at the edge of the placental disc. Table 2.3 summarises the devices that have been used to obtain chorionic villi by aspiration biopsy and direct biopsy. For aspiration biopsy, various permutations and combinations of cannulae and methods of locating them within the uterine cavity have been employed.

Table 2.3 Reported techniques for chorionic villus biopsy

	Device to obtain chorionic villi	Method employed to locate and site device
Aspiration biopsy using 2/20 ml syringes or mechanical suction up to 750 mmHg	Medicut cannula Plastic Portex or Teflon cannulae, with or without malleable metal obturator	None (blind aspiration) Endoscopy Ultrasound
	Metal cannulae — some malleable — some with blunted or bulbous tip	Ultrasound and endoscopy
Direct biopsy	Biopsy forceps	Endoscopy and ultrasound

Success rates

Table 2.4 shows reported success rates for a selection of chorionic villus biopsy methods. Not all series reported have been quoted; some were excluded because the numbers were too small, some because the methods used were too variable or inadequately described and some because no specific information about success rates was given.

It would seem that a long cannula (either of malleable metal or of plastic which can be shaped by bending a malleable obturator) inserted into the extraovular cavity of the uterus under ultrasound control (see Fig. 2.2) offers the best chance of success in terms of obtaining sufficient chorionic villi for laboratory analysis.

Table 2.4 Reported success rates for chorionic villus biopsy

	References	Method	Subjects	Gestational age	Success rates (%)
Aspiration biopsy technique	* Tietung Hospital of Anshan 1975	Blind aspiration with 3 mm rigid metal cannula	100 wanting to know fetal sex	47–100 days	100
	* Horwell et al 1983	Blind aspiration using 16 gauge Medicut cannula	82 pre-termination patients	7–13 weeks	40 (55% at 8 weeks)
	* Liu et al 1983	'Longdwell' 14 gauge teflon i.v. with metal trocar (2 ml syringe)	137	8–14 weeks	33
	Ward et al 1983	16 gauge Medicut or Portex cannula (with obturator) and ultrasound	61 patients pre-termination 7 diagnostic	7–14 weeks	90 for Portex cannula with obturator) 31 otherwise
	Rodeck et al 1983a	17 cm, 16 gauge malleable silver cannula with up to 750 mmHg mechanical suction under real-time ultrasound control	32 pre-termination 8 diagnostic	7–12 weeks	90 (100% in last 23 patients)
	* Simoni et al 1983	Blind aspiration with flexible 1.2 mm cannula with obturator Same cannula with ultrasound	207 pre-termination 103 patients	6–12 weeks 6–12 weeks	65 96

Table 2.4 Continued

References	Method	Subjects	Gestational age	Success rates (%)
Simoni et al 1984	Flexible Portex catheter with ultrasound (up to four attempts)	100 patients (all diagnostic)	7–12 weeks	96
* McKenzie et al 1983	Long soft plastic catheter	60 patients	First trimester	78
Rodeck et al 1983b	Aspiration needle attached to 5 ml syringe with endoscope and real-time ultrasound in eight patients	11 patients yielding 16 biopsies	First trimester	94 overall (100% with ultrasound and needlescope)
Direct biopsy technique Simoni et al 1983	Endoscope and biopsy forceps housed in 3.3 × 4.7 mm oval cannula	62 patients	6–12 weeks	76
Kazy et al 1982	Flexible biopsy forceps and ultrasound	161 patients (135 terminations and 26 at risk of genetic disease)	6–12 weeks	100
Hahnemann 1974	5–7 mm hysteroscope with cylindrical knife biopsy and suction gadget	95 patients before termination	8–15 weeks	60
Kullander & Sandahl 1973	5–7 mm hysteroscope with biopsy forceps	39 pre-termination patients	8–20 weeks	49

* blind aspiration techniques

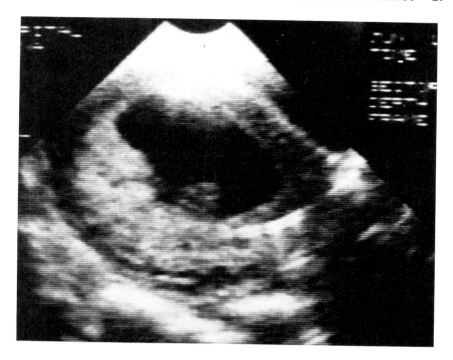

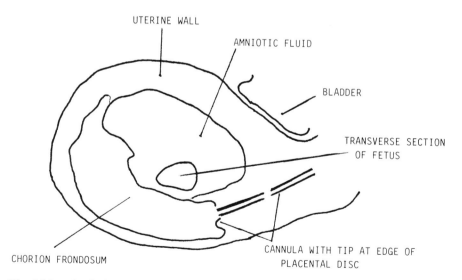

Fig. 2.2 Longitudinal real-time ultrasound sector scan done during chorionic villus sampling at 10 weeks gestation

Immediate complications of chorionic villus biopsy

The immediate complications of chorionic villus biopsy are perforation of the amniotic sac, bleeding, infection (both virus and bacterial) and feto-maternal haemorrhage leading to rhesus isoimmunisation. The last of these can be avoided by giving anti-D to those patients who are rhesus negative. As for bleeding and perforation of the amniotic sac, only few authors give details of the incidence of these occurrences.

Horwell et al (1983) noted some vaginal bleeding in 34 out of 63 patients (54%) having a blind aspiration biopsy and in whom it was possible to pass a cannula into the uterine cavity without preliminary sounding. In 10 of these patients (16%) was the bleeding moderate, while in one (1.6%) was it described as severe. Liu et al (1983) noted moderate bleeding in four out of 137 patients (3%) having a blind aspiration biopsy just before termination of pregnancy. For Simoni et al (1983) the incidence of bleeding in 310 aspiration biopsies done either blind or under ultrasound control was 8.4% (26 patients), the lowest incidence of 4.9% occurring in 103 patients in whom the aspiration cannula was guided by real-time ultrasound. The Chinese group (Department of Obstetrics and Gynecology, Teitung Hospital of Anshan, 1975) obtained some blood (but did not say how much) in 86 of their 100 patients and 'bloody fluid' in a further 11 patients. They reported the aspiration of amniotic fluid in their remaining three patients making the incidence of this complications 3%. Liu et al (1983) encountered perforation of the amniotic sac only once in 137 patients (0.7%). Horwell et al (1983) inadvertently entered the amniotic sac three times in 82 attempted blind aspiration biopsies (3.7%); but two of these patients were at 13 weeks gestational age and probably, therefore, far too advanced for chorionic villus biopsy. There are sporadic reports of infection but no precise and systematically collected information about this complication is known.

From the evidence available, it would seem fair to say that severe bleeding is a rare complication of chorionic villus biopsy, that the incidence of mild or moderate bleeding is probably well under 10% and that the incidence of perforation of the amniotic sac is around 1–2%. Infection remains an unknown quantity. There also seems little doubt that ultrasound guidance of the aspiration cannula not only increases the success of the procedure but also reduces the occurrence of significant bleeding.

Long-term complications of chorionic villus biopsy

The most important complication of chorionic villus biopsy is subsequent miscarriage. Information about the incidence of miscarriage can only be gained by study of the reports of chorionic villus biopsies which were done either at a significant interval before a planned termination of pregnancy or for diagnostic purposes. The information gleaned from such reports is summarised in Table 2.5.

Table 2.5 Outcome of pregnancies allowed to continue after chorionic villus biopsy

Reference	Information about pregnancies allowed to continue	Outcome of those pregnancies	Pregnancy loss rate
	Aspiration biopsy		
Tietung Hospital 1975	70 pregnancies intended to continue to term because fetal sex acceptable	4 spontaneous abortions	4/70
Ward et al 1983	— 3 allowed to continue until termination on some grounds 5 days later	No interim complications	1/10
	— 2 allowed to continue for 3 weeks until termination for diagnosis of fetal thalassaemia	No interim complications	
	— 5 intended to continue till term because fetus judged to be without serious haemogloninopathy	1 missed abortion after 2 days 4 continuing pregnancies	
Rodeck et al 1983a	— 2 allowed to continue for 2 weeks until termination for serious haemoglobinopathy	No interim complications	0/8
	— 2 allowed to continue for 4 days until termination on social grounds	No interim complications Fetuses alive just before termination	
	— 6 pregnancies intended to continue because fetus believed not to have haemoglobinopathy	No reported complications (pregnancies continuing at time of publication of report)	
Simoni et al 1984	88 pregnancies intended to continue	6 post sampling abortions 82 patients in whom there were no publicised details about the outcome of pregnancy	At least 6/88

Table 2.5 Continued

Reference	Information about pregnancies allowed to continue	Outcome of those pregnancies	Pregnancy loss rate
	Forceps biopsy with hysteroscope or ultrasound		
Kullander & Sandahl 1973	19 pregnancies allowed to continue until termination on social grounds 7–43 days later	2 spontaneous abortions associated with Neisserial infection 17 pregnancies apparently intact at the time of termination	2/19
Hahnemann 1974	28 pregnancies allowed to continue for at least 8 days	17 losses by miscarriage within 7 days or fetal death 11 pregnancies presumably progressive at time of termination	17/28
Kazy et al 1982	— 29 allowed to continue for 7–10 days until termination of pregnancy on social grounds — 13 intended to continue to term	No complications Fetuses alive at termination No complications (2 still pregnant at time of report)	0/42

Total pregnancy loss 30 out of 265 (or 11.3%)

It can be seen that there is, as yet, very limited knowledge about the long-term safety of chorionic villus biopsy, with widely divergent reported figures for pregnancy loss rates (see the last column of Table 2.5) and there is a real need for the collection of further data. A noble attempt is being made by Laird Jackson at the Jefferson Medical College in Philadelphia to collect and collate such information from those engaged in chorionic villus biopsy for diagnostic purposes in Europe and the USA. Some results have been distributed 'in confidence' in letters sent to workers in the field, but the information is as yet far too incomplete to allow judgement about the safety of this procedure. There is, however, room for international collection and the publication of detailed results for they must be known as a matter of some urgency.

The other way of obtaining information in this area would be to take chorionic villus biopsies from multiparous patients at 1 or 2 weeks before a termination which is being done because their families are to all intents and purposes complete. If several centres were to collaborate over such a study, if the pregnancies were examined intensively in the interval between biopsy and termination, and if the material obtained at termination was subjected to full biological, bacteriological and histological analysis, soundly-based information about the safety of chorionic villus biopsy would soon come to hand.

THE PRESENT PLACE OF CHORIONIC VILLUS BIOPSY AND FUTURE DEVELOPMENTS

Until the risk of chorionic villus biopsy to the developing fetus is known with certainty, chorionic villus biopsy is a procedure that can only be offered to patients who are:

(a)   at appreciable risk of having a baby with serious genetic disease;
(b)   unwilling to accept amniocentesis or fetoscopy as a method of prenatal diagnosis in the second trimester; and
(c)   keen on the first trimester diagnosis even though the risk of chorionic villus biopsy, as yet not completely known, appears to be around 10% in terms of pregnancy loss.

As for future developments, there are workers who are beginning to test trans-abdominal methods under ultrasound guidance for first trimester chorionic villus biopsy; they hope thus to avoid the risk of introducing bacterial or virus infections to the conceptus as a result of passing a biopsy cannula through the cervical canal into the uterine cavity (Lilford, personal communication). The results of such endeavours are awaited with interest as are developments in the field of DNA technology. If chorionic villus biopsy can be shown to be safe and the list of genetic disorders diagnosable by direct analysis of the DNA in chromosomes grows at the present rate, chorionic villus biopsy could become an important technique for the prenatal diagnosis of genetic disease in the first trimester of pregnancy — a time when termination is a relatively simple and safe procedure. There would then be the ethical problem of what sort of genetic disease constitutes an indication for termination. Would, for example, high risk of the unborn fetus ultimately developing diabetes mellitus or rheumatoid arthritis be an acceptable indication for interrupting a pregnancy? These are dilemmas which society and doctors in future decades may have to face but they are outside the scope of this review which aims to present the status of chorionic villus biopsy in the first half of 1984.

Acknowledgment

I am indebted to Mr David Horwell for his help with the illustrations.

REFERENCES

Boehm C D, Antonarakis S E, Phillips J A, Kazazian H H Jr 1983 Prenatal diagnosis using DNA polymorphism. Report on 95 pregnancies at risk for sickle-cell disease or beta thalassaemia. New England Journal of Medicine 308: 1054–1058

Brambati B, Simoni G 1983 Diagnosis of fetal trisomy 21 in first trimester. Lancet i: 586

Chang J C, Kan Y W 1982 A sensitive new prenatal test for sickle cell anaemia. New England Journal of Medicine 307: 30–32

Davies K E et al 1983 Linkage analysis of myotonic dystrophy and sequences on chromosome 19 using a cloned component 3 gene probe. Journal of Medical Genetics 20: 259–263

Department of Obstetrics and Gynecology Tietung Hospital of Anshan Iron and Steel Company Anshan 1975 Fetal sex prediction by sex chromatin of chorionic villi cells during early pregnancy. Chinese Medical Journal 1: 117–126

Elles R G, Williamson R, Niazi M, Coleman D V, Horwell D H 1983 Absence of contamination of chorionic villi used for fetal gene analysis. New England Journal of Medicine 308: 1433–1435

Evans E P, Burtenshaw M D, Ford C E 1972 Chromosomes of mouse embryos and newborn young: preparations from membranes and tail tips. Stain Technology 47: 229–234

Gianelli F, Choo K H, Winship P R, Ricca C R, Anson D S, Rees D J G, Ferrari N, Brownlee G G 1984 Characterisation and use of an intragenic polymorphic marker for detection of carriers of haemophilia B (Factor IX deficiency). Lancet i: 239–241

Gosden C M 1983 Amniotic fluid cell types and culture. British Medical Bulletin 39: 348–354

Gusella J F et al 1983 A polymorphic DNA marker genetically linked to Huntington's disease. Nature 306: 234–238

Hahnemann N 1974 Early prenatal diagnosis. A study of biopsy techniques and cell culturing from extraembryonic membranes. Clinical Genetics 6: 294

Horwell D H, Loeffler F E, Coleman D V 1983 Assessment of a transcervical aspiration technique for chorionic villus biopsy in the first trimester of pregnancy. British Journal of Obstetrics and Gynaecology 90: 196–198

Kan Y W, Dozy A M, Alter B P, Frigoletto F D, Nathan D G 1972 Detection of sickle cell gene in the human fetus: potential for intrauterine diagnosis of sickle cell anaemia. New England Journal of Medicine 287: 1–5

Kan Y W, Golbus M S, Dozy A M 1976 Prenatal diagnosis of beta-thalassaemia: clinical application of molecular hybridization. New England Journal of Medicine 295: 1165–1167

Kan Y W, Golbus M S, Trecartin R F et al 1977 Prenatal diagnosis of beta-thalassaemia and sickle-cell anaemia: experience with 24 cases. Lancet i: 269–271

Kazy Z, Rosovsky I S, Bakharev V A 1982 Chorion biopsy in early pregnancy: a method of early prenatal diagnosis for inherited disorders. Prenatal Diagnosis 2: 39–45

Kidd V J, Wallace R B, Tan Z-K, Itakura K, Woo S L C 1983 Beta 1-antitrypsin deficiency detection by direct analysis of the mutation site in the gene. Nature 304: 230–234

Kingston H M, Harper P S, Pearson P L, Davies K E, Williamson R, Page D 1983 Localisation of gene for Becker muscular dystrophy. Lancet ii: 1200

Kullander S, Sandahl B 1973 Fetal chromosome analysis after transcervical placental biopsies during early pregnancy. Acta Obstetricia et Gynecologica Scandinavica 52: 355–359

Lau Y-F, Dozy A M, Huang J C, Kan Y W 1984 A rapid screening test for antenatal sex determination. Lancet i: 14–16

Lilford R, Maxwell D, Coleman D, Czepulkowski B, Heaton D 1983 Diagnosis four hours after chorion biopsy, of female fetus in pregnancy at risk of Duchenne muscular dystrophy. Lancet ii: 1491

Liu D T Y, Mitchell J, Johnson J, Wass D M 1983 Trophoblast sampling by blind transcervical aspiration. British Journal of Obstetrics and Gynaecology 90: 1119–1123

McKenzie I Z, Lindenbaum R H, Patel C, Clarke G, Crocker M, Jonasson J A 1983 Prenatal diagnosis of an unbalanced chromosome translocation identified by direct karyotyping of chorionic biopsy. Lancet ii: 1426–1427

Murray J M et al 1982 A cloned DNA sequence on the short arm of the X-chromosome: linkage relationship to Duchenne muscular dystrophy. Nature 300: 69–71

Niazi M. Coleman D V, Loeffler F E 1981 Trophoblast sampling in early pregnancy. Culture of rapidly dividing cells from immature placental villi. British Journal of Obstetrics and Gynaecology 88: 1081–1085

Nussbaum R L, Crowder W E, Nyhan W L, Caskey C T 1983 A three-allele restriction-fragment-length polymorphism at the hypoxanthine phosphoribosyltransferase focus in man. Proceedings of the National Academy of Sciences of the USA 80: 4035–4039

Orkin S H, Little P F R, Kazazian H H Jr, Boehm C D 1982 Improved detection of the sickle mutation by DNA analysis: application to prenatal diagnosis. New England Journal of Medicine 307: 32–36

Patrick A D 1983 Inherited metabolic disorders. British Medical Bulletin 39: 378–385

Peake I R, Furlong B L, Bloom A L 1984 Carrier detection by direct gene analysis in a family with haemophilia B (Factor IX deficiency). Lancet i: 242

Pergament E, Ginsberg N, Verlinsky Y, Cadkin A, Chu L, Trnka L 1983 Prenatal Tay-Sachs diagnosis by chorionic villi sampling. Lancet ii: 286–287

Piratsu M, Kan Y W, Cao A, Conner B J, Teplitz R L, Wallace R B 1983 Prenatal diagnosis of beta-thalassaemia: detection of a single nucleotide mutation in DNA. New England Journal of Medicine 309: 284–287

Pope F M, Cheah K S E, Nicholls A C, Price A B, Grosveld F G 1984 Lethal osteogenesis imperfecta congenita and a 300 base pair gene deletion for an alpha1(I)-like collagen. British Medical Journal 2: 421–424

Prochownik E V, Antonarakis S E, Bauer K, Rosenberg R, Fearon E R, Orkin S H 1983 Molecular heterogeneity of inherited anti-thrombin III deficiency. New England Journal of Medicine 308: 1549–1552

Rodeck C H, Nicolaides K H, Morsman J M, McKenzie C, Gosden C M, Gosden J R 1983a A single-operator technique for first-trimester chorion biopsy. Lancet ii: 1340–1341

Rodeck C H, Morsman J M, Gosden C M, Gosden J R 1983b Development of an improved technique for first-trimester microsampling of chorion. British Journal of Obstetrics and Gynaecology 90: 1113–1118

Simoni G, Brambati B, Danesino C, Rossella F, Terzoli G L, Ferrari M, Fraccaro M 1983 Efficient direct chromosome analysis and enzyme determinations from chorionic villi samples in the first trimester of pregnancy. Human Genetics 63: 349–357

Simoni G, Brambati B, Danesino C, Terzoli G L, Romitti L, Rosella F, Fraccaro M 1984 Diagnostic application of first trimester trophoblast sampling in 100 pregnancies. Human Genetics 66: 252–259

Ward R H T, Modell B, Petrou M, Karagozlu F, Douratsos E 1983 Method of sampling chorionic villi in first trimester of pregnancy under guidance of real time ultrasound. British Medical Journal 2: 1542–1544

Williamson R, Eskdale J, Coleman D V. Niazi M, Loeffler F E, Modell B M 1981 Direct gene analysis of chorionic villi: a possible technique for first trimester diagnosis of haemoglobinopathies. Lancet ii: 1126–1127

Woo S L C et al 1983 Cloned human phenyl alanine hydroxylase gene allows prenatal diagnosis and carrier detection of classical phenylketonuria. Nature 306: 151–155

Fetal therapy

While classical Greek and Roman thinkers conceived the idea of the 'homunculus' — a miniature person living and growing within the mother before birth — it is only during this century with the advances in genetics and molecular biology that the origin and development of the fetus could be explained scientifically. Although molecular biology provided a conceptual framework that demystified fetal development, the concept of the fetus as a patient has only been advanced substantially during the last decade when the techniques of real time ultrasonography and fetoscopy provided the means for detailed anatomical examination of the fetus and fetal tissue sampling respectively. The ill 'homunculus' can now be examined, investigated and in selected cases treated as any other patient would be in postnatal life.

Most medical and correctable surgical abnormalities that can be diagnosed *in utero* are best managed by appropriate therapy after delivery. Prenatal diagnosis improves outcome by allowing the parents and attending doctors to discuss alternatives and choose the appropriate time, mode and place of delivery and to prepare for optimal postnatal care. While vaginal delivery at term will be generally preferred, for certain conditions where continued gestation would have a progressive ill effect on the fetus, induced vaginal or elective Caesarean preterm delivery would be more suitable. However, if the fetus is too immature for extrauterine viability, intrauterine therapy becomes necessary in order to arrest the progressive destructive or deleterious consequences of the underlying defect while allowing further fetal development. At present only a few disorders are amenable to therapy before birth but advances in postnatal treatment coupled with improved techniques for early prenatal diagnosis will ultimately lead to wider possibilities for fetal therapy.

FETAL SURGERY

Although numerous anatomic malformations are detectable before birth, the only ones that warrant consideration for treatment *in utero* are simple structural defects that interfere with organ development and where correction might allow fetal development to proceed normally. Neural tube defects, craniostenoses, congenital diaphragmatic hernia, hydronephrosis and hydrocephalus are potential candidates. The pathophysiology and treatment of these conditions is currently under investigation in animal models. In a few cases of obstructive hydrocephalus and uropathy, fetal therapy has been undertaken by placement of ventriculo- and versico-amniotic shunts. The recent performance of neonatal cardiac transplantation has shown that such therapy is technically possible. Although at present it may seem rather futuristic, *in utero* fetal cardiac and renal transplantation, at a gestational age before the development of immune competence, would have the advantage that a host response against the allogeneic cells would be circumvented by the induction of tolerance obviating the need for immuno-suppressive regimens with all their associated complications.

Obstructive uropathy

Prenatal urethral obstruction produces significant neonatal mortality and morbidity. The critical determinants for immediate extrauterine survival are the degree of associated pulmonary hypoplasia (Reid 1984) and renal insufficiency, that in severe cases is progressive and irreversible despite early postnatal urinary diversion procedures.

Using high resolution real time ultrasound scanners it is now possible to visualise the fetal kidneys and bladder as early as 14 to 15 weeks gestation. The kidneys, located below the level of the stomach on either side and anterior to the spine, are more translucent than the adjacent liver and contain a small echo-free central space, the renal pelvis. In the presence of an obstruction, at or distal to the urethro-vesical junction, there is extensive dilatation of the bladder and ureters while the kidneys demonstrate either hydronephrotic changes, with a dilated calyceal system and a thin cortex of normal translucency, or increased renal parenchymal echogenicity with or without pelvicalyceal distention. Oligohydramnios-anhydramnios are often present but not invariably so.

In order to study the pathophysiology of fetal obstructive uropathy, Beck (1971) ligated the ureters of a series of fetal lambs at various gestational ages and found that obstruction in the last half of gestation resulted in simple hydronephrosis indistinguishable from that seen in adult animals following ureteral ligation. The renal architecture remained well preserved and the tubules were minimally dilated while the glomeruli were essentially free from the deleterious effects of obstruction. However, when unilateral or bilateral ligation was performed during the first half of gestation, the kidneys were contracted, hypoplastic (deficiency in total nephron population) and dysplastic (formation of abnormal nephrons and mesenchymal stroma). In subsequent experiments, Harrison et al (1982a) demonstrated that ligation of the urethra and urachus of fetal lambs in the second half of pregnancy resulted in magacystis, hydroureters, simple hydronephrosis (without dysplasia) and pulmonary hypoplasia. If the obstruction was decompressed, by suprapubic cystostomy at a second operation 3 weeks later, there was significant resolution of the pulmonary hypoplasia and the severe urinary tract dilatation. However, these studies neither addressed nor answered the question as to whether the renal parenchymal dysplasia, which follows urinary tract obstruction in the first half of pregnancy (Beck 1971), can be reversed by such *in utero* decompression. Furthermore, the underlying mechanism for the pulmonary hypoplasia which is associated with renal agenesis (Potter 1946) and bilateral renal dysplasia (Bain & Scott 1960) remains obscure. If the lung changes are secondary to oligohydramnios and thoracic compression (Thomas & Smith 1974), and not due to a primary pulmonary malformation, restoration of normal amniotic fluid volume by fetal urinary tract decompression would reverse the constraint on normal lung growth. However, in human newborns with renal agenesis or dysplasia, the hypoplastic lungs have a decreased number of airway generations reflecting compromised development at between 12 and 16 weeks gestation (Hislop et al 1979, Reid 1984) at which time the source of amniotic fluid is thought to be largely non renal.

With the aim of arresting the progressive destructive consequences of obstruction while allowing further fetal growth and development *in utero,* Harrison et al (1982b) performed bilateral ureterostomies on a 21-week fetus with ultrasonic evidence of severe obstructive uropathy and bilateral hydronephrosis. The lower part of the fetal body was lifted through a hysterotomy incision, the dilated ureters were exposed through bilateral flank incisions, opened through the mid-position and marsupialised to the skin. The fetus was then replaced and the incision closed. Both mother and fetus tolerated the procedure well and the pregnancy was essentially uncomplicated for the next 14 weeks. Following the onset of preterm labour at 35 weeks gestation an infant was delivered by Caesarean section but died after 8 hours despite maximal ventilatory support. At autopsy the lungs were found to be hypoplastic and the kidneys hypo-dysplastic.

Other investigators used a different approach for temporary decompression of the fetal urinary tract by ultrasound guided suprapubic catheterisation and drainage of urine to the mother's exterior (McFadyen et al 1983) or into the amniotic cavity (Rodeck 1983, Rodeck & Nicolaides 1983, Golbus et al 1982, Berkowitz et al 1982, Manning et al 1983). The rationale of the vesico-amniotic shunts is to decompress the urinary tract as well as to allow amniotic fluid formation and prevent the sequelae of oligohydramnios. To date a total of 52 cases of fetal obstructive uropathy treated by *in utero* placement of vesico-amniotic shunts in several centres throughout the world have been reported to the International Fetal Surgery Registry (F. Manning — personal communication). There were six abortions, at least two (4%) as a direct result of the procedure, 23 neonatal deaths, mainly due to pulmonary hypoplasia and the remaining 23 survived, the oldest being 4 years. Neonatal and infant morbidity are not recorded. The underlying pathology was posterior urethral valves in 12 cases, urethral atresia in two, multiple abnormalities of the urinary tract in six, 'Prunebelly' syndrome in two, multicystic kidneys in one and no diagnosis was made or proven in 29 cases. Survival was unrelated to the gestational age at the time of diagnosis and treatment or the degree of associated oligohydramnios but it was most favourable (90%) if the primary pathology for the obstructive uropathy was posterior urethral valves.

These results demonstrate that provided vesico-amniotic shunting is beneficial the relatively low procedure related fetal mortality achieved in specialised centres may be acceptable. They also expose the need for the establishment of reliable criteria for the selection of fetuses who may benefit from such therapy. Some general guidelines have been proposed by a recent conference of obstetricians, surgeons and paediatricians from centres active in fetal therapy (Consensus Report 1982). Unilateral lesions or those causing mild bilateral hydronephrosis with evidence of good renal function do not require treatment *in utero*. The fetus older than 32 weeks may benefit from early delivery and postnatal decompression. Surgical intervention *in utero* may be indicated in second trimester fetuses with bilateral hydronephrosis secondary to urethral obstruction and where there is evidence of progressive bilateral calyceal dilatation in association with increasing oligohydramnios. Our approach to the management of pregnancies with fetal obstructive uropathy (Table 3.1) includes:

1. *Detailed high resolution sonographic* examination for the exclusion of other anatomical defects as up to 50% of these fetuses may have cardiovascular, gastrointestinal, skeletal and central nervous system abnormalities (Potter & Craig 1976). This is often difficult in the presence of severe oligohydramnios-anhydramnios but visualisation is improved by the intra-amniotic instillation of approximately 100 ml of normal saline or Hartman's solution at the time of fetoscopy.

2. *Fetoscopy* and *fetal blood sampling* for rapid karyotyping. Cytogenetic analysis from fetal lymphocytes (Gosden 1984) takes only 3–4 days compared with the 2–4 weeks required for analysis from an amniotic fluid karyotype. This alleviates the parental anxiety associated with the long delay, allows the option of termination should the diagnosis be positive and also helps genetic counselling for future pregnancies. Fetal karyotyping should be performed even in late third trimester because a positive diagnosis would avoid unnecessary obstetric interventions, such as Caesarean section delivery, in the

Table 3.1 Investigation of fetal obstructive uropathy

ULTRASONOGRAPHY
Exclusion of other anatomical defects
Measurement of amniotic fluid volume
Assessment of renal   — architecture
                  — cortical thickness
                  — cortical echogenicity
FETOSCOPY
Rapid fetal karyotyping
INSERTION OF VESICO-AMNIOTIC SHUNT
Biochemical analysis of fetal urine
Assessment of fetal urine production

fetal intrests. We found chromosomal abnormalities in eight of 35 fetuses (23%) with obstructive uropathy where rapid karyotyping was performed; four had Trisomy 18, two Trisomy 13, one triploidy and one had a deletion of the long arm of chromosome 2.

3. *Insertion of a vesico-amniotic shunt* which is performed at the same time as fetoscopy. We consider this as being both diagnostic in terms of assessing the degree of renal damage, and therapeutic. Poor renal function is inferred from the ultrasonic findings of severe oligohydramnios-anhydramnios and increased renal parenchymal echogenicity but more accurately assessed by biochemical analysis of the fetal urine and plasma and by the change in the volume of amniotic fluid, as measured by serial scanning over 2–3 days after insertion of the shunt (in preparation). Thus in all 12 cases of fetal obstructive uropathy where the pregnancy was terminated because of suspected poor renal function (fetal urinary sodium concentration more than 95 mmol/l; no increase in amniotic fluid volume after vesico-amniotic shunting) the fetal kidneys were found to be hypo-dysplastic at postmortem examination. Whereas, in four pregnancies resulting in the delivery of infants with good renal function the fetal urinary sodium concentration was less than 60 mmol/l at the time of the *in utero* catheterisation.

Hydrocephalus

Congenital hydrocephalus, with an incidence of 0.5–1.8/1000 births (Robertson et al 1981), may result from genetic aberrations such as autosomal trisomies, chromosomal deletions and translocations or environmental influences, including cytomegalovirus, toxoplasmosis or rubella infection, but the majority of cases have no clear-cut aetiology and are probably due to a combination of genetic and environmental factors. The risk of recurrence in subsequent pregnancies is in the range of 2–5% but a minority of cases are inherited as X-linked or autosomal recessive traits.

The outlook of congenital hydrocephalus is poor with a high fetal wastage or perinatal death, mainly due to associated severe congenital anomalies (Chervenak et al 1984), whilst amongst the survivors, severe mental retardation is common (Lawrence & Coates 1962, Mealey et al 1973, McCullough & Balzer-Martin 1982). Thus Chervenak et al (1984), found other associated defects in 84% of 50 fetuses with antenatal sonographic diagnosis of ventriculomegaly.

The underlying pathophysiology in many cases is complete or partial obstruction of the aqueduct of Sylvius and consequential cerebral spinal fluid hypertension. This results in progressive enlargement of the ventricles with ependymal effacement, white matter oedema and eventually gliosis, demyelination, and irreversible damage (Milhorat et al 1970, Weller & Schulman 1972). Thus, theoretically, decompression at the earliest possible time should arrest this destructive sequence of events.

Michejda & Hodgen (1981) inserted a ventriculo-amniotic shunt with a one way valve mechanism in a group of fetal rhesus monkeys with corticosteroid induced hydrocephalus. Whereas untreated hydrocephalic neonates rarely survived more than 14 days, manifesting progressive muscular weakness and frequent epileptic seizures, the treated fetal monkeys seldom died, and the neonatal monkeys showed normal growth rates and motor developments.

On the basis of the encouraging results in these animal studies and experience with cerebrospinal fluid diversion procedures in human neonates, that in selected cases are known to be beneficial in improving the outlook of these babies (Foltz & Shurtleff 1963, McCullough & Balzer-Martin 1982), Birnholz & Frigoletto (1981) used ultrasound guided repeated encephalocenteses to decompress the ventricles in one hydrocephalic fetus but were unable to control the ventriculomegaly and the fluid reaccumulated rapidly. Subsequently Clewell et al (1981) introduced percutaneously a silicone rubber ventriculo-amniotic shunt with a one-way valve in a 23 week fetus with hydrocephalus. The function of the shunt was confirmed on serial ultrasonic examinations by an increased cortical mantle thickness, a decreased ventricular to hemisphere ratio (V/H) and a normal biparietal diameter (BPD). However, between 32 and 34 weeks gestation, an increase in BPD and V/H indicated that the shunt had stopped functioning. Following delivery, by Caesarian section, it was found that the shunt was obstructed by an ingrowth of tissue from the ventricular end. The infant had a permanent ventriculo-peritoneal shunt placed on the first day of life. Now, at 4 years of age he has profound psychomotor retardation. Other investigators in several centres have used similar operations, and the total world experience presented in 1984 at the first Fetal Medicine and Surgery Society meeting in Washington amounted to 28 cases. No significant maternal morbidity was reported but there were five fetal deaths due either to the procedure or to other associated fetal abnormalities. Although detailed developmental data is not available, of the 23 survivors 12 have severe retardation while 11 were reported as having essentially normal development. The oldest infant is 4 years of age.

Such limited experience of *in utero* shunting in hydrocephalus does not allow final conclusions to be drawn. The efficacy of treatment cannot be determined until long-term postnatal neurological follow-up is available and until we gain a better understanding of the natural history of the disease. Ventriculo-amniotic shunts can certainly decrease ventricular size and result in an infant with a normal sized head and normal neuro-development. It is also clear that some infants will be grossly retarded even with apparently successful treatment. As there is presently no method of assessing residual brain function *in utero* or excluding an associated extensive intrinsic central nervous system malformation, one must be constantly aware of the very real possibility that intervention may allow survival in a vegetative state of what would have been a non-viable fetus. In the meantime prenatal decompression should not be performed unless:

1. the fetus is too immature to be delivered for postnatal shunting;
2. a detailed ultrasonographic examination is undertaken to exclude other anatomical defects;

3. fetoscopy and pure fetal blood sampling for karyotyping and virological studies are performed;
4. there is evidence of progressive ventricular dilatation and cortical thinning on serial sonographs; and
5. the parents are counselled as to the experimental nature of the procedure prior to giving of consent.

Very few cases fulfill these criteria and the place for this procedure is very limited.

Diaphragmatic hernia

Congenital diaphragmatic hernia (CDH), with an incidence of 1 in 2000 to 3000 births can be diagnosed antenatally by the sonographic demonstration of abdominal viscera in the thorax and the associated mediastinal shift. Polyhydramnios is often present. Although CDH is an anatomically simple defect that is easily correctable by removing the herniated viscera from the chest and closing the diaphragm, 50–80% of neonates do not survive even with prompt surgical correction and optimal neonatal care (Harrison & de Lorimier 1981). The cause of death in both treated and untreated neonates is respiratory insufficiency due to pulmonary hypoplasia resulting from developmental arrest secondary to compression by the herniated viscera.

Recent observations on normal growth and development of the airways and pulmonary vasculature have improved our understanding of how human lung growth is affected by CDH. Thus, the bronchial tree is fully developed by the sixteenth week of gestation whereas alveoli continue to develop even after birth, increasing in number until growth of the chest wall is completed in adulthood. The growth of blood vessels supplying the acinus (intra-acinar vessels) parallels alveolar development, while the growth of pre-acinar vessels follows the development of the airways (Reid 1984). In CDH the pleuroperitoneal canal fails to close by the time the intestines return to the abdomen at 8 to 10 weeks of gestation. The reduced thoracic space available to the developing lung leads to reduction in airways, alveoli and arteries. Furthermore, there is an increase in arterial medial wall thickness and extension of muscle peripherally into the small pre-acinar arteries (Kitigawa et al 1971) offering an explanation for the pulmonary hypertension and persistent fetal circulation observed after neonatal repair. Postnatal surgical correction of CDH decompresses the lung and in the survivors allows development of new alveoli and intra-acinar arteries. However, no new airways can be formed as this stage of development was completed by 16 weeks gestation.

With the use of a fetal lamb model in which diaphragmatic hernias were created by making a hole in the left diaphragm at 100 days of gestation, Harrison and associates (1981) developed a successful *in utero* surgical technique which involved reduction of the viscera from the thoracic cavity into the peritoneal cavity and repair of the diaphragmatic defect. The abdominal contents were accommodated without increased intra-abdominal pressure, that would compromise blood flow in the umbilical vein, by enlarging the abdominal cavity with abdominoplasty which involved the incorporation of an oval silicone rubber patch into the abdominal wall. The repair was performed on 10 lambs at 120 days gestation; four died post-operatively and six were viable after term delivery (140 days).

Although these studies demonstrated that correction of CDH *in utero* is physiologically sound and technically feasible in fetal lambs, correction of CDH has not yet been attempted in a human fetus because of the significant procedure related risks to the fetus and the risks of hysterotomy.

Neural tube defects

Anencephaly is fatal at or within hours of birth but the natural history of spina bifida is variable and surviving infants are often severely handicapped and require frequent surgical interventions (Frank & Fixsen 1980) and institutional care. Handicap typically consists of paralysis or weakness of the lower limbs, urinary and faecal incontinence and hydrocephalus with mental retardation. Without surgical treatment only 20% of infants survive to the age of 2 years (Laurence 1964) and if treatment is delayed to the age of 3 months, survival is little improved (Doran & Guthkelch 1961). If, however, closure is undertaken within 24 hours of birth, the 2 year survival is 60% (Lorber 1971). Furthermore, the results of early and delayed spinal surgery (Sharrard et al 1963) provided evidence that there was improved muscle function with early closure.

The presence of vigorous limb movements commonly observed antenatally by ultrasonography in babies with large spina bifidae (S. Campbell — personal communication) and the assumption that spinal dysraphism leads to progressive neurological deficit, have prompted investigators to assess the effectiveness of *in utero* closure of these defects in the prevention of handicap. With the use of fetal rhesus monkeys induced to develop neural tube defects by administration of synthetic corticosteroids and thalidomide during embryogenesis, Hodgen (1981) was successful in sealing the lesion using a technique in which an agar-based medium containing crushed bone particles was applied as a bone paste over the herniated nerve bundles.

Michejda (1985) induced a spina-bifida-like condition in eight Macaca mulatta fetuses at 110–125 days gestation by intrauterine lumbar laminectomy followed by manual displacement of the spinal cord from the central canal. She subsequently closed the defect with an allogeneic bone paste in five cases. On neurological assessment after delivery at term (160–164 days), the three untreated animals showed severe neurological abnormalities including paraplegia, incontinence and somatosensory loss below the induced lesion. On histological examination of the vertebral column, there was no significant new bone formation or healing, while the exposed spinal cord showed degenerative changes. In contrast, the *in utero* treated animals had completely normal neurological development, complete restoration and remodelling of bone and morphologically normal spinal cords.

Skeletal anomalies

Michejda and coworkers (1981) have successfully performed intrauterine allogeneic bone transplantations in the rhesus monkey at 120–135 days of gestation with the use of either fetus to fetus orthotopic transplantation of the humeral mid-shaft or particles of crushed bone mixed with an agar enriched culture medium. It was of particular interest that the bone paste had strong adhesive properties and could be sculptured into the desired conformation without forfeiting ultimate long bone strength. In some experiments the humeri from two fetuses were osteotomised and the bone segments interchanged during concurrent surgical procedures. Equal success was obtained when bone frozen and stored at –60°C for up to 6 months was used. Accordingly, these investigators concluded that the immune surveillance system of fetal rhesus monkeys may be tolerant of such bone allografts even when performed in the second trimester of pregnancy and suggested that these techniques offer potential for intrauterine surgical repair of human fetal skeletal dysplasias.

In some severe craniofacial syndromes, notably the craniostenoses, in which there is premature closure of one or more cranial sutures with consequent increased intracranial pressure and impairment of cerebral development, the dysmorphogenesis is known to worsen as intrauterine growth proceeds (Poswillo 1982). Early prenatal recognition and *in utero* surgical management, such as craniectomy in Apert or Crouzon syndromes, by allowing subsequent catch-up growth before birth could ameliorate or overcome most of the stigmata of the malformation process.

Facial clefts

In fetal rats horizontal full thickness wounds of the cheeks, from the angle of the mouth, heal within 24 hours with minimal macro- or microscopic evidence of tissue disruption. Similar studies in the orofacial region of Macaca fasicularis monkeys revealed complete healing of wounds after unrepaired incision or excision of tissue. Furthermore, when incised wounds were sutured with a variety of materials, there were minimal signs of perisutural reaction and scarring. In contrast, similar surgical wounds in the lip of the *M. fasicularis* neonate were accompanied, within a few hours, by a considerable inflammatory response which persisted for about 7 days and on healing, there was an obvious linear scar at the site of incision (Poswillo 1982).

The striking similarity between the repair processes of neonatal wounds in *M. fasicularis* and humans, suggests that the patterns of fetal wound healing would be comparable. Indeed, it was noted that when fetal skin biopsy is performed at 18 weeks gestation, there is complete wound healing and no scarring visible at the biopsy site within 2 weeks of the procedure (Rodeck et al 1980). Thus, the prospects for optimal repair of conditions such as severe cleft lip and palate after intrauterine surgery are excellent.

FETAL MEDICINE

Fetal enzyme deficiencies and metabolic derangements or abnormalities of growth and development are potentially treatable by manipulation of the maternal diet for provision of a missing nutrient, vitamin or hormone, or for elimination of potential toxins and teratogens. In some circumstances transplacental drug therapy has been used to treat fetal disorders, for example antiarrhythmic drugs for supraventricular tachyarrhythmias, or to improve the capacity of the fetus for postnatal adaptation.

A more direct approach for medical treatment *in utero* has been attempted by such measures as the intra-amniotic instillation of nutrients in the case of growth retardation due to impaired placental perfusion. Fetal anaemia secondary to severe rhesus isoimmunisation is corrected by transfusing red blood cells into the fetal peritoneal cavity and more recently directly into the fetal intravascular compartment. In non-immune hydrops fetalis, hypo-proteinaemia is correctable by direct intravascular infusion of albumin. Similar techniques will hopefully be used in the near future to infuse stem cell precursors directly into fetal tissues for the correction of genetic disease.

Methylmalonic acidaemia

The first example of *in utero* treatment of a vitamin responsive inborn error of metabolism involved the administration of high doses of vitamin B_{12} to a mother known to have a fetus with B_{12}-responsive methylmalonic acidaemia (Ampola et al 1975). The patient had previously delivered a child who died with severe acidosis and dehydration at the age of 3 months and in whom the diagnosis of methylmalonic acidaemia was made posthumously by chemical analysis of blood and urine. In her subsequent pregnancy a positive prenatal diagnosis was made by the demonstration of high levels of methylmalonic acid in amniotic fluid and maternal urine. In this case prenatal treatment certainly improved fetal and secondarily maternal biochemistry although it is more difficult to assess the clinical benefit to the fetus. However, it seems likely that reducing the fetal burden of methylmalonic acid had some beneficial effect on fetal development.

Multiple carboxylase deficiency

Biotin-responsive multiple carboxylase deficiency, in which affected patients present in the neonatal period or early childhood with severe metabolic acidosis, is another inborn error of metabolism in which prenatal therapy has been attempted. Administration of biotin to two patients during pregnancy prevented the neonatal onset of clinical or chemical manifestations of the disease in their babies (Roth et al 1982, Packman et al 1982). However, it is not possible at this stage to assess the advantages of prenatal therapy as compared to immediate treatment after birth.

Neural tube defects

Maternal diet supplementation with vitamins may have a protective effect on the development of neural tube defects (Smithells 1983, Lawrence 1984). Thus in studies involving women, who had one or more previous pregnancies with neural tube defects, Smithells reported a recurrence rate of 3 in 459 (0.7%) where periconceptual supplementation with a multivitamin preparation was given in contrast to a rate of 24 in 510 (4.7%) amongst unsupplemented pregnancies. Similarly Lawrence in a double blind randomised controlled trial of folate or placebo, given preconceptually and continued throughout the first trimester of pregnancy, found no recurrences amongst 44 women judged to have taken folate, 4 in 51 (7.8%) in the placebo group and 2 in 16 (12.5%) women in the folate group that were considered as non-compliers on the basis of low serum folate levels. Although both these studies demonstrate an apparent protective effect of vitamin supplementation, more definite evidence is awaited from a multi-centre study which is currently being performed by the Medical Research Council.

Maternal phenylketonuria

The toxic effects on the fetus observed in association with either fetal or maternal metabolic diseases are theoretically preventable by restriction of the offending metabolite from the maternal diet. Thus in maternal phenyl-ketonuria and resultant fetal hyperphenylalaninaemia, there is a high incidence of fetal wastage and congenital malformations. In a recent international survey, it was found that the stillbirth rate was approximately 25% and of the surviving children 90% were mentally retarded, 70% were microcephalic and 12% had congenital heart disease (Lenke & Levy 1980). While the results of low phenylalanine diet introduced after the eighth week of gestation have not been encouraging (Smith et al 1979), the pattern of abnormalities indicates that the diet should commence before conception for any reasonable chance of a positive effect on the outcome of pregnancy.

Fetal galactosaemia

In galactosaemia, deficiency of transferase enzyme activity results in intracellular accumulation of the toxic intermediate galactose I-phosphate with widespread involvement of liver, kidney, brain and lens. While signs and symptoms are largely ameliorated by elimination of galactose from the diet soon after birth, long-term reviews of early diagnosed and well treated galactosaemic individuals have shown behavioural disturbances and impaired intelligence, suggesting the possibility of prenatal damage (Komrower & Lee 1970). Furthermore, it has recently been recognised that female galactosaemics have a high frequency of primary or secondary amenorrhoea due to ovarian failure (Chen et al 1981a, Kaufman et al 1981), possibly as a result of an early intrauterine insult (Chen et al 1981b) from transplacentally derived galactose and or its metabolites. It would therefore seem sensible for a mother at risk of having a galactosaemic fetus to start a galactose deficient diet before conception. Prenatal diagnosis can be performed by amniocentesis or chorionic villus sampling and the diet stopped if the fetus is unaffected.

Endrocrinopathies

Theoretical possibilities for *in utero* endocrine therapy include the maternal administration of corticosteroids which might prevent abnormal masculinisation of the external genitalia of a female fetus with congenital adrenal hyperplasia, or testosterone administration for the treatment of male fetuses with testicular enzyme failure, in which, despite anti-Müllerian factor secretion, no testosterone is produced, the Wolffian system does not develop and the external genitalia are female (Beazley 1984). However, for institution of therapy at the correct chronological interval, prenatal diagnosis should be undertaken at a gestational age before the effects of the endocrinopathy on sexual differentiation occur. Furthermore the possible side-effects on the mother and pregnancy have to be considered.

In congenital hypothyroidism (CH) there is poor intellectual and motor function resulting from impaired brain development. While early postnatal detection and treatment can lead to normal or near normal intellectual development (New England Congenital Hypothyroidism Collaborative 1981), it may not prevent poor coordination. This may possibly be due to differences in the critical thyroxine dependent period during the maturation of the cerebrum and cerebellum (Layde 1984). Prenatal diagnosis of CH can be made by fetal blood sampling at 18 weeks gestation and thyroxine supplementation instituted *in utero*. However, since thyroxine crosses the placenta poorly, for treatment to be effective it must be injected into the amniotic fluid (Weiner et al 1980) where it can be swallowed and absorbed by the fetus.

Preterm

Although many agents are being used to arrest preterm labour, both the desirability of their use and their efficacy are questionable (Anderson 1981). Glucocorticoids administered to the mother increase fetal surfactant production, hasten fetal lung maturation and ameliorate the respiratory distress syndrome (Liggins & Howie 1972), while the administration of phenobarbitone can enhance fetal liver microsomal enzyme maturation and prevent neonatal jaundice (Boreus et al 1978).

Intrauterine Growth Retardation (IUGR)

In IUGR, sporadic attempts have been made to improve fetal growth and perinatal outcome by maternal intravenous administration of dextrose and amino acid solutions (Beischer et al 1984) or by the intra-amniotic instillation of nutrients (Renaud et al 1972). However, a more rational approach to the management of this condition should be based on recognition that the population of fetuses with IUGR is heterogeneous, being composed of (a) normal small babies, at no increased risk of mortality or morbidity (70–80% of the cases), (b) dysmature or asymmetrically small fetuses due to uteroplacental insufficiency, associated with a high incidence of perinatal asphyxia and mortality and (c) symmetrical or 'early insult' IUGR, usually observed in fetuses with genetic disease, chromosomal aberrations, congenital malformations and intrauterine infection or chronic maternal vascular disease, malnutrition and hypoxia. Serial ultrasonographic measurements of fetal head to abdomen circumference ratios (Campbell & Thoms 1977) and more recently the study of fetal and utero-placental blood flow characteristics by doppler ultrasound (Griffin et al 1983) should help distinguish between these three types.

In the management of symmetrical IUGR, attention should be directed towards the exclusion of fetal abnormalities by such measures as detailed anatomical examination by sonography and fetal blood sampling for virological studies and rapid karyotyping. In asymmetrical IUGR, with the aim of improving uteroplacental perfusion, we are currently investigating various pharmacological approaches including maternal plasma expansion and vasodilatation. Ultimately, with a better understanding of the mechanisms regulating fetal growth and development, the role played by genetic, maternal, placental and fetal factors (Gluckman & Liggins 1984) and the pathophysiology of abnormal growth patterns, new strategies of management will emerge directed towards the prevention of IUGR.

Rhesus isoimmunisation

During the last 40 years, several innovative therapeutic approaches have been undertaken in the management of severely Rh-isoimmunised pregnancies with the aim of ameliorating the severity of the disease and preventing intrauterine fetal death (Table 3.2).

Neutralisation of maternal Rh-antibodies and prevention of erythroblastosis by the administration of an Rh-hapten has been claimed (Carter 1947) but not

Table 3.2 In utero therapy in RH isoimmunisation

1. Reduction or alteration of maternal RH antibodies
2. Prevention of fetal haemolysis
3. Increase in fetal red cell production
4. Fetal marrow transplantation
5. Fetal top-up or exchange blood transfusion

substantiated. 'Desensitisation' of a woman, who had previously delivered a hydropic infant, was attempted by repeated injections of her husband's blood but rather than becoming 'desensitised', she became hyperimmunised, with an increase in her serum antibody levels. However, she delivered an infant that was only mildly affected (East & Mair 1949) and this was presumably due to an alteration in the maternal immune response from the production of IgG antibody (which crosses the placenta) to IgM (which does not). In a subsequent study of four patients receiving the same treatment, delivery of hydropic infants was not prevented (Allen & Diamond 1959). More recently, maternal 'desensitisation' by the daily ingestion of gastric acid resistant capsules containing Rh(D)-positive red blood cell membranes has been reported to be beneficial (Bierme et al 1979) but further controlled studies are necessary to confirm these findings. Intensive plasmapheresis (Powell 1968, Clarke et al 1970, Fraser et al 1976) whereby large volumes of anti-D containing plasma are removed from the pregnant woman, usually biweekly, is a controversial method of management and there are no randomised controlled trials to demonstrate its efficacy. Although there is a transient decrease in the amount of circulating anti-D after treatment, this is often followed by a rebound increase in antibody production.

Prevention or modification of the haemolytic process of antibody-coated fetal red cells has been attempted by immunosuppression with corticosteroids (Hunter 1955, Caritis et al 1977, Anderson & Cordero 1980, Navot et al 1982) and promethazine hydrochloride (Gusdon & Witherow 1973, Charles & Blumenthal 1982). While corticosteroids have become the mainstay of treatment in autoimmune haemolytic anaemia, exerting a number of beneficial effects including decreased antibody production, impairment of antibody-red cell interaction and inhibition of macrophage binding of antibody-coated red cells (Murphy & LoBuglio 1976), they have not been conclusively shown to be effective in the treatment of severe Rh-isoimmunisation despite theoretical alterations at the maternal site of antibody production, as well as effects at the level of fetal cellular destruction. Promethazine hydrochloride has been shown in *in vitro* and animal experiments to stabilise antibody-coated fetal erythrocytes and to inhibit their destruction by phagocytosis in the reticulo-endothelial system. Gusdon & Witherow (1973) reported equivocal evidence of a beneficial effect from this treatment in 13 patients, but this was not substantiated in studies using untreated matched controls (Stenchever 1978).

The accepted cause of fetal anaemia in Rh-isoimmunisation is the decrease in the lifespan of antibody-coated erythrocytes. However, a further possibility that may be important in some cases is relative failure of erythropoiesis or of haemopoiesis in general. Thus, a megaloblastic crisis, where there is arrest of haemopoiesis due to folic acid or vitamin B_{12} deficiency is a recognised complication of autoimmune haemolytic anaemias (Allgood & Chaplin 1967). Although in theory this could apply in some cases of erythroblastosis, in one study the administration of high doses of vitamin B_{12}, folic acid and other known haematinics to a group of women who had previously had erythroblastotic stillbirths, did not result in any improvement in the outcome of pregnancy (Allen 1963).

In 1957 bone marrow transplantation from Rh-negative donors was attempted in four erythroblastotic fetuses at 12 to 16 weeks gestation by injection of the donor material into the fetal peritoneal cavity (Allen 1963). However, many technical problems were encountered and the author was certain of correct placement of the graft in only two of the cases. After abortion of the fetuses, within 3 weeks of the procedure, no evidence of viable donor tissue could be obtained. Nevertheless, the theoretical basis for this attempt is valid because transplantation at a gestational age before the development of fetal immune competence would result in the induction of tolerance to the graft and possibly lead to a state of stable erythropoietic chimerism. This would ameliorate the severity of the disease since even a modest production of Rh-negative cells would prevent severe anaemia and its sequelae. Since the technical difficulties encountered in the early sixties have been overcome by the advent of real-time ultrasonography and fetoscopy, the feasibility of bone marrow transplantation should now be reconsidered. This would not only benefit fetuses in severe Rh-disease, but also those with various haematological disorders including the haemoglobinopathies.

Following the first transabdominal intrauterine fetal blood transfusion (Liley 1963), Freda & Adamsons (1964), performed successfully an 'open' intrauterine exchange transfusion. The leg of a 27 week fetus was delivered up to the groin through a hysterotomy incision and a 22 gauge polyethylene catheter was inserted into the femoral artery. An exchange transfusion with a total of 220 ml of fresh O Rh-negative blood was performed over a 2 hour period by removing and replacing 5 ml of blood at a time. Although both mother and fetus tolerated the procedure well, on the second post-operative day, premature labour resulted in the delivery of an 800 g infant who died in the neonatal period from respiratory distress. Asensio et al (1966), used a similar technique and successfully performed an exchange transfusion through the saphenous vein of a 31 week fetus. The post-operative period was uneventful and the infant, who was delivered after spontaneous labour at 34 weeks, survived.

The various therapeutic approaches discussed above have largely remained experimental. The traditional management of Rh-isoimmunised pregnancies, evolved over the last 20 years, has been well reviewed by Whitfield in Volume 2 of this series (1982). This includes (a) prediction of whether the fetus is severely affected, and if so at what stage of gestation hydrops will develop or intrauterine death will occur. This is based on the patient's previous obstetric history, the levels and trend of maternal Rh-antibody levels and the amniotic fluid bilirubin concentration, as determined by the deviation it produces in the optical density at 450 nm wavelength — $\triangle OD450$ (Liley 1961, Whitfield 1970) and (b) planned early delivery or if the fetal lungs are immature, intrauterine intraperitoneal blood transfusion. Although many centres have enthusiastically endorsed this approach reporting good survival rates in severely affected pregnancies (Whitfield et al 1972, Hobbins et al 1976, Frigoletto et al 1981,

Harman et al 1983, Scott et al 1984), Whitfield (1983) has estimated that in patients who had at least one previous Rh death, the currently achievable Rh survival rate is approximately 60%. Furthermore, the outlook for fetuses developing hydropic changes at an early gestational age remains extremely poor.

In 1981, a technique for direct intravascular fetal blood transfusion by fetoscopy was described (Rodeck et al 1981). Under direct vision an umbilical cord artery is punctured and a pure fetal blood sample obtained for haematological and biochemical analysis including blood grouping, haemoglobin, reticulocyte count, antibody level and bilirubin estimation. With the tip of the needle in the lumen of the vessel, fresh packed (haematocrit 60–80%) Rh-negative blood compatible with the mother is infused manually through a 5 ml syringe at a rate of 1–3 ml/min. The quantity transfused is determined by consideration of the estimated feto-placental blood volume, the pre-transfusion haematocrit and the haematocrit of the transfused blood. Fetal haematocrit is checked approximately two-thirds of the way through the transfusion and the volume transfused is adjusted to bring the final value to the normal 35–45% range. Transfusions can be started as early as 18 weeks gestation and repeated at 1–3 weekly intervals up to 30 to 32 weeks. Depending on fetal lung maturity, and in close collaboration with a neonatal paediatric team experienced in dealing with the particular problems of the rhesus-affected newborn, delivery is planned for 32 to 34 weeks. While vaginal delivery is preferable, the threshold for Caesarian section should be low (Rodeck & Nicolaides 1983, Rodeck et al 1985). Using this approach for the management of 34 severely rhesus isoimmunised pregnancies, referred before 25 weeks gestation and including 15 with ultrasonic evidence of fetal hydrops the overall survival rate achieved was 85%; 13 out of 15 (87%) of the hydropic fetuses and 16 of 19 (84%) of those with no antenatal evidence of hydrops survived.

Unexplained fetal hydrops

Hydrops fetalis is a non-specific finding in a wide variety of fetal and maternal disorders (Potter 1943). With the decline in the incidence of Rh-isoimmunisation, 'non-immune' causes have become responsible for at least 75% of the cases (Machin 1981) and make a greater contribution to perinatal mortality (Anderson et al 1983). While in many instances the underlying cause can be determined by detailed ultrasound scanning (Fleischer et al 1981), quite often the abnormality remains unexplained, even after post-mortem examination (Keeling et al 1983).

The ability to obtain pure fetal blood samples by fetoscopy (Rodeck & Campbell 1978), has given us the opportunity to study the cytogenetic, haematological, virological and biochemical status of 30 fetuses with unexplained hydrops with the aim of gaining a better understanding of the pathophysiology of this condition (Nicolaides et al 1984). In one fetus, paroxysmal tachyarrhythmia was noted on routine real-time ultrasound scanning 24 hours after fetoscopy and this was corrected by administration of digitalis to the mother. Ten (33%) of the fetuses had chromosomal abnormalities, one an erythroblastic process, possibly erythroleukaemia, one α-thalassaemia and one cytomegalovirus infection. Fetal hypoalbuminaemia and hypoproteinaemia in association with high protein levels in the serous cavities and amniotic fluid was found in all cases where biochemical analysis was performed. Although hypoproteinaemia may result from decreased synthesis, it seems more likely that in these fetuses it was secondary to a generalised capillary endothelial defect causing leakage of colloids into the extravascular space and the serous cavities and through the kidneys into the amniotic fluid. The cause of this defect could be intrauterine infection by an as yet unidentified organism. This is supported by our finding of neutrophilia or eosinophilia, which certainly in post-natal life are commonly associated with infection or inflammatory conditions, in a large proportion (62%) of these fetuses.

Based on these findings our current management of pregnancies with non-Rhesus fetal hydrops (Table 3.3) includes detailed real-time ultrasound examination of the external and internal anatomy of the fetus, assessment of fetal scalp or generalised skin oedema and measurement of pleural effusions and ascites. The fetal heart is evaluated by two dimensional scanning (Allan 1984) for structural defects, arrhythmias and pericardial effusion. As fetal tachyarrhythmias are often paroxysmal, prolonged periods of heart rate monitoring are necessary for their detection. If no anatomical defect is found to explain the hydrops, fetoscopy and blood sampling are performed. In the treatment of fetal hydrops mere ultrasound guided repeated paracenteses and thoracenteses for drainage of peritoneal, or pleural effusions are unlikely to be successful and may possibly be detrimental as it has been our experience that under these circumstances the fluid re-accumulates in the various body cavities within 24–48 hours of drainage, causing further loss of protein and exacerbating the condition. Although fetal hypoproteinaemia is likely to be a secondary phenomenon we are currently investigating the value of correcting the hypoalbuminaemia, in cases where other abnormalities have been excluded, by repeated fetoscopic intravascular infusions of albumin (Rodeck 1984). However, treatment is likely to be most successful when the underlying defect has been identified and corrected.

Table 3.3 Investigation of non-Rhesus hydrops

ULTRASONOGRAPHY
Assessment of severity
Exclusion of anatomical defects
CARDIOTOCOGRAPHY
Diagnosis of dysrrhythmias
FETAL BLOOD SAMPLING
Karyotyping
Virology screen
Blood film and indices
Biochemistry

CONCLUSION

At present fetal surgery is mainly confined to experimental studies in animals. Its value in the few situations where it has been applied to the human fetus, remains unproven and controversial. However, in the case of fetal medicine, as the model of rhesus isoimmunisation has shown, understanding of the pathophysiology of a fetal disease process can lead to innovative therapeutic approaches for *in utero* correction.

REFERENCES

Allan L D 1984 The prenatal detection of congenital heart disease. In: Rodeck C H, Nicolaides K H (eds). Prenatal Diagnosis. Proceedings of the eleventh study group of the Royal College of Obstetricians & Gynaecologists. pp 285–296

Allen F H 1963 Attempts at prevention of intrauterine death in erythroblastosis fetalis. New England Journal of Medicine 269: 1344–1349

Allen F H Jr, Diamond L K 1959 Erythroblastosis fetalis: attempts at prevention by desensitization. Journal of Diseases of Childhood 98: 505

Allgood J W, Chaplin H 1967 Idiopathic acquired autoimmune haemolytic anaemia. American Journal of Medicine 43: 254–273

Ampola M G, Mahoney M J, Nakamura E, Tanaka K 1975 Prenatal therapy of a patient with vitamin B_{12} — responsive methylmalonic acidemia. New England Journal of Medicine 293: 313–317

Anderson A B M 1981 Second thoughts on stopping labour. In: Studd J (ed) Progress in Obstetrics and Gynaecology, vol. 1, pp 125–138. Churchill Livingstone, Edinburgh

Anderson C W, Cordero L 1980 Changes in amniotic fluid optical density at 450 μm in Rh-sensitised patients after hydrocortisone treatment. American Journal of Obstetrics and Gynecology 137: 820–822

Andersen H M, Drew J H, Beischer N A, Hutchinson A A, Fortune D W 1983 Non-immune hydrops fetalis: changing contribution of perinatal mortality. British Journal of Obstetrics and Gynaecology 90: 636–639

Asensio S H, Figueroa-Longo J G, Pelegrina I A 1966 Intrauterine exchange transfusion. American Journal of Obstetrics and Gynecology 95: 1129–1133

Bain A D, Scott J S 1960 Renal agenesis and severe urinary tract dysplasia. A review of 50 cases with particular reference to the associated anomalies. British Medical Journal 1: 841–846

Beazley J M 1984 Doubtful gender at birth. In: Studd J (ed) Progress in Obstetrics and Gynaecology, Vol. 4, pp 257–271. Churchill Livingstone, Edinburgh

Beck A D 1971 The effect of intra-uterine urinary obstruction upon the development of the fetal kidney. Journal of Urology 105: 784–789

Beischer N A, Abell D A, Drew J H 1984 Intra-uterine growth retardation. In: Studd J (ed) Progress in Obstetrics and Gynaecology, Vol. 4, pp 82–91. Churchill Livingstone, Edinburgh

Berkowitz R L, Glickman M G, Smith G J W, Siegel N J, Weiss R M, Mahoney M J, Hobbins J C 1982 Fetal urinary tract obstruction: what is the role of surgical intervention in utero? American Journal of Obstetrics and Gynecology 144: 367–375

Bierme S J, Blanc M, Abbal M, Fournie A 1979 Oral Rh treatment for severely immunized mothers. Lancet i; 604–605

Birnholtz J C, Frigoletto F D 1981 Antenatal treatment of hydrocephalus. New England Journal of Medicine 303: 1021–1023

Boreus L O, Jalling B, Wallin A 1978 Plasma concentrations of phenobartital in mother and child after confirmed prenatal and postnatal administration for prophylaxis of hyperbilirubinemia. Journal of Pediatrics 93: 695–698

Campbell S, Thoms A 1977 Ultrasound measurement of the fetal head to abdomen circumference ratio in the assessment of growth retardation. British Journal of Obstetrics and Gynaecology 84: 165–174

Caritis S, Mueller-Heubach E, Edelstone D 1977 Effect of betamethasone on analysis of amniotic fluid in the Rhesus sensitised pregnancy. American Journal of Obstetrics and Gynecology 127: 529–532

Carter B 1947 Preliminary report of a substance which inhibits anti-Rh. serum. American Journal of Clinical Pathology 17: 646–649

Charles A G, Blumenthal L S 1982 Promethazine hydrochloride therapy in severely Rh-sensitised pregnancies. Obstetrics and Gynecology 60: 627–630

Chen Y T, Mattison D R, Schulman J D 1981a Hypogonadism and galactosemia. New England Journal of Medicine 305: 464

Chen Y T, Mattison D R, Feigenbaum L, Fukui H, Schulman J D 1981b Reduction in oocyte number following prenatal exposure to a high galactose diet. Science 214: 1145–1147

Chervenak F A, Duncan C, Ment L R, Hobbins J C, McClure M, Scott D, Berkowitz R L 1984 Outcome of fetal ventriculomegaly. Lancet ii: 179–181

Clarke C A, Elson C J, Bradley J, Donohoe W T A, Lehane D, Hughes-Jones N C 1970 Intensive plasmapheresis as a therapeutic measure in rhesus-immunised women. Lancet i: 793–798

Clewell W H, Johnson M L, Meier P R, Newkirk J B, Hendee R W J, Bowes W A J, Zide S L, Hecht F, Henry G, O'Keeffe D 1981 Placement of ventriculoamniotic shunt for hydrocephalus in a fetus. New England Journal of Medicine 305: 955

Concensus Report 1982 Fetal treatment. New England Journal of Medicine 307: 1651–1652

Doran P A, Guthkelch A N 1961 Studies in spina bifida cystica. 1. General survey and reassessment of the problem. Journal of Neurology, Neurosurgery and Psychiatry 24: 331–345

East E N, Mair C M 1949 Intensive immunization of already sensitised Rh-negative women: birth of mildly diseased baby. Journal of Laboratory and Clinical Medicine 34: 983–991

Fleischer A C, Killam A P, Boehm F H, Hutchison A A, Jones T B, Shaff M I, Barret J M, Lindsey A M, James A E Jr 1981 Hydrops fetalis: sonographic evaluation and clinical implications. Radiology 141: 163–168

Foltz E L, Shurtleff D B 1963 Five year comparative study of hydrocephalus in children with and without operation (113 cases). Journal of Neurosurgery 20: 1064–1078

Frank J D, Fixsen J A 1980 Spina bifida. British Journal of Hospital Medicine 24: 422–437

Fraser I, Bothamley J A, Bennett M O, Airth G R, Lehane D, McCarthy M, Roberts F M 1976 Intensive antenatal plasmapheresis in severe rhesus isoimmunisation. Lancet i: 6–9

Freda V F, Adamsons K J 1964 Exchange transfusion in utero. American Journal of Obstetrics and Gynecology 89: 817–821

Frigoletto F D, Umansky I, Birnholz J, Acker D, Easterday C L, Harris G B, Griscom N T 1981 Intrauterine fetal transfusion in 365 fetuses during 15 years. American Journal of Obstetrics and Gynecology 139: 781–790

Gluckman P D, Liggins G C 1984 Regulation of fetal growth. In: Beard R W, Nathanielsz P W (eds) Fetal physiology and medicine, 2nd ed, pp 511–557. Butterworths, London

Golbus M S, Harrison M R, Filly R A, Callen P W, Katz M 1982 In utero treatment of urinary tract obstruction. American Journal of Obstetrics and Gynecology 142: 383–388

Griffin D, Cohen-Overbeek T, Campbell S 1983 Fetal and utero-placental blood flow. Clinics in Obstetrics and Gynaecology 10: 565–602

Gosden C M 1984 The recognition of clinically significant chromosome abnormalities in prenatal diagnosis: problem cases. In: Rodeck C H, Nicolaides K H (eds) Prenatal diagnosis. Proceedings of the eleventh study group of the Royal College of Obstetricians and Gynaecologists. pp 65–84

Gusdon J P, Witherow C C 1973 Possible ameliorating effects of erythroblastosis by promezathine hydrochloride. American Journal of Obstetrics and Gynecology 117: 1101–1108

Harman C R, Manning F A, Bowman J M, Lange I R 1983 Severe Rh-disease — poor outcome is not inevitable. American Journal of Obstetrics and Gynecology 145: 823–829

Harrison M R, deLorimier A A 1981 Congenital diaphragmatic hernia. Surgical Clinics of North America 61: 1023–1035

Harrison M R, Ross N A, deLorimier A A 1981 Correction of congenital diaphragmatic hernia in utero. III. Development of a successful surgical technique using abdominoplasty to avoid compromise of umbilical blood flow. Journal of Pediatric Surgery 16: 934–942

Harrison M R, Nakayama D K, Noall R, deLorimier A A 1982a Correction of congenital hydronephrosis in utero. II. Decompression reverses the effects of obstruction on the fetal lung and urinary tract. Journal of Pediatric Surgery 17: 965–974

Harrison M R, Golbus M S, Filly R A, Callen R W, Katz M, deLorimier A A, Rosen M, Jensen A R 1982b Fetal surgery for congenital hydronephrosis. New England Journal of Medicine 306: 591–593

Hislop A, Hey E, Reid L 1979 The lungs in congenital renal agenesis and dysplasia. Archives of Disease in Childhood 54: 32–38

Hobbins J C, Mahony M J, Goldstein L A 1974 New methods of intrauterine evaluation by the combined use of fetoscopy and ultrasound. American Journal of Obstetrics and Gynecology 118: 1069–1072

Hodgen G D 1981 Antenatal diagnosis and treatment of fetal skeletal malformations with emphasis on in utero surgery for neural tube defects and limb bud regeneration. Journal of the American Medical Association 246: 1079–1083

Hunter O B Jr 1955 Cortisone in the management of haemolytic disease of the newborn. New York State Journal of Medicine 55: 1136–1140

Kaufman R R, Kogut M D, Donnell G N, Goebelsmann U, March C, Loch R 1981 Hypogonadotrophic hypogonadism in female patients with glactosaemia. New England Journal of Medicine 304: 994–998

Keeling J W, Gough D J, Illiff P 1983 The pathology of non-Rhesus hydrops. Diagnostic Histopathology 6: 89–111

Kitigawa M, Hislop A, Boyden E A, Reid L 1971 Lung hypoplasia in congenital diaphragmatic hernia. A quantitative study of airway, artery and alveolar development. British Journal of Surgery 58: 342–346

Komrower G M, Lee D H 1970 Long-term follow up of galactosaemia. Archives of Disease in Childhood 45: 367–373

Laurence K M 1964 The natural history of spina bifida cystica: detailed analysis of 407 cases. Archives of Disease in Childhood 39: 41–57

Laurence K M 1984 Prevention of neural tube defects. In: Rodeck C H, Nicolaides K H (eds) Prenatal diagnosis. Proceedings of the eleventh study group of the Royal College of Obstetricians and Gynaecologists, pp 261–277

Laurence K M, Coats S 1962 The natural history of hydrocephalus: detailed analysis of 182 unoperated cases. Archives of Disease in Childhood 37: 345–362

Layde P M 1984 Congenital hypothyroidism. In: Wald N J (ed) Antenatal and Neonatal Screening, pp 239–257. Oxford University Press, Oxford

Lenke R R, Levy H L 1980 Maternal phenylketonuria and hyperphenylalalinaemia. New England Journal of Medicine 303: 1202–1208

Liggins G C, Howie R N 1972 A controlled trial of antepartum glucocorticoid treatment for prevention of the respiratory distress syndrome in premature infants. Pediatrics 50: 515–525

Liley A W 1961 Liquor amnii analysis in the management of the pregnancy complicated by Rhesus sensitization. American Journal of Obstetrics and Gynecology 82: 1359–1370

Lorber J 1971 Results of treatment of myelomenigocele. An analysis of 524 unselected cases, with special reference to possible selection for treatment. Developmental Medicine and Child Neurology 13: 279–303

Machin G A 1981 Differential diagnosis of hydrops fetalis. American Journal of Medical Genetics 9: 341–350

Manning F A, Harman C R, Lange I R, Brown R, Decter A, MacDonald N 1983 Antepartum chronic fetal vesico-amniotic shunts for obstructive uropathy: a report of two cases. American Journal of Obstetrics and Gynecology 145: 819–822

Murphy S, LoBuglio A F 1976 Drug therapy of autoimmune hemolytic anemia. Seminars in Haematology 13: 323–334

McCullough D C, Balzer-Martin L A 1982 Current prognosis in overt neonatal hydrocephalus. Journal of Neurosurgery 57: 378–383

McFadyen I R, Wigglesworth J S, Dillon M J 1983 Fetal urinary tract obstruction: is active intervention before delivery indicated? British Journal of Obstetrics and Gynaecology 90: 342–349

Mealey J, Gilmor R, Bubb M P 1973 The prognosis of hydrocephalus overt at birth. Journal of Neurosurgery 39: 348–355

Michejda M 1985 Intrauterine treatment of spina bifida: primate model. Zeitschrift fur kinderchirugie (in press)

Michejda M, Hodgen G D 1981 In utero diagnosis and treatment of non-human primate fetal skeletal anomalies. I. Hydrocephalus. Journal of the American Medical Association 246: 1093–1097

Michejda M, Bacher J, Kuwabara T, Hodgen G D 1981 In utero allogeneic bone transplantation in primates. Roentgenographic and histological observations. Transplantation 32: 96–100

Milhorat T H, Clark R G, Hammock M K, McGrath P P 1970 Structural, ultrastructural and permeability changes in the ependyma and surrounding brain favouring equilibrium in progressive hydrocephalus. Archives of Neurology 22: 397–407

Navot D, Rozen E, Sadovsky E 1982 Effect of dexamethasone on amniotic fluid absorbance in Rh-sensitised pregnancy. British Journal of Obstetrics and Gynaecology 89: 456–458

New England Congenital Hypothyroidism Collaborative. (1981). Effects of neonatal screening for hypothyroidism: prevention of mental retardation by treatment before clinical manifestations. Lancet ii: 1095–1098

Nicolaides K H, Rodeck C H, Lange I, Watson J, Gosden C M, Miller D, Mibashan R S, Moniz C, Morgan-Capner P, Campbell S 1984 Fetoscopy in the evaluation of unexplained fetal hydrops. British Journal of Obstetrics and Gynaecology (in press)

Packman S, Cowan M J, Golbus M S, Caswell N M, Sweetman L, Burri B J, Nyhan W L, Baker H 1982 Prenatal treatment of biotin-responsive multiple carboxylase deficiency. Lancet i: 1435–1438

Poswillo D E 1982 Prospects for fetal surgery. In: Barson A J (ed) Fetal and Neonatal Pathology. The Royal College of Pathologists, pp 131–142. Praeger Scientific, Eastbourne

Potter E L 1943 Universal oedema of the fetus unassociated with erythroblastosis. American Journal of Obstetrics and Gynecology 46: 130–134

Potter E L 1946 Bilateral renal agenesis. Journal of Pediatrics 29: 68–76

Potter E L, Craig J M 1976 Pathology of the Fetus and Infant, Ch. 22, Year Book Medical Publishers Inc, pp 434–475

Powell L C Jr 1968 Intense plasmapheresis in the pregnant Rh-sensitized woman. American Journal of Obstetrics and Gynecology 101: 153–170

Reid L 1984 Lung growth in health and disease. British Journal of Diseases of the Chest 78: 105–126

Renaud R, Vincendon G, Boog G 1972 Injections intraamniotiques d'acides amines dans les eaus de malnutrition foetale. Journal de Gynecologie, Obstetrique et Biologie de la Reproduction 1: 231–241

Robertson R D, Sarti D A, Brown W J, Crandall B F 1981 Congenital hydrocephalus in two pregnancies following the birth of a child with neural tube defect: aetiology and management. Journal of Medical Genetics 18: 105–107

Rodeck C H 1983 Invasive fetal therapy. In: Bovicelli L, Hobbins J C, Rizzo N, Pilu G (eds). Nuovi Concetti di Terapia Fetale. Proceedings of the international meeting on new concepts in intrauterine therapy, Bologna 1982. Co. Fe. Se. Palermo pp 89–96

Rodeck C H 1984 Fetal therapy. In: Rodeck C H, Nicolaides K H (eds) Prenatal Diagnosis. Proceedings of the eleventh study group of the Royal College of Obstetricians and Gynaecologists, pp 331–341

Rodeck C H, Campbell S 1978 Sampling pure fetal blood by fetoscopy in the second trimester of pregnancy. British Medical Journal 2: 728–730

Rodeck C H, Eady R A J, Gosden C M 1980 Prenatal diagnosis of epidermolysis bullosa letalis. Lancet i: 949–952

Rodeck C H, Kemp J R, Holman C A, Whitmore D N, Karnicki J, Austin M A 1981 Direct intravascular fetal blood transfusion by fetoscopy in severe Rhesus isoimmunisation. Lancet i: 625–628

Rodeck C H, Nicolaides K H 1983 Ultrasound guided invasive procedures in obstetrics. Clinics in Obstetrics and Gynaecology 10: 529–539

Rodeck C H, Nicolaides K H, Warsof S L, Fysh W J, Gamsu H R, Kemp J R 1985 The management of severe Rhesus isoimmunization by fetoscopic intravascular transfusions. American Journal of Obstetrics and Gynecology 150: 769–774

Roth K S, Yang W, Allan L et al 1982 Prenatal administration of biotin in biotin-responsive multiple carboxylase deficiency. Pediatric Research 16: 126–129

Scott J R, Kochenour N K, Larkin R M, Scott M J 1984 Changes in the management of severely Rh-immunized patients. American Journal of Obstetrics and Gynecology 149: 336–341

Sharrard W J W, Zachary R B, Lobrer J, Bruce A M 1963 A controlled trial of immediate and delayed closure of spina bifida cystica. Archives of Disease in Childhood 38: 18–22

Smith I, Erdohazi M, Macartney F J, Pincott J R, Wolff O H, Brenton D P, Biddle S A, Fairweather D V I, Dobbing J 1979 Fetal damage despite low-phenylalanine diet after conception in a phenylketonuric woman. Lancet i: 17–19

Smithells R W 1983 Diet and congenital malformation. In: Campbell D M, Gillmer M D G (eds) Nutrition in pregnancy. Proceedings of the tenth study group of the Royal College of Obstetricians and Gynaecologists, pp 155–163

Stenchever M A 1978 Promethezine hydrochloride: use in patients with Rh-isoimmunization. American Journal of Obstetrics and Gynecology 130: 665–668

Thomas I T, Smith D W 1974 Oligohydramnios, cause of the non-renal features of Potter's Syndrome, including pulmonary hypoplasia. Journal of Pediatrics 84: 811–814

Weiner S, Scharf J L, Bolognese R J, Librizzi R J 1980 Antenatal diagnosis and treatment of a fetal goiter. Journal of Reproductive Medicine 24: 39–42

Weller R O, Schulman K 1972 Infantile hydrocephalus: clinical, histological and ultrastructural study of brain damage. Journal of Neurosurgery 36: 255–265

Whitfield C R 1983 Haemolytic disease of the newborn — a continuing problem. In: Chiswick M L (ed) Recent Advances in Perinatal Medicine No. 1, pp 95–115. Churchill Livingstone, Edinburgh

Whitfield C R 1970 A three year assessment of an Action Line method of timing intervention in Rhesus isoimmunisation. American Journal of Obstetrics and Gynecology 108: 1239–1244

Whitfield C R 1982 Future challenges in the management of Rhesus disease. In: Studd J (ed) Progress in Obstetrics and Gynaecology, Vol. 2, pp 48–59. Churchill Livingstone, Edinburgh

Whitfield C R, Thompson W, Armstrong M J, Reid H McC 1972 Intrauterine fetal transfusion for severe Rhesus haemolytic disease. Journal of Obstetrics and Gynaecology of the British Commonwealth 79: 931–940

Fetal growth

Being a fetus is about growing and developing, but not all fetuses grow or develop equally. To a farmer retarded fetal growth produces 'runts' — small poorly developed animals which do not thrive after birth. This is a straightforward visual diagnosis in animals but in man significant fetal growth retardation is less easy to define. Inspection of the baby is not sufficient; gestational age and other factors associated with birthweight, such as maternal size, must also be included in the assessment of fetal growth and development at birth. An accurate diagnosis of reduced fetal growth is important because those who are significantly retarded are at increased risk of neonatal problems and developmental retardation. In this chapter the definition and assessment of growth retardation are first reviewed, then ethnic differences are discussed, and the relevance of changes in the maternal cardiovascular system to fetal growth are considered.

DEFINITION OF FETAL GROWTH RETARDATION

Many human variables, such as height, are normally distributed but birthweight is not. About 95% of birthweights form a normal bell-shaped gaussian curve but the remaining 3–5% form a prolonged tail of low weights (Fig. 4.1), and these babies are different from the rest (Wilcox & Russell 1983). This is true for both animals and humans. Among horses (Platt 1979) and other animals, runts account for 2–3% of deliveries. In pigs and others with large litters these light fetuses have been shown statistically to form a separate population whether conceived naturally (Royston et al 1982) or after super-ovulation (McLaren & Michie 1960a). Among humans also it has been shown that the lightest 3–5% are different.

Perinatal mortality among those weighing less than the third centile was at least 5 times greater than those who were born heavier (Usher & McLean 1974). Cerebral palsy was considerably more common among those who were below the fifth centile than in the higher centiles (Fig. 4.2). Blood glucose and haematocrit of neonates under the third centile were significantly different from those above the tenth centile and also from those between the third and tenth centiles (Haworth et al 1967).

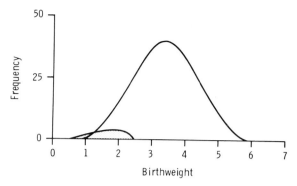

Fig. 4.1 Birthweight has a bimodal distribution. The majority of birthweights are normally distributed but there is a residual population (shaded area) which is 2–5% of all births. (after Wilcox & Russell 1983)

From such animal and human studies it is apparent that a definition of regarded fetal growth which includes all of those below the tenth centile of birthweight will include many normals. If only those under the fifth centile are included there will be few babies who are not truly growth retarded, and if the line is drawn at the third centile (corresponding to 2 standard deviations below the mean which also may be used) definition will be almost perfect, and certainly as precise as is necessary clinically.

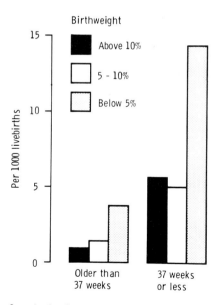

Fig. 4.2 The incidence of cerebral palsy per 1000 live births is greater in those children whose birthweight was below the fifth centile than in those born heavier, both premature and mature (after Hagberg 1978)

To determine whether or not a birthweight is truly below the third or fifth centile it has to be placed on a reference range of birthweights. Several of these have been published: to find the most appropriate and to use it with confidence you should be aware of differences in the populations from which they were derived as these may affect the range of weights. Some are the range of a single ethnic group (Thomson et al 1968), but others mix Caucasian and Negroid (Gruenwald 1966a) or other races. The social class of the population also is important since birthweight falls with falling social class (Butler & Alberman 1969, Dowding 1981) so a range constructed from a predominantly indigent population may have lower birthweights than a population of wider social class distribution.

Where the population lived may also be relevant: many of the ranges published were from populations living at sea level but one which is widely used (Lubchenco et al 1966) is from Denver, Colorado which is 5000 feet above sea level and one-third of these children were born to mothers who lived at 10 000 feet: since birthweight is reduced by 100 g for every 1000 m above sea level (McCulloch et al 1977) this range is not applicable to most populations. It has another drawback which is not uncommon — it was constructed from delivery at a referral centre and is biased by the inclusion of neonates referred because of their low birthweight.

Most reference ranges of birthweight exclude some of the children born during the period reviewed. Twins invariably are excluded since their birthweights are not comparable with singletons. Most omit stillbirths both because the actual date of death is uncertain and because the changes which take place after death alter fetal weight: some exclude only macerated fetuses since a fresh stillbirth's weight is taken to be an accurate measure of the true weight (Thomson et al 1968). The exclusion of neonatal deaths also was suggested by Naeye & Dixon (1978) since many who die in the first week of life are light-for-dates. Such exclusion of neonatal deaths would be appropriate in the construction of a normal range of birthweight but not in a reference range for clinical use which should include all accurate birthweights. For the same reason babies born after induced labour or elective Caesarean section are included even though their gestational age is therapeutically shortened. Illegitimate pregnancies are excluded by some since these pregnancies frequently are poorly documented, particularly the gestational age.

Apart from the actual birthweight gestational age is the most important piece of information in constructing reference ranges and may be the most difficult to obtain accurately. Birthweight, gravidity, maternal height and weight and the baby's sex are recorded with accuracy but even with the most co-operative mother giving the maximum of information there is always the uncertainty of the date of conception in calculating the estimated date of delivery. Most authors ascertained the accuracy of gestational age by review of the obstetric records, but Usher & McLean (1969) included assessment of neonatal maturity to increase precision. Now that ultrasonic measurement of fetal size in early pregnancy is common gestational age is less of a problem and this will increase the accuracy of a range (McFadyen et al 1984a). The bimodal distribution of birthweight which frequently is found at 28–34 weeks (Neligan 1965, Battaglia et al 1966, Gruenwald 1966a) has been interpreted as meaning that the heavier group of babies had inaccurate gestational ages and were several weeks more advanced in pregnancy than was calculated: they were omitted from further consideration by some (Lubchenco et al 1963, Gruenwald 1966a). These heavy babies may however have been prematurely born rhesus-affected or the infants of diabetic mothers, or the bimodality could have been due to ethnic differences in patterns of fetal growth which will be described later. These heavy babies discarded by some have a perinatal mortality five times that of mature babies of the same birthweight (Battaglia et al 1966) which suggests that many are born at the gestational age which was estimated from their menstrual data and should not be discarded. Abnormal fetuses also are excluded from some ranges. Since congenital anomaly tends to be associated with reduced birthweight omission of these babies will tend to raise the mean birthweight.

Adjustments to birthweight

Birthweight varies not only with gestational age but also with maternal size and other factors. For the most accurate assessment of the appropriateness of a baby's weight for its maturity adjustments have to be made to its birthweight to allow for these variables (Thomson et al 1968). Failure to do so may lead to light babies from small mothers labelled being 'light-for-dates' when their adjusted weights are close to the mean, and to growth retardation being ignored in relatively heavy babies born to large mothers. An extreme example is a boy of 3.1 kg born at 40 weeks to a mother in her second pregnancy, 180 cm tall weighing 80 kg: this apparently normal birthweight when adjusted lies on the third centile. Maternal size was most important in this adjustment, but the other information in her description was also relevant. Boys are heavier than girls from 32 weeks, the difference increasing with gestational age until it reaches 150 g at term, which is a significant proportion of many a newborn's weight. Second (and subsequent) fetuses are 100 g heavier than the first from 32 weeks. What constitutes a first pregnancy is not unanimously agreed: Thomson et al (1968) found that the weights of first children were not affected by the presence or absence of a previous abortion, but there is some more recent evidence (Alberman et al 1980) that a first pregnancy which aborts is associated with birthweight in the next pregnancy being very similar to that of second babies who were preceded by a normal first pregnancy.

Adjusted birthweights are more useful clinically than the raw data. The Aberdeen range (Thomson et al 1968) which was derived from 52 004 legitimate single births, with its adjustments which can be used confidently after 37 weeks is the best for white populations living at sea level. One adjustment which is not included is cigarette smoking but it is worth consideration (particularly in comparing populations in whom a large proportion smoke with non-smokers) since smoking tends to reduce birthweight by 150–200 g (McFadyen et al 1984a).

Patterns of fetal growth

Birthweight reflects the fetal condition at only one point in the pregnancy. Ultrasound, however, can assess the growth of several organs as they develop before delivery, and this is clinically useful. Some fetuses which are growth retarded have symmetrical reduction in the size of all organs; this tends to occur in fetal abnormality or in severe nutritional deprivation from early in pregnancy (Winick et al 1973). Where there is 'placental insufficiency' however, the pattern is different: the growth of liver, thymus and subcutaneous fat are reduced early, whereas brain and bone are last and least affected. This is consistent in naturally occurring and in experimentally induced growth retardation in animals (Verges 1939, Widdowson 1971, Myers et al 1971) and humans (Gruenwald 1963, Naeye 1970). Since brain growth can be assessed by serial measurements of the biparietal diameter and liver size by measurement of the abdominal circumference the pattern of fetal growth can be followed and if this is retarded symmetrical and asymmetrical retardation can be differentiated, and whether or not there is continuing deterioration.

Ethnic variation in birthweight and fetal growth

Humanity is the sum of its different races. Identified and defined by differences in body size, by the proportions and shapes of bones, by skin colour and hair texture, by the distribution of blood groups and biochemical differences, and by other measurable characteristics, the number of races ranges from three to 20 or more according to the method of classification used. One describes five principal races and subdivides them (Table 4.1). Within the races are ethnic groups which have common cultural and linguistic characteristics so that for

Table 4.1 Ethnic classification after Coon (1981). For brevity this does not include all populations

Mongoloid	northern: China, Korea, Tibet
	southern: Burma, Thailand
	Ainu
Congoid	Negro
	Pygmy
Caucasoid	Europe
	West Asia
	North Africa
	India
Capoid	Bushman
	Hottentot
Australoid	Melanesia, Micronesia, Polynesia
	Papua
	Australian aborigine

example the Caucasoid race contains ethnic groups from both Europe and India. Birthweight shows considerable racial and ethnic variation, but also geographically localised differences within these divisions. In Africa, Gambians have lower mean birthweights than Nigerians (Thomson & Baird 1957), but differences may be considerable even in individual countries. In England babies born to Irish mothers have heavier mean birthweights than the English (Barron & Vessey 1966, Grundy et al 1978). In Singapore the mean birthweights to Chinese and Malays were both 225 g less than to Europeans but were 160 g greater than to Indians (Cheng et al 1972). In Indonesia Chinese infants were heavier than the native Indonesians even when allowance was made for maternal stature, social class and birth rank (Barron 1976). Town and country dwellers often show differences in the same population: Finns who live in Helsinki have babies which are lighter than those who live in the surrounding country (Rantakalio 1969). Immigration also affects birthweight. Indians and Pakistanis who have come to any part of the United Kingdom not only have birthweights which are 150–300 g lighter than white British births (Arthurton 1972, Alvear & Brooke 1978, Grundy et al 1978, Haines et al 1982) but where the mother was herself born affects the weight of her children. Asian mothers born in East Africa have lighter babies than mothers born in India (McFadyen et al 1984a). Similarly Jewish mothers from North Africa have heavier babies than Israelis; but when they move to Israel birthweight comes closer to Israelis, and the longer they live in Israel the closer to Israelis do the birthweights come (Yudkin et al 1983).

Patterns of fetal growth and subsequent development

The best documented differences in patterns of fetal growth are between North American Negros and whites from similar social circumstances. Negros consistently have heavier mean birthweights up to 34–35 weeks, then the whites' birthweights catch up so that by term they have heavier babies (Freeman et al 1970, Fujikara & Froehlich 1972, Penchaszadehet et al 1972). This is not due to differences in the overall rate of organ maturation: renal glomerular maturity in peri-natal deaths is the same in both of these racial groups (Fujikara & Froehlich 1972). Ethiopian birthweights show a similar pattern (Gebre-Medhuin et al 1978): mean birthweights being greater than Swedish up to 33–36 weeks, but increasing little thereafter. This may well have a nutritional basis since rich Ethiopians have a mean birthweight almost 500 g greater than poor, but the mean gestational age at delivery for these two groups is not recorded. Body length, however, is known for both Swedes and Ethiopians; among the latter birthweight and body length run almost in parallel suggesting a symmetrical reduction which could be, at least in part, genetic.

Earlier studies of fetal growth were dependent on the weights of delivered babies which certainly for the premature birth may have differed in fetal growth from those not delivered at term. More recently longitudinal studies of growth *in utero* with ultrasound have produced more physiological data. Such a study has shown different patterns of growth between Indians and Europeans of similar social background (Meire & Farrant, 1980). There was an increased incidence of asymmetrically growth retarded fetuses, and also an increased proportion of small fetuses. There was no obvious reason for this, but the authors suggested that this may be partly genetic and partly environmental. Further studies of such populations are needed to resolve the relative importance of causative factors. Follow-up studies of the children may help to do this. Accelerated 'catch-up' growth infers intrauterine malnutrition and such 'catch-up' growth indeed occurred in another Indian population although these Indian babies were still 1 kg lighter than whites when they were a year old (Brooke & Wood 1980). Comparison of African, Indian, Chinese and European children born in Guyana and Jamaica (Ashcroft & Desai 1976) showed that Indians and Chinese remained lighter than Africans and Europeans for the first 9 years of life, and that these differences were independent of social class. They possibly reflect ethnic difference in body proportion rather than in malnutrition. Behavioural development in this population also showed similar differences.

Possible causes of ethnic variation

Some differences in birthweight and growth patterns are genetic. In-breeding is important: this is common in some communities and religions, it is found among Muslims, and among some Hindu groups in South India; where this occurs birthweight is reduced (Sibert et al 1979), being greater in uncle-niece marriages than in those between first cousins. A similar reduction with marriage between relatives has also been found both in Japan (Schork 1964) and in Jerusalem (Fried & Davis 1974). Such reduction might be due in part to an increase in the rate of fetal abnormality (Barnes 1981) but among the Tamil of South India 80% of marriages are between first cousins or closer relatives and the number of malformations recognised at birth is not increased; nor is the stillbirth rate (Rao & Imbarj 1977): it may be that since such in-breeding has continued for many generations all severe malformations have been bred out of the population as they have no survival advantage. An alteration in sex ratio with in-breeding would also alter birthweight, but this has probably not occurred. Some pregnancy complications such as hypertension may be partly genetic (Sutherland et al 1981); certainly different rates of complications in pregnancy may affect birthweight and the genetic element in these is uncertain and not well documented.

Environment is an important determinant of birthweight. Two unavoidable environmental factors are climate and altitude. Altitude is the more straightforward of these: for every 1000 m rise in altitude mean birthweight falls by 100 g (Lichty 1957, McCulloch et al 1977). Climate is more complex since it frequently is associated with patterns of work and of disease. Warm climates tend to be associated with reduced birthweights which may be due to diversion of blood to the skin from the uterus (Rowell 1974). In many tropical countries the warm wet season is a time of hard work and reduced calorie intake, which can reduce birthweight by 200 g (Prentice et al 1983) or more (Thomson & Baird 1967) part of which may be due to a rise in premature deliveries. Work not only diverts blood flow from the uterus to the limbs and elsewhere in the body, it also reduces the circulating volume (Kaltreider & Mendly 1940) which aggravates the reduction in utero-placental flow. Training may minimise this reduction: it does in sheep (Curet et al 1976) and women with a high physical work capacity after training have heavier babies (Errkkola 1976): in the Gambia birthweights in multigravid patients are not reduced in the wet season to the same extent as in primigravida and this may be due not only to the improved blood flow in the uterus which has already carried a pregnancy (Becker 1948) but to a more efficient pattern of work by the multigravida (Thomson & Baird 1967).

The rainy season not only coincides with harvesting but also with increasing malarial infection which reduces birthweight. Malaria is the most common severe infection likely to affect birthweight. It is well known that maternal immunity to malaria decreases during pregnancy and this change may be reflected in the reduction of 8 oz in birthweight associated with placental colonisation with the parasite (Bruce-Chwatt 1952, Cannon 1958). Possibly the reduction in birthweight is in part due to altered maternal immunity (Scott 1977) but preventive treatment of malaria raised baby weight by 0.35 lb which suggests that the infection itself contributes to the reduction (Morley et al 1964). There are other factors associated with infection which may reduce birthweight: competition for nutrients by the infecting organisms; reduction in absorption of nutrients, less effective utilisation or increase in their excretion: release of bacterial toxins which affect the uterus: such mechanisms as these may reduce birthweight. Treatment of pregnant animals with antibiotics increases birthweight possibly by eliminating subclinical infection: man responds similarly, apparently-healthy pregnant women given tetracycline for 6 weeks had heavier babies than women given a placebo (Elder et al 1971) probably because the tetracycline group had longer pregnancies. Infection may not only reduce fetal growth, it can precipitate premature labour.

Maternal diet can restrict fetal growth by reduction of total calorie intake or by lack of specific nutrients. Acute starvation reduces birthweight by 300–400 g due to loss of fat rather than protein, the fetuses are lean not stunted (Hytten 1979). Supplementation of the calorie content of the diet increases birthweight only when the mother is in chronic negative energy balance (Viegas et al 1982, Prentice et al 1983). Absorption of the food obviously affects its value to the mother and disease such as tropical sprue may reduce this. High fibre content in the diet also may interfere with the absorption of trace elements such as zinc which are required for fetal growth. Dietary fibre has other relevant effects: metabolism of the fibre in the lumen of the gut produces fatty acids which are absorbed and can depress glucose production by the liver. Also, fibre-rich foods such as beans and other leguminous seeds contain starch which may resist enzymic breakdown (Jenkins et al 1980).

The relevance of these observations to fetal growth is that fetal insulin is an important hormone in the regulation of that growth (Milner 1981, Khouzami et al 1981): its secretion by the fetal pancreas is stimulated by glucose passing across the placenta from the mother. The higher the concentration of glucose in the fetus the greater the section of insulin and the more the fetus grows, so depression of maternal glucose levels may depress fetal insulin secretion and so depress its growth. Other constituents of the diet may have similar effects: Karela (bitter-gourd) is one of these. It is a vegetable which is commonly used in Indian salads, but also in the treatment of diabetes because it reduces the rise in blood sugar with the ingestion of carbohydrate (Jenkins et al 1980). The lack of zinc reduces fetal growth in animals and man (Campbell Brown et al 1982): how this is mediated is not known but an interesting speculation is that it could be due to excessive production of vasoconstrictor prostaglandins (Cunnane et al 1983) which might interfere with utero-placental blood flow. The relationship of maternal diet to birthweight in man is becoming better established (Hytten 1979) but ethnic differences in its content may introduce uncertainties such as those mentioned in this partly hypothetical paragraph which require further investigation. They may explain part of the ethnic differences in birthweight.

Other substances which are eaten, drunk or inhaled may reduce birthweight and some of these are used by different ethnic groups or their effects are modified by the mother's origin. Tobacco smoking occurs world-wide and reduces birthweight at term by 150–200 g, the more the mother smokes the greater being the reduction in birthweight (Butler & Alberman 1969, Andrews & McGarry 1972). This effect is greater in Negros than in whites (Lubs 1973). Tobacco may be chewed as well as smoked: some Indian women do chew tobacco and this too reduces birthweight (Krishna 1978). The effects of smoking tobacco are complex but part of the reduction in birthweight which accompanies smoking is due to a reduction in maternal calorie intake, the fall being minimised when the maternal diet is increased (Papoz et al 1982). Other drugs taken by the mother also reduce birthweight: marijuana (Hingson et al 1982) and alcohol (Clarren & Smyth 1978) are both known to do so. Drugs frequently are taken in combination and their effects may also be combined. While a mother's smoking habits usually are known, whether or not she drinks excess alcohol or takes other drugs frequently is not, and yet this information is also relevant to fetal growth.

Social class differences affect birthweight, the lower the social class of the mother the lighter are her babies. Differences in maternal size and parity, in length of gestation and in smoking habits account for much of the difference but when these factors are allowed for a social class effect remains (Butler & Alberman 1969, Dowding 1981). This is true for the Registrar General's social classification of Europeans in Britain but not for Asian immigrants to the United Kingdom whose birthweight is not so related. The Registrar General's method is to classify by husbands' occupation (and hence income) which is valid for the European nuclear family but may not be for the extended Asian family in which earnings tend to be pooled and shared which perhaps helps to compensate for some inequalities. Nonetheless a simple classification of families in Pakistan by their income did show a direct relationship between income and birthweight (Rahimtoola et al 1968). Social status, however defined, is related to birthweight worldwide. It accounts for some of the differences between and within ethnic groups but is only one of the many factors influencing birthweight.

CARDIOVASCULAR CHANGES

Birthweight is related to changes in both maternal and fetal cardiovascular systems. Some affect fetal growth directly, others reflect the poor maternal adaptation to pregnancy which results in low birthweight. The fetal changes may be secondary to the maternal, but they directly affect transport from the placenta and fetal growth.

Maternal hypertension

Maternal hypertension is associated with reduction in birthweight. The higher the diastolic pressure rises above 90 mmHg or the systolic above 130 mmHg (Fig. 4.3), or the higher the mean arterial pressure, the greater is the reduction in birthweight (Baird et al 1957, Gruenwald 1966b, Butler et al 1969, Tervilla et al 1973, Page & Christiansson 1975, Lin et al 1981. If the mother also has proteinuria the reduction is even greater (Fig. 4.4) particularly if it rises over 3.5 g per litre (Baird et al 1957, Tervila et al 1973, Page & Christiansson 1975, Lin et al 1981) (Fig. 4.4). In one series of severely hypertensive women with

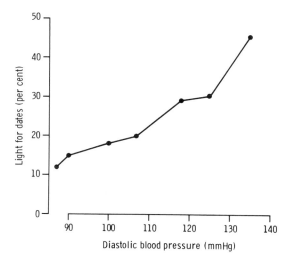

Fig. 4.3 The incidence of birthweights below the 10th centile increases as the diastolic blood pressure rises in pre-eclampsia (after Tervilla et al 1973)

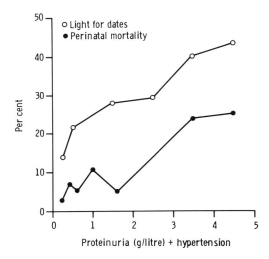

Fig. 4.4 If hypertension is accompanied by proteinuria both the incidence of birthweights below the 10th centile and the perinatal mortality rate rise as proteinuria increases (after Tervilla et al 1973)

proteinuria 39% of birthweights were under the tenth centile and 96% under the 50th centile (Brazy et al 1982). This reduction in birthweight is greater in subsequent than in first infants (Hendricks & Brenner 1971), and the earlier in pregnancy the hypertension appears the more is fetal growth affected (Hendricks & Brenner 1971, Long et al 1980, Redin et al 1980, Lin et al 1981), with retardation being greatest in those with hypertension before the pregnancy (Hendricks & Brenner, 1971). This is not unexpected as 80% of multiparous patients with hypertension have underlying renal pathology (McCartney 1966). Fetal growth retardation in hypertension has another association: there is an increased incidence of accidental haemorrhage in maternal hypertension if fetal growth is retarded (Hendricks & Brenner 1971, Long et al 1980, Naeye 1981).

As well as the maximal blood pressure in pregnancy the mean arterial pressure at 5–6 months is related to birthweight, the higher it is the lower is the birthweight (Page & Christiansson, 1976). This is in accord with the clinical observation that fetal growth frequently is retarded before hypertension appears, and observed changes in circulating volume and electrolytes also may start before the blood pressure rises (Bletga et al 1970, MacGillivray et al 1975, Gallery et al 1979).

An apparent anomaly is that some mothers with mild hypertension in whom the diastolic pressure remains below 100 mmHg (particularly if they were hypertensive before conception) have babies whose mean birthweight is increased (Baird et al 1957, Walters & Adel 1966, MacGillivray 1979). This may be due to a rise in cardiac output increasing uterine blood flow, thus improving fetal nutrition and growth.

Renal disease without hypertension is associated with fetal growth retardation (Studd 1975, Katz et al 1980) but the addition of raised blood pressure makes low birthweight more likely. In an intensively investigated group of 157 severely hypertensive women the incidence of fetal growth retardation varied with the underlying renal pathology (Lin et al 1982): in those with nephrosclerosis only 9% of babies were below the tenth centile but if pre-eclampsia was superimposed 39% fell below this level; in primigravida with pre-eclampsia alone 18% were below the tenth centile, but with glomerulonephritis in addition this rose to 46%.

Ethnic differences in the effect of hypertension have been found. Birthweight at any particular level of raised blood pressure is reduced more in North American blacks than whites (Page & Christiansson 1976). There are, however, resemblances between different races: in both Europeans and Africans proteinuria rarely is found below 140/90 mmHg (Baird et al 1957). More research is required to differentiate the effects of hypertension on birthweight from other ethnic effects.

Myometrial and placental blood flow

Blood flow to myometrium and placenta is directly related to fetal weight in experimental animals (Wootton et al 1977) and in man (Claverol-Nunz et al 1977, Lunell et al 1979). Flow to myometrium and placenta are independent but related, the placenta tending to have short-term preference (Curet et al 1976). Since uterine blood flow is not autoregulated (Greiss, 1966; Speroff et al 1977) and since peripheral resistance rises in hypertension with little change in cardiac output (Freund et al 1977) a moderate rise in blood pressure may increase uterine flow and with this improvement in fetal nutrition there is an increase in fetal growth (Walters, 1966).

In more severe hypertension this blood flow is reduced and is lower still if proteinuria is present (Dixon et al 1963, Nylund et al 1983). Although the placenta appears to have a safety margin so that fetal health is not threatened until flow is less than 50% of normal (Dixon et al 1963), this reserve may be taken up by diversion of flow in exercise due to vasoconstriction.

In healthy pregnant women exercise produces the expected increase in cardiac output (Bader et al 1955). Training increases flow to the placenta (at the expense of the myometrium) in sheep (Curet et al 1976), and in man it may increase birthweight (Erkkola 1976). If the fetus is unhealthy maternal exercise can produce pathological changes in its ECG (Pomerance et al 1974) possibly by diverting blood from the uterus to the active muscles: rest increases uterine flow by 10% (Morris et al 1956). The effects of exercise when both mother and fetus are not healthy is not known, but when regular during pregnancy may well reduce birthweight.

Cigarette smoking added to hypertension and exercise will tend to reduce fetal growth even more. A single cigarette smoked by a woman accustomed to doing so reduces intervillous flow for 15 min (Lehtoviza & Foss 1978). These are good reasons for advising a hypertensive pregnant woman to rest and to cut down smoking as much as possible.

Placental bed vessels

The condition of the vessels in the maternal placental bed also help to determine fetal growth. Pregnancies with retarded fetal growth may be accompanied by failure of normal physiological changes to appear, or by pathological degeneration in the vessels. In normal pregnancies the walls of the spiral arteries are invaded by trophoblast which replaces their musculo-elastic wall with an amorphous tissue and extends into the myometrial segments of these arteries by 16 weeks. The process is complete by 20 weeks converting these previously vasoactive arteries into passive voluminous ducts which can cope with the much increased flow of blood necessary for adequate fetal nutrition (Brosens et al 1977). These physiological changes do not take place in some pregnancies so that the vessels of the placental bed remain relatively narrow and may be able to respond to vasoconstrictive stimuli, although hypertension is not necessarily present (Brosens et al 1977, Gerretsen et al 1981, McFadyen et al 1984b).

Occasionally a degenerative atherotic lesion appears in the wall of spiral arteries which have not undergone physiological change. Most observations of this lesion have been made in cases of severe albuminuric hypertension (Zeek & Assali 1950, Brosens et al 1977) but it has also been observed in normotensive pregnancies (Sheppard & Bonnar 1981). Even if this atherotic change is not accompanied by maternal hypertension it is almost always associated with fetal growth retardation (Brosens et al 1977, Sheppard & Bonnar 1981, McFadyen et al 1984b).

The relationship of fetal growth to absence of physiological change in the placental bed vessels is less well agreed, varying between 25 and 75% of growth retarded fetuses in mothers without this physiological change (Brosens et al 1977, Gerretson et al 1981, McFadyen et al 1984b). Differences in fetal growth rates in this group may depend not only on the presence of hypertension, but also on the viscosity of the blood circulating through the vessels which is determined partly by the physiological haemodilution of pregnancy.

Circulating volume

Plasma volume and red cell mass both increase in pregnancy, but since the plasma volume increases by 50% while the red cell mass by only 30% (Paintin, 1962) the blood tends to become less viscous. The volume increase is greater in multigravida than in primigravida (Campbell & MacGillivray 1972), and in twins it is almost doubled (Rovinsky & Jaffin, 1965). Birthweight and plasma volume increase are directly related, the greater the increase the heavier the baby (Hytten & Paintin 1963, Arias 1965). The volume increase is 30% less than normal in women who have aborted frequently, and in pregnancies with idiopathic retarded fetal growth (Gibson 1973).

Hypertensive women are more likely to have a stillborn baby if their plasma volume increase is reduced (Sibai et al 1981). Although the expansion is not generally related to the non-pregnant plasma volume (Hytten & Paintin, 1963) there is an association between recurrent birthweight below the fifth centile and low non-pregnant plasma volume (Croal et al 1978).

Smokers (Pirani 1978), women who take diuretics for a large part of their pregnancies (Campbell & MacGillivray 1975) and hypertensive women (Gallery et al 1979) all have smaller than normal increase in plasma volume and this too is associated with lighter babies. Chronic hypertensives have a reduced increment in blood volume throughout pregnancy, whereas women developing hypertension during pregnancy may have a normal increase until the third trimester and then contract their plasma volume before the blood pressure rises (Gallery et al 1979). Among diuretic-takers, although birthweight is reduced, there is more 'catch-up' growth than in the infants of these mothers not taking this medication so possibly some of this reduction in birthweight is due to reduced feto-placental circulating volume (Blumenthal 1976).

Blood viscosity

This is related to more than the circulating volume. Changes in plasma proteins, in deformability of red cells and in other factors also affect it. Changes in viscosity have been measured in normal and hypertensive pregnancies. Viscosity is increased in pre-eclampsia, more due to changes in plasma than in the red cells; it may rise before the blood pressure does, and returns to normal within a day of delivery. Increased viscosity is directly related to maternal hypertension and to reduced birthweight (Buchan 1982, Hobbs et al 1982).

Treatment of maternal hypertension with hypotensive drugs does not improve fetal growth. Neither increased birthweight nor an improved pattern of growth has been produced by reserpine (Landesman et al 1957), methyldopa (Redman 1980) or labetalol (McFadyen et al 1984b) started before 28 weeks. Oxyprenolol did appear to increase fetal and placental weights (Gallery et al 1979) but this drug was started at any stage in pregnancy and the significance of this apparent improvement is difficult to assess. Hypotensive drugs tend to reduce placental perfusion (although they may relieve vasospasm in the placental bed), and do not affect the physiological adaptations to pregnancy. Methyldopa does reduce the incidence of midtrimester abortion (Redman et al 1976) but the principal effect of the use of hypotensives is to improve neonatal health by keeping the mother fit enough to allow the pregnancy to continue until the baby is sufficiently mature to survive. They do not improve fetal growth.

Fetal circulation

The depressant effects of acute hypoxia on the fetal myocardium are well documented, but the state of the circulation in fetal growth retardation is less satisfactorily established. Clinical examination suggests that there is peripheral vasoconstriction and this is in accord with the blood velocity wave forms in growth retardation (Stuart et al 1980). There also is myocardial hyperplasia (Naeye, 1965) which may be a consequence of the extra work which is required of the heart by the increased peripheral resistance and by hyperviscosity of the blood which frequently is present in light for dates fetuses. Plasma viscosity is raised in 15% of those born under the tenth centile at 38–42 weeks and in 17% of those born light for dates after 42 weeks (Wirth et al 1979). Such hyperviscosity is increased by maternal smoking (Buchan 1983). In the neonate it is associated with complications due to reduced flow in the kidneys and central nervous systems, and with necrotising enterocolitis, as well as with reduced birthweight. The fetal myocardium contains less glycogen than normal, other sources of energy may be deficient, and amino acids or other substances which affect cardiovascular function adversely present in greater concentrations than normal. Factors such as these suggest that the feto-placental circulation is less efficient than normal when the fetus is growth retarded (Brambati & Bonsignore 1982).

Maternal hypertension, placental bed pathology and failure of circulatory adaptation to pregnancy have defined relationships with fetal growth retardation but why they occur is not yet known. Ethnic differences in birthweight are real, and are clinically important: their recognition is relevant not only to paediatric and obstetric practice but to the light which they may shed on the basics of fetal growth. Definition of retarded fetal growth is essential before any of these, or any other factors related to fetal growth, can be examined: hence the space given to discussion of both man and animals at the beginning of this chapter.

REFERENCES

Alberman E, Roman E, Pharoah P O D, Chamberlain G 1980 Birth weight before and after a spontaneous abortion. British Journal of Obstetrics and Gynaecology 87: 275–280

Andrews J, McGarry J M 1972 A community study of smoking in pregnancy. Journal of Obstetrics and Gynaecology of the British Commonwealth 79: 1057–1073

Arias F 1975 Expansion of intravascular volume and fetal outcome in patients with chronic hypertension and pregnancy. American Journal of Obstetrics and Gynecology 123: 610–616

Ashcroft M T, Desai P 1976 Ethnic differences in growth potential of children of African, Indian, Chinese and European origin. Transactions of the Royal Society of Tropical Medicine and Hygiene 70: 433–438

Bader R A. Bader M E, Rose D J, Braunwald E 1955 Haemodynamics at rest and during exercise in normal pregnancy as studied by cardiac catheterisation. Journal of Clinical Investigation 34: 1524–1536

Baird D, Thomson A M, Billewicz W Z 1957 Birthweights and placental weights in pre-eclampsia. Journal of Obstetrics and Gynaecology of the British Empire 64: 370–372

Bamford F N 1971 Immigrant mother and her child. British Medical Journal i: 276–280

Barnes A C 1981 The repercussion of population growth. Journal of Reproductive Medicine 26: 433–437

Barron S L 1976 Perinatal Mortality and birthweight in Makassar, Indonesia. Journal of Obstetrics and Gynaecology of British Commonwealth 81: 187–195

Barron S L, Vessey M P 1966 Immigration — a new social factor in obstetrics. British Medical Journal i: 1189–1197

Battaglia F C, Frazier T M, Hellegers A E 1966 Birthweight, gestational age, and pregnancy outcome with special reference to high birthweight — low gestational age infants. Pediatrics 37: 417–422

Beker J C 1948 Aetiology of eclampsia. Journal of Obstetrics and Gynaecology of British Empire 55: 756–765

Blekta M, Hlavaty V, Tenkova M, Bendl J, Bendova L, Chytil M 1970 Volume of whole blood and absolute amount of serum proteins in the early stage of late toxemia of pregnancy. American Journal of Obstetrics and Gynecology 106: 10–13

Blumenthal I 1976 Diet and diuretics in pregnancy and subsequent growth of offspring. British Medical Journal ii: 733

Buchan P C 1982 Preeclampsia — A hyperviscosity syndrome. American Journal of Obstetrics and Gynecology 142: 111–112

Buchan P C 1983 Cigarette smoking in pregnancy and fetal hyperviscosity. British Medical Journal 286: 1315

Butler N R, Alberman E D 1969 Maternal factors affecting duration of pregnancy, birthweight and fetal growth. In: Butler N R, Alberman E D (eds) Perinatal Problems, pp 53–67 Churchill Livingstone, Edinburgh

Brambati B, Bonsignore L 1982 Intra-ventricular conduction time in fetuses born with growth retardation. British Journal of Obstetrics and Gynaecology 89: 900–903

Brazy J E, Grimm J K, Little V A 1982 Neonatal manifestations of severe maternal hypertension occurring before the thirty-sixth week of pregnancy. Journal of Pediatrics 100: 265–271

Brooke O G, Wood C 1980 Growth in British Asians: longitudinal data in the first year. Journal of Human Nutrition 34: 355–359

Brosens I, Dixon H G, Robertson W B 1977 Fetal growth retardation and the arteries of the placental bed. British Journal of Obstetrics and Gynaecology 83: 656–663

Bruce-Chwatt L J 1952 Malaria in African infants and children in Southern Nigeria. Annals of Tropical Medicine and Parasitology 46: 173–200

Campbell D M, MacGillivray I 1972 Comparison of maternal response in first and second pregnancies in relation to baby weight. Journal of Obstetrics and Gynaecology of the British Commonwealth 79: 684–693

Campbell D M, MacGillivray I 1975 The effect of a low calorie diet or a thiazide diuretic on the incidence of pre-eclampsia and on birth weight. British Journal of Obstetrics and Gynaecology 82: 572–577

Campbell Brown M, Cashmore G C, Ward R J, Abraham R, King J C, Turnlund J R, McFadyen I R 1982 Trace elements in a pregnant Asian population. In: McFadyen I R, MacVicar J (eds) Obstetric Problems of the Asian Community in Britain, pp 133–145. Royal College of Obstetricians and Gynaecologists, London

Cannon D S H 1958 Malaria and prematurity in the western region of Nigeria. British Medical Journal 2: 877–878

Cheng M C E, Chew P C T, Tatnam S S 1972 Birthweight distribution of Singapore Chinese, Malay and Indian infants from 34 weeks to 42 weeks gestation. Journal of Obstetrics and Gynaecology of British Commonwealth 79: 149–153

Clarren S K, Smith D W 1978 The fetal alcohol syndrome. New England Journal of Medicine 298: 1063–1067

Clavero-Munez J A, Ortiz-Quintana L 1977 Utero-placental blood flow index. Its relationship with the placental histology and fetal hypoxia. Journal of Perinatal Medicine 6: 268–273

Coon C S 1981 Populations, Human. In: Encyclopedia Britannica 14: 839–848

Croall J, Sherrif S, Matthews J 1978 Non-pregnant maternal plasma volume and fetal growth retardation. British Journal of Obstetrics and Gynaecology 85: 90–95

Cunnane S C, Majid E, Senior J, Mills C F 1983 Uteroplacental dysfunction and prostaglandin metabolism in zinc deficient pregnant rats. Life Sciences 32: 2471–2478

Curet L B, Orr J A, Rankin J H G, Ungerer T 1976 Effect of exercise on cardiac output and distribution of uterine blood flow in pregnant ewes. Journal of Applied Physiology 40: 725–728

Dixon H G, McClure Browne J C, Davey D A 1963 Choriodecidual and myometrial blood-flow. Lancet ii: 369–373

Dowding V M 1982 Distributions of birth weight in seven Dublin maternity units. British Medical Journal 284: 1901–1904

Elder H A, Santamarina B A G, Smith S, Kass E H 1971 The natural history of asymptomatic bacteriuria during pregnancy: The effect of tetracycline on the clinical course and the outcome of pregnancy. American Journal of Obstetrics and Gynecology 111: 441–462

Errkkola R 1976 The influence of physical training during pregnancy on physical work capacity and circulatory parameters. Scandinavian Journal of Clinical and Laboratory Investigation 36: 747–754

Freeman M G, Graves W L, Thompson R L 1970 Indigent Negro and Caucasian birth weight-gestational age tables. Pediatrics 46: 9–15

Freund M, French W, Carlson R W, Weil M H, Shubin H 1977 Haemodynamic and metabolic studies of a case of toxemia of pregnancy. American Journal of Obstetrics and Gynecology 127: 206–208

Fried K, Davies A M 1974 Some effects on the offspring of uncle-niece marriages in the Moroccan Jewish Community in Jerusalem. American Journal of Human Genetics 26: 65–72

Fujikura T, Froehlick L A 1972 Birth weight, gestational age, and renal glomerular development as indices of fetal maturity. American Journal of Obstetrics and Gynecology 113: 627–631

Gallery E D M, Hunyor S N, Györy A Z 1979 Plasma volume contraction: A significant factor in both pregnancy-associated hypertension (pre-eclampsia) and chronic hypertension in pregnancy. Quarterly Journal of Medicine, New Series XLVIII 192: 593–602

Gebre-Medhin M, Sterky G, Taube A 1978 Observations on intrauterine growth in urban Ethiopia. Acta Paediatrica Scandinavica 67: 781–789

Gerretsen G, Huisjes H J, Elema J D 1981 Morphological changes of the spiral arteries in the placental bed in relation to pre-eclampsia and fetal growth retardation. British Journal of Obstetrics and Gynaecology 88: 876–881

Gibson H M 1973 Plasma volume and glomerular filtration rate in pregnancy and their relation to differences in fetal growth. Journal of Obstetrics and Gynaecology of the British Commonwealth 80: 1067–1074

Greiss F C 1966 Pressure-flow relationship in the gravid uterine vascular bed. American Journal of Obstetrics and Gynecology 96: 41–46

Gruenwald P 1963 Chronic fetal distress and placental insufficiency. Biology of the Neonate 5: 215–265

Gruenwald P 1966a Growth of the human fetus. I. Normal growth and its variation. American Journal of Obstetrics and Gynecology 94: 1112–1119

Gruenwald P 1966b Growth of the human fetus. II. Abnormal growth in twins and infants of mothers with diabetes, hypertension, or isoimmunization. American Journal of Obstetrics and Gynecology 94: 1120–1132

Grundy M F B, Hood J, Newman G B 1978 Birth weight standards in a community of mixed racial origin. British Journal of Obstetrics and Gynaecology 85: 481–486

Hagberg G 1978 Children with IQs of 50–70. In: Major Mental Handicap: Methods and costs of prevention, Ciba Foundation Symposium 59, p. 211. Elsevier Excerpta Medica, Amsterdam

Haines A P, McFadyen I R, Campbell Brown M, North W R S, Abraham R 1982 Birthweight and complications of pregnancy in an Asian Population. In: McFadyen I R, MacVicar J (eds) Obstetric Problems of the Asian Community in Britain, pp 119–126. Royal College of Obstetricians and Gynaecologists, London

Haworth J C, Dilling L, Younoszai M K 1967 Relation of blood-glucose to haematocrit, birthweight, and other body measurements in normal and growth-retarded newborn infants. Lancet ii: 901–905

Hendricks C H, Brenner W E 1971 Toxaemia of pregnancy: relationship between fetal weight, fetal survival, and the maternal state. American Journal of Obstetrics and Gynecology 109: 225–233

Hingson R, Alpert J J, Day N, Dooling E, Kayne H, Morelock S, Oppenheimer E, Zuckerman B 1982 Effects of maternal drinking and marijuana use on fetal growth and development. Pediatrics 70: 409

Hobbs J B, Oats J N, Palmer A A, Long P A, Mitchell G M, Lou A, McIver M A 1982 Whole blood viscosity in preeclampsia. American Journal of Obstetrics and Gynaecology 142: 288–292

Hytten F E 1979 Nutrition in pregnancy. In: Thalhammer O, Baumgarten K, Pollak A (eds) Perinatal Medicine, pp 34–43. Georg Thieme Publishers, Stuttgart

Hytten F E, Paintin D B 1963 Increase in plasma volume during normal pregnancy. Journal of Obstetrics and Gynaecology of the British Commonwealth 70: 402–407

Jenkins D J A, Wolever T M S, Taylor R H, Barker H M, Fielden H 1980 Exceptionally low blood glucose response to dried beans: comparison with other carbohydrate foods. British Medical Journal 2: 578–580

Kaltreider N L, Meneely G R 1940 The effect of exercise on the volume of the blood. Journal of Clinical Investigation 19: 627–634

Katz A I, Davison J M, Hayslett J P, Singson E, Lindheimer M D 1980 Pregnancy in women with kidney disease. Kidney International 18: 192–206

Khouzami V A, Ginsburg D S, Daikoku N H, Johnson J W C 1981 The glucose tolerance test as a means of identifying intrauterine growth retardation. American Journal of Obstetrics and Gynecology 139: 423–426

Krishma K 1978 Tobacco chewing in pregnancy. British Journal of Obstetrics and Gynaecology 85: 726–728

Koch G 1979 Cardiovascular dynamics after acute and long term α- and β- adrenoceptor blockade at rest, supine and standing, and during exercise. British Journal of Clinical Pharmacology 8: (Suppl 2): 101S–105S

Landesmann R, McLarn W D, Ollstein R N, Mendelsohn B 1957 Reserpine in toxaemia of pregnancy. Obstetrics and Gynecology 9: 377–383

Lehtovita P, Forss M 1978 The acute effect of smoking on the intervillous blood flow of the placenta. British Journal of Obstetrics and Gynaecology 85: 729–731

Lichty J A, Ting R Y, Bruns P D and Dyar E 1957 Studies of babies born at high altitude. American Journal of Diseases of Children 93: 666–678

Lin C-H, Lindheimer M D, River P, Moawad A H 1982 Fetal outcome in hypertensive disorders of pregnancy. American Journal of Obstetrics and Gynecology 142: 255–260

Long P A, Abell D A, Beischer N A 1980 Fetal growth retardation and pre-eclampsia. British Journal of Obstetrics and Gynaecology 87: 13–18

Lubchenco L O, Hansman C, Dressler M, Boyd E 1963 Intrauterine growth as estimated from liveborn birth-weight data at 24 to 42 weeks of gestation. Pediatrics 32: 793–800

Lubs M E 1973 Racial differences in maternal smoking effects on the newborn infant. American Journal of Obstetrics and Gynecology 115: 66–76

Lunell N O, Sarby B, Levander R, Uylund L 1979 Comparison of uteroplacental blood flow in normal and in intrauterine-growth-retarded pregnancy. Measurement with Indium-113m and a computer-linked gamma camera. Gynecologic and Obstetric Investigation 10: 106–118

McCartney C P 1964 Pathological anatomy of acute hypertension of pregnancy. Circulation 30 (Suppl 2): 37–42

McCullough R E, Reeves J T, Liljegren R L 1977 Fetal growth retardation and increased infant mortality at high altitude. Archives of Environmental Health 32: 36–39

McFadyen I R, Campbell Brown M, Abraham R, North W R S, Haines A P 1984a Factors affecting birthweight in Hindus, Moslems and Europeans. British Journal of Obstetrics and Gynaecology 91: 968–972

McFadyen I R, Geirsson R T, Stacey T E 1984b Hypertension discovered in the first or second trimester and treated with labetalol. Unpublished observations

McLaren A, Michie D 1960a Congenital Runts. In: Wolstenholme G E W, O'Connor M (eds) Congenital Malformations (Ciba Foundation Symposium), pp 178–194. Churchill Livingstone, Edinburgh

McLaren A, Michie D 1960b Control of prenatal growth in mammals. Nature 187: 363–365

Meire H B, Farrant P 1981 Ultrasound demonstration of an unusual fetal growth pattern in Indians. British Journal of Obstetrics and Gynaecology 88: 260–263

Milner R D G 1981 Role of the fetal endocrine pancreas in metabolic control. In: van Assche F A, Robertson W B (eds) Fetal Growth Retardation, pp 163–172. Churchill Livingstone, Edinburgh

Morley D, Woodland M, Cuthbertson W J F 1964 Controlled trial of pyrimethamine in pregnant women in an African village. British Medical Journal 2: 667–668

Morris N, Osborn S B, Wright H P, Hart A 1956 Effective uterine blood flow during exercise in normal and pre-eclamptic pregnancies. Lancet ii: 481–484

Myers R E, Hill D E, Holt A B, Scott R E, Mellits E D, Cheek D B 1971 Fetal growth retardation produced by experimental placental insufficiency in the Rhesus monkey. Biology of the Neonate 18: 379–394

Naeye R L 1965 Cardiovascular abnormalities in infants malnourished before birth. Biology of the Neonate 8: 104–113

Naeye R L 1970 Structural correlates of fetal undernutrition. In: Waisman H A, Kerr G R (eds) Fetal Growth and Development, pp 242–252. McGraw-Hill, New York

Naeye R L 1981 Maternal blood pressure and fetal growth. American Journal of Obstetrics and Gynecology 131: 780–787

Naeye R L, Dixon J B 1978 Distortions in fetal growth standards. Pediatric Research 12: 987–991

Neligan G 1965 A community study of the relationship between birthweight and gestational age. In: Dawkins M, MacGregor W G (eds) Gestational age, Size and Maturity, pp 28–32. Spastics Society and Heinemann Medical Books Ltd, London

Page E W, Christianson R 1976 The impact of mean arterial pressure in the middle trimester upon the outcome of pregnancy. American Journal of Obstetrics and Gynecology 125: 740–745

Paintin D B 1962 The size of the total red cell volume in pregnancy. Journal of Obstetrics and Gynaecology of the British Commonwealth 69: 719–723

Papoz L, Eschwege E, Peqnignot G, Barrat J, Schwartz D 1982 Maternal smoking and birthweight in relation to dietary habits. American Journal of Obstetrics and Gynecology 142: 870–876

Penchaszadeh V B, Hardy J B, Mellits E D, Cohen B H, McKusick V A 1972 Growth and development in an 'inner city' population: an assessment of possible biological and environmental influences. I. Intra-uterine growth. Johns Hopkins Medical Journal 130: 384–389

Pirani B B K 1978 Smoking during pregnancy. Obstetrical and Gynecological Survey 33: 1–13

Platt H 1978 Growth and maturity in the equine fetus. Journal of the Royal Society of Medicine 71: 658–661

Pomerance J J, Gluck L, Lynch V A 1974 Maternal exercise as a screening test for uteroplacental insufficiency. Obstetrics and Gynecology 44: 383–387

Prentice A M, Whitehead R G, Watkinson M, Lamb W H, Cole T J 1983 Prenatal dietary supplementation of African women and birth-weight. Lancet i: 489–492

Rahimtoola R J, Mir S, Baloch S 1968 Low birth weight, the 'small for dates' syndrome and perinatal mortality in a low family income group. Acta Paediatrica Scandinavica 57: 534–536

Rantakallio P 1969 Groups at risk in low birth weight infants and perinatal mortality. Acta Paediatrica Scandinavica (Suppl 193): 5–71

Rao P S S, Inbaraj S G 1977 Inbreeding effects on human reproduction in Tamil Kadu of South India. Annals of Human Genetics 41: 87–98

Redman C W G 1980 Treatment of hypertension in pregnancy. Kidney International 18: 267–278

Redman C W G, Beilin L J, Bonnar J, Ounsted M K 1976 Fetal outcome in trial of antihypertensive treatment in pregnancy. Lancet ii: 753–756

Rovinsky J J, Jaffin H 1965 Cardiovascular hemodynamics in pregnancy. I. Blood and plasma volumes in multiple pregnancy. American Journal of Obstetrics and Gynecology 93: 1–13

Royston J P, Flecknell P A, Wootton R 1982 New evidence that the intrauterine growth-retarded piglet is a member of a discrete subpopulation. Biology of the Neonate 42: 100–104

Schork M A 1964 The effects of inbreeding on growth. American Journal of Human Genetics 16: 292–299

Scott J R 1977 Fetal growth retardation associated with maternal administration of immunosuppressive drugs. American Journal of Obstetrics and Gynecology 128: 668–676

Sheppard B L, Bonnar J 1981 An ultrastructural study of utero-placental spiral arteries in hypertensive and normotensive pregnancy and fetal growth retardation. British Journal of Obstetrics and Gynaecology 88: 695–705

Sibai B M, Abdella T N, Anderson G D, McCubbin J H 1981 Plasma volume determination in pregnancies complicated by chronic hypertension and intrauterine fetal demise. Obstetrics and Gynecology 60: 174–178

Sibert J R, Jadhav M, Inbaraj S G 1979 Fetal growth and parental consanguinity. Archives of Disease in Childhood 54: 317–319

Speroff L, Haning R V, Levin R M 1977 The effect of angiotensin II and indomethacin on uterine artery blood flow in pregnant monkeys. Obstetrics and Gynecology 50: 611–614

Stuart B, Drumm J, Fitzgerald D, Duignan N 1980 Fetal blood velocity waveforms in pregnancy, p. 121. Proceedings of the 22nd British Congress of Obstetrics and Gynaecology, Edinburgh

Studd J 1973 The origin and effects of proteinuria in pregnancy. Journal of Obstetrics and Gynaecology of the British Commonwealth 80: 872–883

Sutherland A, Cooper D W, Howie P W, Liston W A, MacGillivray I 1981 The incidence of severe pre-eclampsia amongst mothers and mothers-in-law of pre-eclamptics and controls. British Journal of Obstetrics and Gynaecology 88: 785–791

Tervila L, Goecke C, Timonen S 1973 Estimation of gestosis of pregnancy (EPH-gestosis). Acta Obstetricia et Gynecologica Scandinavica 52: 235–243

Thompson B, Baird D 1967 Some impressions of childbearing in tropical area. Part II. Pre-eclampsia and low birthweight. Journal of Obstetrics and Gynaecology of the British Commonwealth 74: 499–509

Thomson A M, Billewicz W Z, Hytten F E 1968 The assessment of fetal growth. Journal of Obstetrics and Gynaecology of the British Commonwealth 75: 903–916

Usher R, McLean F 1969 Intrauterine growth of liveborn Caucasian infants at sea level: standards obtained from measurement in 7 dimensions of infants born between 25 and 44 weeks of gestation. Journal of Pediatrics 74: 901–910

Usher R H, McLean F H 1974 Normal fetal growth and the significance of fetal growth retardation. In: Davis J A, Dobbing J (eds) Scientific Foundation of Paediatrics, pp 69–80. Heinemann, London

Verges J B 1939 Yearb, Suffolk Sheep Society, Ipswich, quoted by Hammond J 1944 Physiological factors affecting birth weight. Proceedings of the Nutrition Society 2: 8–12

Viegas O A C, Scott P H, Cole T J, Mansfield H N, Wharton P, Wharton B A 1982 Dietary protein energy supplementation of pregnant Asian mothers at Serrento, Birmingham. I. Unselective during second and third trimesters. British Medical Journal 285: 589–595

Walters W A W, Adel M B 1966 Effects of sustained maternal hypertension on foetal growth and survival. Lancet ii: 1214–1217

Wharton B 1982 Food, Growth and the Asian Fetus. In: McFadyen I R, MacVicar J (eds) Obstetric Problems of the Asian community in Britain, pp 67–76. Royal College of Obstetricians and Gynaecologists, London

Widdowson E R 1971 Intra-uterine growth retardation in the pig. 1. Organ size and cellular development at birth and after growth to maturity. Biology of the Neonate 19: 329–340

Wilcox A J, Russell I T 1983 Birthweight and Perinatal Mortality: 1. On the frequency distribution of birthweight. International Journal of Epidemiology 12: 314–325

Winick M. Brasel J A, Velasco E G 1973 Effects of prenatal nutrition upon pregnancy risk. Clinical Obstetrics and Gynecology 16: 184–198

Wirth F H, Goldberg K E, Lubchenco L O 1979 Neonatal hyperviscosity. I. Incidence. Pediatrics 63: 833–836

Wootton R, McFadyen I R, Cooper J E 1977 Measurement of placental blood flow in the pig and its relation to placental and fetal weight. Biology of the Neonate 31: 333–339

Yudkin P L, Harlap S, Baras M 1983 High birthweight in an ethnic group of low socio economic status. British Journal of Obstetrics and Gynaecology 90: 291–296

Zeek P M, Assali N S 1950 Vascular changes in the decidua associated with eclamptogenic toxemia of pregnancy. American Journal of Clinical Pathology 20: 1099–1109

Pre-pregnancy health and counselling

A leading article in the British Medical Journal (12 September 1981) concluded:

> 'If obstetric care is to reduce further fetal wastage and the incidence of malformation, a better understanding of the first trimester of pregnancy is vital. Only by encouraging women to attend preconception clinics and thereby early pregnancy clinics can we hope to improve our knowledge of and clinical management of this vital, and as yet largely ignored, period of human development.'

By the end of the eighth week of gestation, when the embryo is renamed the fetus, most anomalies that are going to affect the fetus and newborn are already present.

PREVENTING REPETITIONS OF THE DISAPPOINTING OUTCOME

After a disappointing pregnancy the obstetrician is often faced with the question: 'What is the danger of this happening again next time?' Chamberlain now of St George's Hospital, London, writing about the pre-pregnancy clinic which he ran at Queen Charlotte's Hospital, suggested that the obstetrician should be able to give reasonably valid probabilities when women ask about risks, and referred to 'the large number of women and their doctors who are concerned about a previous premature labour or late spontaneous abortion' (Chamberlain 1980). Subsequent correspondence in the British Medical Journal emphasised that preconception care should begin in general practitioner or family planning clinics but that clinics were also needed in major obstetric departments for referral of difficult problems. Chamberlain listed over 30 types of problem brought to his pre-pregnancy clinic. Some of the most serious of these problems, including perinatal mortality, low birthweight and early abortions are frequently associated with exogenous factors, particularly toxins and nutritional imbalances.

PRE-PREGNANCY NUTRITION AND PERINATAL MORTALITY

Studies of laboratory, domestic and wild animals have shown that good nutrition before conception is necessary for a successful outcome of pregnancy.

78

A series of papers from Nelson and colleagues at the University of California published between 1946 and 1953, showed that the outcome of animal pregnancy is most sensitive to a range of nutritional deficiencies during the days and weeks immediately before mating (seven references in Wynn & Wynn 1983). Females who, before mating, are deficient in thiamine, pyridoxine, folic acid or pantothenic acid or protein caused a cluster of adverse effects including infertility, faulty implantation, resorptions, low birthweight, perinatal death and short life of survivors. Deprivation of Nelson's rats beginning only at mating had a less serious effect on pregnancy outcome, and deprivation during the latter part of pregnancy had little effect on the offspring. Animal experiments point to the great importance of maternal nutritional stores at the time of conception. However, other studies by Nelson and Warkany in the USA, by Giroud in France, and by many others showed that critical levels of many essential nutrients for a short time during the embryonic period could also seriously damage the progeny. A shortage of zinc for only 4 days during the embryonic period can, for example, cause pregnancy failure in animals (Hurley 1981).

There are historical records going back to the last century showing that human reproduction is also most susceptible to defective nutrition during the weeks immediately before and after conception. There was, for example, a food shortage over a large part of Holland which began about October 1944 and continued until May 1945. A study of this Dutch Hunger Winter was published in 1975 (Stein et al 1975, Wynn & Wynn 1981). Negative nutritional balances are cumulative and nutritional status was at its lowest at the beginning of May 1945 immediately before the Allies restored food supplies. The highest perinatal mortality of 65 per 1000 live and still births was recorded during December 1945, 8 or 9 months *after* the worst month of the food shortage, as shown in Figure 5.1, among babies *conceived* during the food shortage. The highest stillbirth rate of 42 and the highest early neonatal death rate of 23 were also recorded in December 1945 for the same babies, *conceived* during the food shortage. In the light of modern understanding it would be expected that the food shortage would have affected the reproductive capacity of both men and women.

The reproductive capacity of the Dutch population as reflected in perinatal death rates recovered completely from the effects of the food shortage, but took about 5 months to do so. This is not unexpected as it is known that many specialised body cells, for example lymphocytes, take many months to recover from deficiencies of some essential nutrients such as folic acid or cobalamin.

It follows that couples should be counselled on the importance both of good nutrition during the months before conception to build up nutritional stores and also on the importance of a good day to day diet.

INFERTILITY, NUTRITION AND BODY WEIGHT

The periods of food shortage in Holland, Germany and Eastern Europe following the two world wars were accompanied by epidemics of infertility.

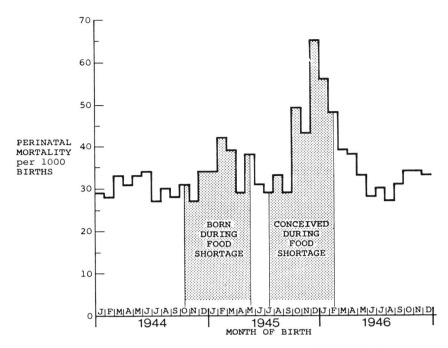

Fig. 5.1 Food shortage and perinatal mortality: babies born or conceived during the Dutch Hunger Winter 1944–45 (154 356 babies) Source: Wynn & Wynn, 1981, p. 8

The birth-rate in Holland fell to only about 40% of the level before the food shortage in November 1946, 7 months after the restoration of food supplies.

All male and female mammals become infertile if diet is inadequate. The reproductive system is inactivated by a reduction in gonadotrophin secretion by the pituitary, which is mainly controlled by the luteinising-hormone releasing-hormone (LHRH) secreted by the hypothalamus. The hypothalamic-pituitary-gonadal axis in animals has been reported to be sensitive to a wide range of nutrient deficiencies including low intakes of protein and individual amino acids, fats, individual vitamins and minerals.

In humans the relationship between maternal body weight and fertility is best documented, but certainly hides a much more complicated relationship between the quality of nutrition and fertility. However, voluntary weight reduction is among the important causes of infertility (Nillius 1978). Frisch and colleagues of the Harvard Center for Population Studies show the 50th percentile of the ponderal index for the onset or restoration of menstrual cycles at about 20.8 kg/m^2 for white American women (Frisch 1977). The mean ponderal index of American women aged 25 to 34 is close to 24 kg/m^2. This is just above the upper 10% confidence limit of the Harvard infertility threshold. The American 50th percentile for the onset of amenorrhoea of 20.8 kg/m^2 is somewhat higher than calculated from British data of 20.1 kg/m² (Crisp 1979) or from Swedish data of 18.4 kg/m² (Fries 1974).

A low body weight or excessive slimming before conception increases the risk of infertility and of an unfavourable pregnancy outcome. Average weights of women of reproductive age appear to provide a satisfactory target for counselling and are published for American women by the US National Center for Health Statistics. A ponderal index of 24 kg/m² may also be used.

PERICONCEPTIONAL NUTRITION AND MALFORMATIONS

Hurley, one time President of the Teratology Society and of the University of California, hypothesised that any factor that reduces embryonic deoxy-ribonucleic acid (DNA) synthesis increases the risk of malformations (Eckhert & Hurley 1977, Hurley 1981). Any reduction in the rates of cell replication below the genetically programmed level appears to increase the risk of asynchronous or disorganized differential growth. Spiers of the University of Washington has reported on the close association of growth retardation and congenital malformations of different types in monozygotic twins and in a variety of other special circumstances and arrived at conclusions similar to Hurley (Spiers 1982):

> 'According to the hypothesis proposed here, overall growth retardation constitutes a state of increased susceptibility to congenital malformations. For this reason it is the causes of growth retardation that must be understood if the incidence of the more serious malformations is to be reduced.'

The European experience points to a deficient diet as an important cause of embryonic growth retardation and the more serious malformations. The prevalence of neural tube defects or of other malformations did not increase in Berlin during the war in spite of the nervous stress caused by allied bombing, evacuation of women and children into improvised and overcrowded accommodation, and the high wartime casualties. The Berlin epidemic of malformations only began after the defeat of the German armies when the war was over and there was a food shortage caused by a breakdown in communications with countries that had been supplying food.

Lethal malformations of the neural tube increased in pregnancy among the babies *conceived* during the food shortage in Holland by 175% as shown in Table 5.1. The risk of 'other' malformations increased by 143% which suggests that the risk of many types of malformation is increased by poor nutrition. The epidemics of malformations in Holland continued among babies conceived for over 4 months after restoration of food supplies in May 1945, a recovery period similar to that noted above for perinatal mortality.

In conformity with the Hurley and Spiers hypothesis the same babies conceived during the Dutch Hunger Winter showed evidence of embryonic growth retardation. Of 197 deaths of babies less than 7 days old from November 1946 to February 1947 95, or 48%, were stated to have died of 'prematurity',

Table 5.1 Deaths from malformations of babies under 1 year born before and conceived during and after the Dutch food shortage October 1944 to May 1945

	Number of births	Neural tube malformations		Other malformations	
		Deaths	Rate per 1000 births	Deaths	Rate per 1000 births
Babies born Jan–July 1944 *before* shortage	26 888	24	0.89	38	1.41
Babies *conceived* during shortage and born from July '45–Feb '46	16 130	35 $\chi^2 = 11.1$	2.17 P<0.001	53 $\chi^2 = 15.9$	3.29 P<0.001
Babies *conceived* during 4 months *after* shortage and born March to June 1946	25 330	62 $\chi^2 = 18.2$	2.45 P<0.001	87 $\chi^2 = 21.5$	3.43 P<0.001
Babies conceived 5 to 12 months after shortage	42 527	49 $\chi^2 = 1.02$	1.15 N.S	104 $\chi^2 = 8.1$	2.45 P<0.01

Source: based on Stein et al, 1975 (pp 188–191)

which meant simply low birthweight. Among babies conceived during the food shortage embryonic growth retardation was a major cause of death and was part of a cluster of adverse consequences including malformations. Food shortage had caused a slow-down in DNA synthesis.

Statistics for England and Wales today show the death-rate attributed to congenital anomalies as increasing from 0.6 per 1000 at birthweights in the range 3501–4000 g to 89.8 per 1000 at birthweights under 1500 g. The death rate attributed to congenital anomalies increased about 50 times when the birthweight was halved. This close association of death from malformation and low birthweight is consistent with the Hurley and Spiers hypothesis.

Measurement of fetal size by ultrasound both in primates (Sabbagha et al 1975) and in human pregnancy (Sabbagha et al 1976, Moore et al 1976) has shown that fetal growth-retardation generally has its origin early in pregnancy. There are important exceptions when growth retardation begins later in pregnancy, generally associated with maternal illness. Ultrasonic measurement therefore also points to much, but not all, fetal growth retardation as originating in reduced rates of embryonic cell replication so that the fetus and placenta begin the later weeks of pregnancy with a reduced cell complement.

Nutrition counselling as a means of preventing the repetition of neural tube defects and spontaneous abortion was the subject of study by Laurence and colleagues in Cardiff. When the nutrition counselling succeeded in persuading the patients to consume a 'good diet' there was no repetition of a neural tube malformation or occurrence of a spontaneous abortion, but when the nutrition-counselling failed there were repetitions as shown in Table 5.2.

Table 5.2 Association of poor diet, spontaneous abortion and neural tube malformations (South Wales, 1980) in 186 women with a previous neural tube malformation

	Quality of diet			Significance of difference
	Good	Fair	Poor	
Normal births	53	85	22	
Spontaneous abortion	0	3	15	$P<0.001$
Repeat neural tube malformation	0	0	8	$P<0.001$

Source: Laurence et al, 1980

The 'poor' diets in Table 5.2 were those with 'a deficient intake of first-class protein, usually no fruit or vegetables, and generally a severe imbalance with excessive amounts of carbohydrates'. It may be inferred from Table 5.2 that only women with rather grossly deficient diets had a repeat neural tube malformation and that women on a good diet prior to conception have a low risk of bearing a baby with a neural tube malformation. 'Good diet' meant no more than a diet apparently conforming to the accepted norms of a balanced diet.

It may also be inferred from the study of Laurence and colleagues that dietary recall using a check-list, although only providing crude data, is enough to produce a short list of patients including many of those at risk of a repeat malformation or spontaneous abortion. Simple computer analysis greatly facilitates interpretation of dietary data sheets. Suitable programmes are used in Canada (Bonham 1983). Dietary recall with computer interpretation has also been found to be a valuable part of educational programmes for patients.

There is some evidence on the nutrient deficiencies in the British Isles associated with the occurrence of malformations or slow-down in DNA synthesis. These include: Folic acid and vitamin C (Smithells et al 1976); zinc (Meadows et al 1981, Soltan & Jenkins 1982); pyridoxine (Doyle 1982). American nutrition surveys have shown that in the developed world of today there are great variations, often exceeding 20 to 1, in the intakes of particular essential nutrients. The Cardiff study suggests that the parents who are at particular risk of bearing a malformed baby have diets that are a long way from the norm with intakes of important nutrients at the low end of the distributions of intake. Much more knowledge is needed of the prevalence of such deficiencies to guide nutrition counselling.

Smithells et al (1981) reported apparent reductions in recurrence of neural tube defects in mothers given periconceptional multivitamin supplementation. An apparent reduction in the recurrence of cleft lip following periconceptional multivitamin supplementation has also been reported (Tolarova 1982). There must be many circumstances when such blind supplementation of a patient's diet with physiological quantities of vitamins is desirable. However the remedying of actual, diagnosed nutrient deficiencies is obviously preferable, and such supplementation can be no substitute for improvement by education of the patient's diet.

When a slow-down in embryonic growth is suspected, any mother of a baby of low birthweight should have her diet assessed by recall. If a mother has had a seriously malformed baby or following an unexplained stillbirth a biochemical assessment of nutritional status should be considered.

EARLY SPONTANEOUS ABORTION

Ebbs and colleagues of the University of Toronto reported as long ago as 1941 that women on 'poor diets' had five times the abortion rate of women on 'good diets'. Epidemics of early spontaneous abortion were reported during the European food shortages. The association of spontaneous abortion with a poor maternal pre-pregnancy diet, reported by Laurence and colleagues in South Wales in 1980, is summarised in Table 5.2. This association has been reported many times in the literature. Nutrient deficiency has also been shown experimentally to cause spontaneous abortion and resorption in animals.

From 30 to 60% of cases of early spontaneous abortion are reported to suffer from chromosomal defects (Alberman et al 1976, Boué & Boué 1973); many of the spontaneous abortions with apparently normal chromosomes are thought to be a result of genetic defects (Simpson 1980). It may then be asked whether the slow-down in the synthesis of DNA postulated by Hurley as increasing the risk of malformations of the embryo does not extend to the period before conception to cause chromosomal and genetic defects. The importance of this question is increased by reports that deficiencies of folic acid, cobalamin, zinc and magnesium not only slow down DNA synthesis but can also cause chromosomal damage (Bell et al 1975, Das & Herbert 1978).

If poor nutrition can result in a damaged gamete before conception it is improbable that the damage is confined to the female.

Counselling the male partner

The proportion of morphologically abnormal sperm is reported to be directly related to the number of cigarettes smoked daily. Smoking more than 30 cigarettes per day appears to double approximately the risk of producing morphologically abnormal sperm (Viczian et al 1969). Smoking is also reported to reduce sperm number and motility. Smoking by the male partner is one of the causes of reduced fertility of couples. The male is reported solely responsible in about 45% of cases of infertility (Ansbacher 1982). There is a tight correlation between chromosomal abnormality of sperm and low sperm count (Alexander 1982).

Morphological abnormalities in sperm are known to be caused by mutagens (DeMarini 1983). Some 30 different mutagens have been identified in tobacco smoke distributed between the particulate and gas phases (Bridges et al 1979). Tobacco smoke is reported to cause chromosomal aberrations in human subjects and animals and point mutations in standard tests. Smoking by men might, therefore, be expected to increase the risk of reproductive casualties. Only one German study has been found of 5200 pregnancies which included male smoking in a multifactorial study of perinatal mortality (Mau & Netter 1974). A significant association was found between paternal consumption of more than 10 cigarettes a day and perinatal mortality and frequency of major congenital malformations. There was also a statistically non-significant increase in spontaneous abortion among the wives of smoking fathers. This single study is an inadequate basis for very firm conclusions and further work is desirable. American dose response estimates for women show 20 cigarettes a day as increasing spontaneous abortion rates by a factor of 1.61 (Kline et al 1981).

Techniques are available for estimating the mutagenicity of urine, and have been used for detecting suspected mutagens. Their use has been proposed for monitoring the mutagenicity of human populations (Yamasaki & Ames 1977). Mutagenicity of smokers' urine rises during the day to twice or more the value in early morning, but is substantially higher than the mutagenicity of non-smokers even in the morning. While the mutagenicity of urine is evidence of systemic mutagenicity, many mutagens such as acetaldehyde, the first mutagenic metabolite of alcohol, are not voided.

The mutagenicity of alcohol is well-established (Obe & Ristow 1979). Regular consumption of alcohol for 8 to 10 years in non-smokers is reported to be associated with an approximate doubling of the number of peripheral lymphocytes with chromosomal aberrations (Obe et al 1980). Dose-response estimates for women show that 'alcohol consumption every day' increases spontaneous abortion by a factor of 2.53 (Kline et al 1981). In neither of these studies was it clear how much alcohol had to be consumed to produce these results. Both these studies show the effects of smoking and alcohol as approximately additive on a logarithmic scale, and the latter study showed a substantial inverse association of the effects of smoking with maternal education, probably reflecting differences in diet, which is shown to be correlated with education in other studies.

Magenis et al (1977) averaging the results from 18 series of cases of Down's syndrome found that in 24 out of 97 cases, or about 25%, the chromosomal aberration was of paternal origin. Paternal responsibility for Down's syndrome in different series varies up to about 35%. British statistics for the occupational and social class of the father of reported cases of Down's syndrome by mother's age have been published in 1982 for the first time by the Office of Population Censuses & Surveys. The figures show a steep social class gradient in the incidence of Down's syndrome pointing to the likelihood of major environmental factors in the aetiology.

The damage to male sperm may originate as much as 12 weeks before conception. The dividing spermatogonia are highly susceptible to radiation damage and are most sensitive to toxins soon after their last mitotic division at the time of maximum DNA synthesis immediately preceding meiosis. The stem cells, spermatids and spermatozoa are not so easily damaged. This timetable suggests that men planning a family should be particularly careful of their health for 3 or 4 months at least before risking a conception.

In animals some nutrient deficiencies are reported to affect the male gonads directly while others affect spermatogenesis primarily through the endocrine system. Four nutrients reported to be essential for spermatogenesis in rats independently of the endocrine system are linoleic acid, vitamin A, vitamin E and zinc (Leathem 1975). This is certainly not a complete list of nutrients essential to spermatogenesis which must include all nutrients needed for DNA synthesis. However, a deficiency of many other nutrients, such as pyridoxine, depresses secretion of gonadotrophins, also essential for spermatogenesis. Animal studies show that defective diet can cause abnormal sperm (Komatsu et al 1982).

The health of the male gonads depends upon the biochemical environment containing a normal satisfactory balance of essential nutrients and hormones, as well as upon low enough levels of toxins. As in the female a sufficiently serious nutrient deficiency in the male causes the endocrine system to produce infertility. The casualties are caused by a marginal imbalance in nutrients and hormones, or by toxins, which do not prevent spermatogenesis but cause sperm to be damaged. One paper says that in between infertility caused by damage to sperm and healthy reproduction in which sperm are not damaged there is an 'intermediate zone' in which conception is possible but defects in the sperm prejudice the embryo (Viczian et al 1969).

There is much that is not known about the interaction of nutrition, endocrine activity and spermatogenesis. There are, however, good reasons for inferring that nutritional normality may be as important as freedom from toxins in ensuring male reproductive health. There is evidence enough to make pre-pregnancy health and counselling of the male partner a necessary function of every pre-pregnancy clinic.

REFERENCES

Alberman E D, Creasy M, Elliott M, Spicer C 1976 Maternal factors associated with fetal chromosomal anomalies in spontaneous abortions. British Journal of Obstetrics and Gynaecology 83: 621–627

Alexander N J 1982 Male evaluation and semen analysis. Clinical Obstetrics and Gynecology 25: 463–482

Ansbacher R (ed) 1982 Male infertility. Clinical Obstetrics and Gynecology 25: 461–541

Bell L T, Branstrator M, Roux C, Hurley L S 1975 Chromosomal abnormalities in maternal and fetal tissues of magnesium-and-zinc-deficient rats. Teratology 12: 221–226

Bonham G H 1983 Strategies for nutritional fitness in pregnancy: selections from Canadian experience. Nutrition and Health 1: 219–226

Boué J G, Boué A 1973 Increased frequency of chromosomal anomalies in abortions after induced ovulation. Lancet i: 679–680

Bridges B A, Clemmesen J, Sugimura T 1979 Cigarette smoking — does it carry a genetic risk? Mutation Research 65: 71–81

Chamberlain G 1980 The prepregnancy clinic. British Medical Journal 281: 29–30

Crisp A H 1979 Psycho-pathology of weight-related amenorrhoea. In: Advances in Gynaecological Endocrinology. Royal College of Obstetricians and Gynaecologists, London

Das K C, Herbert V 1978 The lymphocyte as a marker of past nutritional status: persistence of deoxyuridine (dU) suppression and chromosomes in patients with past deficiency of folate and vitamin B_{12}. British Journal of Haematology 38: 219–233

DeMarini D M 1983 Genotoxicity of tobacco smoke and tobacco condensate. Mutation Research 114: 59–89

Doyle W, Crawford M A, Laurence B M, Drury P 1982 Dietary survey during pregnancy in a low socio-economic group. Human Nutrition: Applied Nutrition 36A: 95–106

Eckhert C D, Hurley L S 1977 Reduced DNA synthesis in zinc deficiency: regional differences in embryonic rats. Journal of Nutrition 107: 855–861

Fries H 1974 Secondary amenorrhoea self-induced weight reduction and anorexia nervosa. Acta Psychiatrica Scandinavica Suppl. 249

Frisch R 1977 Food intake fatness and reproductive ability. In: Vigersky R A (ed) Anorexia Nervosa. Raven Press, New York

Hurley L S 1981 Teratogenic aspects of manganese zinc and copper nutrition. Physiological Reviews 61: 249–295

Kline I, Levin B, Stein Z, Susser M, Warburton D 1981 Epidemiologic detection of low dose effects on the developing fetus. Environmental Health Perspectives 42: 119–126

Komatsu H, Kakizoe T, Niijima T, Kawachi T, Sugimura T 1982 Increased sperm abnormalities due to dietary restriction. Mutation Research 93: 439–446

Laurence K M, James N, Miller M, Campbell H 1980 Increased risk of recurrence of pregnancies complicated by fetal neural tube defects in mothers receiving poor diets, and possible benefit of dietary counselling. British Medical Journal 281: 1592–1594

Leathern J H 1975 Nutritional influences on testicular composition and function in animals. In: Handbook of Physiology Sec 7, pp 225–232 American Physiological Society, Washington

Magenis P E, Overton K M, Chamberlin J, Brady T, Lourien E 1977 Parental origin of the extra chromosome in Down's syndrome. Human Genetics 37: 7–16

Mau G, Netter P 1974 Die Auswirkungen des väterlichen Zigarettenkonsums auf die perinatale Sterblichkeit und die Missbildungshäufigkeit. Deutsche medizinische Wochenschrift 99: 1113–1118

Meadows N J, Ruse W, Smith M F, Day J, Keeling P W N, Scopes J W, Thompson R P H, Bloxam D L 1981 Zinc and small babies. Lancet ii: 1135–1136

Moore W M O, Jones V P, Ward B S 1976 Fetal growth retardation in the second trimester. European Journal of Obstetrics Gynaecology and Reproductive Biology 6: 121–123

Nillius S J 1978 Epidemiology and endocrinology of weight loss-related amenorrhoea. In: Advances in Gynaecological Endocrinology. Royal College of Obstetricians and Gynaecologists, London

Obe G, Ristow H 1979 Mutagenic, carcinogenic and teratogenic effects of alcohol. Mutation Research 65: 229–259

Obe G, Göbel D, Engeln J, Herha J, Natargan A T 1980 Chromosomal aberrations in peripheral lymphocytes of alcoholics. Mutation Research 73: 377–386

Sabbagha R E, Turner J H, Chez R A 1975 Sonar biparietal diameter growth standards in the rhesus monkey. American Journal of Obstetrics and Gynecology 121: 371–374

Sabbagha R E, Barton F B, Barton B A 1976 Sonar biparietal diameter; analysis of percentile growth differences in two normal populations using same methodology. American Journal of Obstetrics and Gynecology 126: 479–484, 485–490

Simpson J L 1980 Genes, chromosomes and reproductive failure. Fertility and Sterility 33: 107–116

Smithells R W, Sheppard S, Schorah C J 1976 Vitamin deficiencies and neural tube defects. Archives of Disease in Childhood 51: 944–950

Smithells R W, Sheppard S, Schorah C J, Seller M J, Nevin N C, Harris R, Read A P, Fielding W 1981 Apparent prevention of neural tube defects by periconceptional vitamin supplementation. Archives of Disease in Childhood 56: 911–918

Soltan M H, Jenkins D M 1982 Maternal and fetal plasma zinc concentration and fetal abnormality. British Journal of Obstetrics and Gynaecology 89: 56–58

Spiers P S 1982 Does growth retardation predispose the fetus to congenital malformation? Lancet i: 312–314

Stein Z, Susser M, Saenger G, Marolla F 1975 Famine and Human Development. Oxford University Press, Oxford

Tolarova M 1982 Periconceptional supplementation with vitamins and folic acid to prevent recurrence of cleft lip. Lancet ii: 217

Viczian M, Hancsok M, Czeizel E 1969 Bedeutung der Spermuntersuchungen bei den Gatten habituell abortierenden Frauen. Zentralblatt für Gynäkologie 91: 277–284

Wynn M, Wynn A 1981 The prevention of handicap of early pregnancy origin. Foundation for Education and Research in Child-Bearing, London

Wynn M, Wynn A 1983 Effects of nutrition on reproductive capability. Nutrition and Health 1: 165–178

Yamasaki E, Ames B N 1977 Concentration of mutagens from urine by adsorption with the non-polar resin XAD-2: Cigarette smokers have mutagenic urine. Proceedings of the National Academy of Sciences of the United States of America 74: 3555–3559

Hypertensive disorders of pregnancy

Hypertension is one of the commonest complications of pregnancy and may be associated with proteinuria though proteinuria only occurs in about 10% of women with hypertension in pregnancy. In the past hypertension was also thought to be associated with oedema though oedema normally occurs in 80% of pregnant women (Robertson 1971) and has been shown to be of no diagnostic or prognostic significance (Friedman & Neff 1977a). The concept of one disease peculiar to pregnancy characterised by a triad of hypertension, proteinuria and oedema is therefore not valid and should be abandoned. Hypertension in pregnancy is more correctly regarded as the chief clinical manifestation or end result of a number of different diseases or disorders which may be either incidental or peculiar to pregnancy. The disorders are best known as 'The Hypertensive Disorders of Pregnancy' and include all conditions which present in pregnancy with hypertension and/or proteinuria.

DIAGNOSIS OF PRE-ECLAMPSIA, GESTATIONAL AND ESSENTIAL HYPERTENSION AND CHRONIC RENAL DISEASE

At the present time at least three different entities may be distinguished in addition to the rarer causes of hypertension such as coarctation of the aorta and phaechromocytoma.

1. Pre-eclampsia

Some women who have normal blood pressures at the beginning of pregnancy develop hypertension and proteinuria, usually in the last trimester, which disappears after delivery suggesting one type of disease peculiar to pregnancy. This disease is often designated as 'pre-eclampsia'. 'True pre-eclampsia' is defined by the characteristic changes in the renal glomeruli on renal biopsy and is almost invariably associated with albuminuria. Patients who do not have albuminuria do not have the glomerular lesions (Sheehan and Lynch 1973a). Albuminuria or proteinuria, in the absence of chronic renal disease, may thus be regarded as diagnostic of 'true pre-eclampsia'.

True pre-eclampsia is primarily a disease of primigravidae but may recur in subsequent pregnancies and tends to run in families. It is not associated with an increased incidence of hypertension in later life except where the pre-eclampsia develops in a woman with pre-existing hypertension (Reid & Teel 1939, Chesley 1978a). Because true pre-eclampsia occurs primarily in primigravidae an abnormal immunological reaction to a first pregnancy is thought to play a key part in its aetiology (Petrucco 1981).

2. Gestational hypertension and chronic essential hypertension

Chesley (1980) has made a strong case for at least a second form of hypertension in pregnancy known as gestational hypertension. Gestational hypertension is characterised by the development of hypertension (but not proteinuria) in women who are apparently normotensive at the beginning of pregnancy but who have a strong family history of hypertension. The condition occurs in both primigravidae and multigravidae but is more common in multigravidae. It increases in frequency with increasing age, and is most common in women over the age of 30 (Nelson 1955). Gestational hypertension is postulated to be due to an inherited latent tendency to hypertension which becomes overt in pregnancy. The blood pressure usually returns to normal in the puerperium and the condition is analogous to gestational diabetes. The hypertension, however, usually recurs in subsequent pregnancies, becomes more severe with increasing age and sooner or later manifests as established essential hypertension. On follow-up women who develop gestational hypertension in pregnancy have a much higher incidence of essential hypertension in later life and women who remain normotensive in pregnancy have a much lower incidence (Adams & MacGillivray 1961). Gestational hypertension and chronic essential hypertension are thus in all probability two phases of the same disorder.

The concept of hypertension in pregnancy being an expression of latent essential hypertension is by no means new and was put forward almost 50 years ago by Herrick & Tillman (1936) and Fishberg (1939). These authors however believed that all hypertension in pregnancy, including eclampsia, were forms of latent or established essential hypertension. In a classic paper Nelson (1955) stated quite clearly that mild and severe pre-eclampsia may not be the same diseases, particularly in women over the age of 30. Nelson defined mild pre-eclampsia as a diastolic blood pressure of 90 mmHg or more (which would correspond to gestational hypertension) and severe pre-eclampsia as 'more than a trace of albumin' (which would correspond to pre-eclampsia under the present definitions).

There is good epidemiological evidence that women with gestational hypertension have an inherited latent tendency to hypertension which has the same basis as essential hypertension. The nature of this inherited tendency is not known, but there is increasing evidence that hypertensive patients and their close relatives have a defect or impairment of sodium and potassium co-transport or counter transport in erythrocytes, leucocytes and probably all tissues of the body including vascular smooth muscle (Blaustein 1977, Kaplan 1982a).

3. Chronic renal diseases

These are characterised by the fact that they are present before and persist after pregnancy though they may be only diagnosed for the first time at booking. They are most commonly recognised by the occurrence of proteinuria which is out of proportion to the level of blood pressure or by proteinuria with a normal blood pressure. They are essentially incidental diseases, and the aetiological and pathological mechanisms which are responsible for the diseases continue to act throughout the pregnancy and are probably entirely different from those causing gestational hypertension or pre-eclampsia.

DISTINCTION BETWEEN TRUE PRE-ECLAMPSIA AND GESTATIONAL HYPERTENSION

The distinction between true pre-eclampsia and gestational hypertension is important for a number of reasons:

1. true pre-eclampsia with proteinuria is associated with a higher perinatal mortality;
2. true pre-eclampsia is more likely to progress to eclampsia than gestational hypertension (eclampsia is very rare without proteinuria) and is consequently associated with a higher maternal morbidity and mortality;
3. true pre-eclampsia is primarily a disease of primigravidae but may recur in second pregnancies in women who have had true pre-eclampsia in a first pregnancy. It rarely occurs for the first time in second or subsequent pregnancies except with a new father (Ikedife 1980). Gestational hypertension, in contrast, frequently occurs for the first time in second, third or subsequent pregnancies, particularly in women over the age of 30, and recurrence of gestational hypertension is the rule rather than the exception;
4. true pre-eclampsia is not associated with essential hypertension in later life (unless it develops as superimposed pre-eclampsia on essential or gestational hypertension). Gestational hypertension on the other hand is associated with a much higher incidence of essential hypertension in later life and thus carries a more serious connotation in the long term;
5. true pre-eclampsia may be associated with more widespread pathological changes including disseminated intra-vascular coagulation and fibrin deposition, renal and liver lesions and other generalised organ damage;

6. the hypertension in true pre-eclampsia may have a different aetiology and a different pathophysiological basis to the hypertension of gestational and essential hypertension and may therefore require different anti-hypertensive and other treatment.

The main distinguishing features between gestational hypertension and pre-eclampsia are as follows:

1. Proteinuria

Proteinuria is the main clinical distinguishing feature of pre-eclampsia to the extent of being pathognomonic in the absence of chronic renal disease (Sheehan & Lynch 1973a). Patients with pre-eclamptic glomerular lesions almost invariably have an associated albuminuria. Patients who do not have albuminuria do not have glomerular lesions. Proteinuria is also the chief diagnostic feature of pre-eclampsia superimposed on essential hypertension, and the occurrence of proteinuria in a woman with essential hypertension in pregnancy indicates the occurrence of a separate superimposed pre-eclamptic disease process and not worsening of the essential hypertension (Altchek 1964).

2. Renal biopsy findings

The diagnosis of true pre-eclampsia can only be confirmed by the finding of characteristic changes in the renal glomeruli on renal biopsy (Chesley & Valenti 1958), though the occurrence of proteinuria in the absence of chronic renal disease appears to be pathognomic (Sheehan & Lynch 1973a). Gestational or essential hypertension appears to be associated with normal appearances of the kidney on renal biopsy. The findings on renal biopsy in a series of 214 unselected cases of acute hypertension in pregnancy (McCartney 1964) are shown in Table 6.1. It will be noted that in the 62 primipara the incidence of true pre-eclampsia was 71%, chronic renal disease 25%, normal (essential or gestational hypertension) 4%. In the 152 multipara in contrast, the incidence of true pre-eclampsia was 3%, chronic renal disease 44% and essential or gestational hypertension 53%. Pre-eclampsia is thus common in primiparae with hypertension (approximately 70%) but is rare in multiparae (less than 3%). Renal biopsy is not generally performed in pregnancy but the parity of the patient and the occurrence of proteinuria in the absence of chronic renal disease provides a reliable indicator of the presence of true pre-eclampsia.

3. Serum Urate

Pollak & Nettles (1960) showed that the level of serum uric acid increases significantly with increasing severity of the glomerular lesions in women with pre-eclampsia and suggested that serum uric acid may be useful in recognising pre-eclampsia and distinguishing it from hypertensive vascular disease in pregnancy. Other workers (Redman et al 1976) have regarded raised serum urate as a specific diagnostic feature and have based the whole diagnosis of pre-eclampsia on the basis of increased serum urate levels. Serum urate levels are raised early when the kidney is affected in hypertensive disorders of pregnancy and provide a valuable guide to the assessment of severity and prognosis of fetal outcome. Serum urate however is also frequently raised in essential hypertension (Breckenridge 1966). Uric acid is filtered through the glomeruli but is primarily excreted through the tubules and its secretion is directly related to renal blood flow (Messerli et al 1980). Raised serum urate levels are therefore probably better regarded not as a diagnostic or specific feature of pre-eclampsia, but as an early and sensitive indicator of impaired renal function and of renal blood flow. Serum urate levels furthermore appear to provide a useful prognostic guide to fetal outcome not only in pre-eclampsia but in all patients with hypertension in pregnancy (Wood 1977).

Table 6.1 Acute hypertension of pregnancy: renal biopsies

Renal History	No of Cases	Normal	T L	T L and C R D	C R D
Primipara	62	3 (4.8%)	43 (69.4%)	1 (1.6%)	15 (24.2%)
Multipara	152	81 (53.3%)	5 (3.3%)	16 (10.5%)	50 (32.9%)

T L = Toxemic lesion; C R D = Chronic renal disease. (Adapted from McCartney 1964)

NOMENCLATURE AND CLASSIFICATION OF HYPERTENSIVE DISORDERS OF PREGNANCY

More than 100 names have been used in the English and German literature to describe the different hypertensive diseases of pregnancy and there have been almost as many classifications (Rippmann 1969). In the past hypertensive disorders were regarded as one of the 'toxaemias of pregnancy'. In the last 20 to 30 years a considerable number of new names have been introduced including pre-eclamptic toxaemia (PET), pre-eclampsia (PE), EPH gestosis, pregnancy induced hypertension (PIH), pregnancy associated hypertension (PAH) and gestational hypertension (GH). As the underlying aetiology and pathology of the different disorders is not known a new classification based solely on clinical criteria is proposed (Table 6.2). This classification though based on clinical criteria should nevertheless for reasons given in this chapter provide an indicator of probable underlying pathology and aetiology as well as providing a guide to prognosis and management. The classification follows those of Chesley (1971) and Gant & Worley (1980) but with some important differences in nomenclature as follows:

Table 6.2 Clinical classification of hypertensive disorders of pregnancy

---

A. *Pregnancy-induced hypertension (PIH):* Hypertension developing during pregnancy in a known normotensive, non-proteinuric woman; one of
   1. Gestational hypertension (GH) (without proteinuria)
   2. Pre-eclampsia (PE) (with proteinuria)
   3. Eclampsia (with eclamptic fit)
B. *Chronic hypertension;* Hypertension occurring in pregnancy with or without proteinuria in a woman known to have hypertension or chronic renal disease present before or persisting after pregnancy; one of
   1. Essential hypertension (usually *without* proteinuria)
   2. Chronic renal disease (usually *with* proteinuria)
   3. Other known hypertensive disease (e.g. coarctation of the aorta, phaechromocytoma)
C. *Pre-eclampsia or eclampsia superimposed on gestational or chronic hypertension:* Proteinuria or eclamptic fit occurring in a woman with gestational or chronic hypertension
D. *Transient intrapartum hypertension:* Hypertension occurring for the first time during labour or puerperium and returning to normal within 48 h of delivery
E. *Late Hypertension:* Hypertension with or without proteinuria present in a patient at booking after 20 completed weeks of pregnancy (if hypertension is found at booking before 20 weeks patient is presumed to have essential hypertension unless other obvious cause present)
F. *Unclassified hypertension:* Hypertension in a patient in whom there is insufficient information to permit classification

---

Pregnancy induced hypertension (PIH)

Includes all normotensive women who develop hypertension in pregnancy.

Gestational hypertension (GH)

Includes all normotensive women who develop hypertension *without proteinuria* and in most cases results from an inherited latent tendency to hypertension which becomes overt in pregnancy, and is in general associated with a relatively good fetal outcome.

Pre-eclampsia (PE)

Includes all normotensive women who develop hypertension *with proteinuria*, is a condition peculiar to pregnancy, occurs mainly in primigravidae, may go on to eclampsia and is associated with a relatively poor fetal outcome.

Pre-eclampsia superimposed on essential or chronic hypertension

The reported incidence of superimposed true pre-eclampsia (as evidenced by proteinuria or by renal biopsy) varies from 4% (Chesley 1978b) to 37% (Sheeham & Lynch 1973b). It nevertheless appears that true pre-eclampsia may develop as a superimposed disease and is more common in patients with essential or gestational hypertension. This suggests that some factor associated with essential hypertension, such as ischaemia of the uterus or feto placental unit may be an aetiological factor in true pre-eclampsia.

Transient hypertension

Occurring for the first time in labour and the puerperium and returning to normal within 48 h of delivery is separated from other causes because in the majority of women the raise in blood pressure in labour is due to excitement, exertion or stress and in most cases is probably a normal response. Rises in blood pressure may also occur as a normal phenomenon at delivery because of the haemodynamic changes at this time. Transient hypertension occurs in about 20% of labours and may lead to an over-diagnosis of hypertension in pregnancy if not placed in a separate category.

Late hypertension

In some women who book late with hypertension it is impossible to say whether they had been normotensive earlier in pregnancy and became hypertensive, or whether they had chronic essential hypertension and had been hypertensive throughout the pregnancy. In these patients it is not possible to distinguish between pregnancy-induced and chronic hypertension during pregnancy and it is better to put such patients in a separate category of 'late hypertension in pregnancy'. It may be possible to reclassify such patients in the puerperium as the blood pressure will remain raised in patients with chronic hypertension whereas in those with pregnancy induced hypertension the blood pressure will revert to normal.

Unclassified hypertension.

In some instances insufficient information is available to permit classification and it is better to put these patients in a separate category rather than to make an arbitrary assignment or to confuse existing categories.

MEASUREMENT OF BLOOD PRESSURE, BLOOD PRESSURE CHANGES AND DIAGNOSIS OF HYPERTENSION IN PREGNANCY

1. Measurement of blood pressure (see Appendix)

Arterial blood pressure is nearly always measured in clinical practice by sphygmomanometry and the precise technique used and the conditions under which observations are made significantly affect the measurements. It is essential that the technique and conditions of measurement should be standardised if consistent results are to be obtained (O'Brien & O'Malley 1979). In interpreting blood pressure measurements in pregnancy it is also essential that due allowance is made for the changes in blood pressure in normal pregnancy. Lastly, precise and agreed criteria for the definition of hypertension in pregnancy are essential if the incidence of hypertension and the effects of treatment in different centres are to be compared and mutual understanding is to be achieved.

(a) Diastolic blood pressure (DBP).

In non-pregnant patients it is generally agreed that the point of disappearance of the Korotkoff sounds (Point V) corresponds most closely to the true DBP as measured by intra-arterial catheter. In pregnant patients, however, the ausculated Korotkoff sounds may persist to zero due to the marked peripheral vasodilatation and therefore the point of muffling (Point IV) provides a better measure of true DBP in pregnancy and should be used in all BP measurements during pregnancy and labour.

(b) Conditions of measurement and posture.

Exercise, posture and stress tend to affect the systolic more than the diastolic blood pressure and the resting DBP provides the most reproducible and best guide to prognosis and measurement. It is recommended that the blood pressure should always be measured with the patient resting comfortably and lying on the R side at 30° to the horizontal and with the sphygmomanometer cuff at the level of the heart. The R side is suggested as most obstetricians take the blood pressure in the R arm. The practice of taking the blood pressure on the L or R side with one arm uppermost or turning patients into this position is to be condemned as this leads to falsely low blood pressure readings due to the difference in hydrostatic pressure between the level of the sphygmomanometer cuff and the level of the heart. This error may be as much as 15 or 20 mmHg.

(c) Repeated and average measurement

The blood pressure varies greatly during the day, and isolated readings must be checked after a period of rest. For the diagnosis of hypertension it is accepted practice to require two consecutive abnormally high measurements made at least 4 to 6 hours apart. A useful measurement for management of in-patients is to calculate the mean of the 4 hourly or 6 hourly measurements for each 24 hour period.

2. Blood pressure changes in normal pregnancy

The blood pressure normally falls at the beginning of pregnancy and reaches its lowest level in the second trimester when the DBP is on average 15 mmHg lower and the SBP 5 mmHg lower in the lying position than pre-pregnancy levels (Fig. 6.1) (MacGillivray et al 1969, Friedman & Neff 1977b). What is perhaps not sufficiently appreciated is that the blood pressure normally rises in the third trimester and may reach pre-pregnancy levels by term. This relative rise in BP to pre-pregnancy levels is associated with other changes such as a

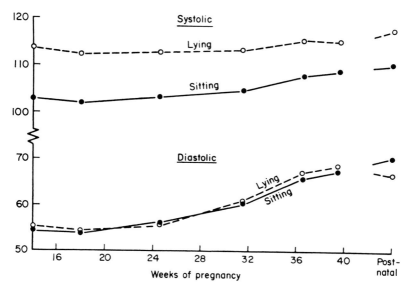

Fig. 6.1 Blood pressure trends (sitting and lying) during pregnancy (from MacGillivray et al 1969)

reduction in renal blood flow and glomerular filtration rate in the last weeks of pregnancy (Davison et al 1980). As it does not appear to be associated with any deleterious effects on fetus or mother it should be regarded as a normal phenomenon. This means that definitions of hypertension in pregnancy based on a rise in blood pressure irrespective of absolute levels probably include some patients in whom the blood pressure has risen as a normal phenomenon. MacGillivray (1961) has shown that the level of BP attained in late pregnancy is more important than the amount of rise of BP in pregnancy and it is therefore recommended that the use of a rise in BP as a criterion for the diagnosis or definition of hypertension in pregnancy should be discontinued. It has been suggested that different ranges of blood pressure should be used to define the different limits of 'normality' at the different stages of pregnancy particularly as it has been shown that women with slightly elevated levels of BP in mid-pregnancy do tend to develop hypertension later (Page 1976). Whilst this approach has considerable merit it would nevertheless cause problems in practice because the exact gestational age is uncertain in many patients and it would be difficult to decide precisely which criteria should be applied at which stage of the pregnancy.

3. Definition of hypertension

Any definition of hypertension is inevitably arbitrary but the use of diastolic blood pressure (Point IV Korotkoff) of 90 mmHg or more throughout pregnancy as originally proposed by Nelson (1955) has a number of advantages:

(a)   it is simple and precise, and overcomes the difficulties of using combined criteria based on systolic and diastolic measurements and of the calculation of the mean arterial pressure. The use of criteria based on systolic and diastolic or on mean arterial pressure moreover does not offer any advantage as the DBP has been shown to be the best predictor of fetal outcome (Friedman & Neff 1977c);

(b)   in the first 2 trimesters of pregnancy it corresponds with 3 s.d. above the mean (MacGillivray et al 1969) and in the third trimester of pregnancy it corresponds with 2 s.d. above the mean (MacGillivray et al 1969) (Table 6.3).

(c)   it corresponds with the point of inflexion of the curve relating DBP to perinatal mortality (Fig. 6.2). Above a DBP of 85 mmHg there is a significant increase in perinatal mortality (Friedman & Neff, 1977d) (Fig. 6.2).

As the occurrence of proteinuria with hypertension is associated with a significant increase in perinatal mortality Nelson (1955) proposed that the proteinuria should be used as the criterion for the definition of *severe* pre-eclampsia. For reasons given above, however, the occurrence of proteinuria is

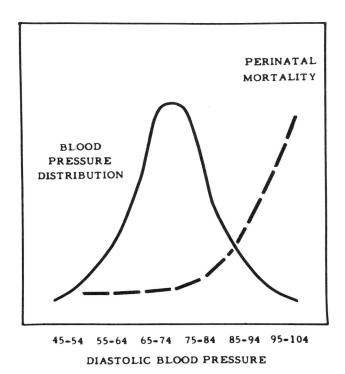

DIASTOLIC BLOOD PRESSURE

Fig. 6.2 Relationship between diastolic blood pressure and perinatal mortality (from Friedman 1976)

better used to define the occurrence of pre-eclampsia and to adopt other criteria for the classification and definition of severity. Suggested criteria for the definition of *'severe'* hypertension and proteinuria in pregnancy and of *imminent eclampsia* are set out in Table 6.3, and are based as far as possible on general accepted indicators of fetal and maternal risk and are guides and indications for particular forms of management.

Table 6.3 Criteria of 'severity' of hypertension in pregnancy

---

A. *'Mild hypertension'* (not necessarily requiring admission or immediate treatment)
  1. 'Spot' DBP* 100 mmHg or more but less than 120 mmHg
  2. Repeated or average 24 h DBP 90 mmHg or more but less than 110 mmHg
  3. No proteinuria
  4. No impairment renal function
  5. No impairment fetal condition or growth
  6. No maternal complication.
B. *'Severe hypertension'* (requiring admission to hospital and probably anti-hypertensive treatment)
  1. 'Spot' DBP 120 mmHg or more
  2. Repeated or average 24 h DBP 110 mmHg or more
  3. Any significant proteinuria (greater than 300 mg/24 h)
  4. Impairment renal function (raised serum creatinine, urate or urea)
  5. Impairment fetal condition or growth
  6. Any maternal complication
C. *'Imminent eclampsia' or eclampsia* (requiring intensive care and probably anti-convulsive therapy)
  1. Eclamptic fit
  2. Imminent eclampsia — epigastric pain, headache, visual symptoms
  3. Hyper-reflexia
  4. Rapidly developing generalised oedema
  5. Oliguria less than 500 ml/24 h (or 20 ml/h)
  6. Rapidly deteriorating renal function

---

*'Spot' DBP is a diastolic blood pressure reading taken in a clinic, consulting room or ward and checked after resting for 2–3 min but not necessarily repeated in 4–6 h. A repeated DBP measurement is one found to be raised on a second consecutive reading after an interval of at least 4/6 h. Average 24 h DBP is the average of the 4/6 readings taken over previous 24 h period and represents the best criterion in practice for the assessment of severity of hypertension in pregnancy.

PHYSIOLOGICAL BASIS OF TREATMENT OF HYPERTENSION IN PREGNANCY

Objectives

The objectives of treatment are:

  1. to lower the blood pressure and reduce the degree of vasospasm to 'safe' levels so that the danger of direct damage to the blood vessels such as necrosis and rupture and of major complications such as cerebral haemorrhage are eliminated;
  2. to increase the blood flow in the uterus, kidneys and other organs to normal pregnancy levels and to prevent or reverse any pathological changes;
  3. to remove, reverse, or control the primary initiating cause of the hypertension.

Mechanisms

The blood pressure may be lowered in several ways:

1. by reducing cardiac output (e.g. with beta adrenergic blocking agents);
2. by producing vasodilatation (e.g. with hydralazine);
3. by increasing sodium excretion and reducing the mean circulating filling pressure (e.g. with diuretics).

1. Cardiac output.

It is claimed that a small sustained increase in cardiac output as occurs in the early acute stages of hypertension may produce a relatively large increase in peripheral resistance (Guyton 1980a) and it might be predicted that a reduction in cardiac output to normal levels and lowering the blood pressure by this means would be advantageous. On the other hand any lowering of cardiac output would tend to reduce blood flow to uterus and kidneys unless at the same time there is at least a compensatory vasodilatation in these organs.

If cardiac output falls and there is no adequate compensatory vasodilatation then blood flow through organs such as the uterus and kidney must be reduced. This would be a serious disadvantage as one of the main objectives of treatment is to increase renal and uterine blood flow. Any treatment which acts primarily by reducing cardiac output (such as beta adrenergic blocking agents) is therefore not to be recommended unless there is evidence of any abnormally increased cardiac output or it can be shown that uterine blood flow is at least maintained if not increased.

2. Vasodilatation

Most anti-hypertensive agents lower the blood pressure by producing a decrease in peripheral resistance, principally by vasodilatation in the limbs and to a lesser degree by vasodilatation in the splanchnic region. This means that when the blood pressure is lowered with these agents the blood flow tends to be deviated away from the splanchic organs including the kidneys and uterus and that the renal and uterine blood flow may be reduced. Fortunately in most instances auto-regulating mechanisms in the kidney and uterus appear to compensate for the fall in blood pressure so that unless the fall in blood pressure is precipitous blood flow is at least maintained (Ferris et al 1976). Nevertheless what is really required in the treatment of hypertension in pregnancy is an agent which will produce a relative vasodilatation in the splanchic area and in the kidneys and uterus in particular. Such an agent should also reset the auto-regulating vascular mechanisms in these organs so that the blood flow at any given level of blood pressure is relatively increased.

The blood flow through any organ is determined by two main factors: (a) the vascular resistance in the organ and (b) the perfusing pressure. In the case of the uterine arteries the perfusing pressure is virtually the same as the arterial blood pressure which is in turn determined by the cardiac output and total peripheral resistance.

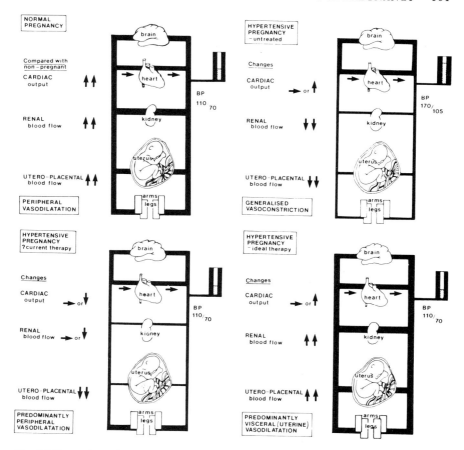

Fig. 6.3 Haemodynamic changes in normal and hypertensive pregnancy and probable effect of current anti-hypertensive therapy and ideal anti-hypertensive therapy on uterine, renal and peripheral vascular resistance and blood flow

These relationships may be expressed by the two standard formulae:

$$\text{Blood pressure} = \text{Cardiac output} \times \text{Total peripheral resistance}$$

$$\text{Uterine blood flow} = \frac{\text{Uterine perfusing pressure}}{\text{Uterine vascular resistance}}$$

As the arterial blood pressure and uterine perfusing pressure are the same, the equations may then be combined and re-written as

$$\text{Uterine blood flow} = \text{Cardiac Output} \times \frac{\text{Total peripheral resistance}}{\text{Uterine vascular resistance}}$$

Expressed in this way it will be seen that the uterine blood flow is dependent upon the cardiac output and upon the ratio of the total peripheral resistance to the uterine vascular resistance. The main need in hypertension in pregnancy is in fact not so much to lower pressure (except when hypertension is severe) but to increase the uterine blood flow. Much more attention therefore needs to be paid to the relative effects of anti-hypertensive agents on the uterine vascular resistance and on the total peripheral resistance. To improve fetal outcome in hypertension in pregnancy, any anti-hypertensive drug must produce a relative uterine vasodilatation. The changes in vascular resistance in hypertension as compared with normal pregnancy and the effects of current anti-hypertensive therapy and of ideal therapy are illustrated in Fig. 6.3.

3. Salt and water excretion and mean circulatory filling pressure

Many different mechanisms control the level of blood pressure, and these mechanisms act with different time courses of action. In the long-term (several days), the main mechanism is the renal blood volume pressure relationship and the main determinant of blood pressure is the mean circulatory filling pressure (Guyton 1980b) (Fig. 6.4). According to Guyton salt and water are retained and the mean circulatory pressure and the blood pressure rise until the renal blood flow is such as to maintain a balance between salt output and intake. When anti-hypertensive drugs are given vasodilatation is produced and the mean circulatory pressure falls. If renal blood flow also falls and salt excretion is inadequate, salt will be retained and the blood pressure will rise again until renal blood flow and salt excretion are adequate. In chronic hypertension one of the most effective ways of lowering the blood pressure is to give a diuretic which will enhance salt and water excretion and reduce the mean circulatory filling pressure and hence the blood pressure. Diuretics, however, may also produce a reduction in total blood volume and plasma volume. In hypertension in pregnancy the blood volume is already reduced and further reduction in blood volume may reduce the venous return to the heart and hence the cardiac output and the blood flow to vital organs. Because diuretics tend to reduce blood volume they are not currently recommended in the treatment of acute hypertension in pregnancy.

In long term treatment of hypertension with diuretics, however, the blood volume returns to normal, whilst the anti-hypertensive effect appears to remain (Kaplan 1982b). In long-term treatment it must also be remembered that when any anti-hypertensive vasodilator agent is given, though the blood pressure may be lowered initially, unless the agent at the same time promotes salt and water excretion, then after a few days salt and water will be retained and the mean circulating filling pressure and the blood pressure will rise. Salt and water will then continue to be retained and the blood pressure will continue to rise until salt intake and output are in balance. This is probably why most anti-hypertensive agents have been found to be relatively ineffective in long-term treatment unless given with a diuretic (Dustan et al 1972). In the treatment of

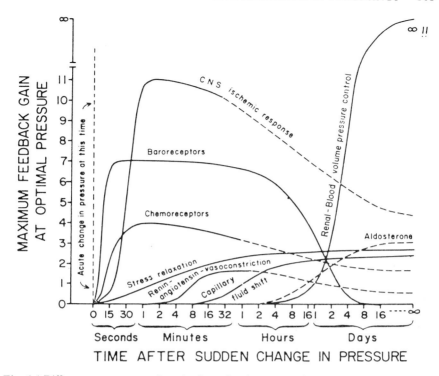

Fig. 6.4 Different pressure control mechanisms showing degree of activation and feedback gain following a sudden change in arterial pressure (from Guyton 1980b)

hypertension in pregnancy it is frequently found that anti-hypertensive drugs appear to become progressively less effective and this may well be due to salt and water retention in the same way as in non-pregnant hypertensive patients. It may thus be necessary to reconsider the use of diuretics in combination with other anti-hypertensive agents particularly in the long-term treatment of hypertension of pregnancy.

CONCLUSIONS

Hypertension in pregnancy is best regarded as the chief clinical manifestation of a number of different disorders of pregnancy, known as 'The Hypertensive Disorders of Pregnancy', which include pre-eclampsia and gestational hypertension. 'True pre-eclampsia' is characterised by typical renal glomerular lesions, proteinuria, primiparity and relative infrequency of essential hypertension in later life. Gestational hypertension is characterised by absence of glomerular lesions and proteinuria, occurrence in both primigravid and multigravid patients, recurrence in successive pregnancies, increase in frequency with increasing age, strong family history of hypertension and subsequent development of essential hypertension. Patients with gestational hypertension may have an inherited familial tendency to hypertension due to an inherited defect in cellular transport of sodium and potassium. This defect may be exacerbated in pregnancy, may increase with age and may then manifest as gestational hypertension in pregnancy and as essential hypertension in later life. A new classification of hypertension in pregnancy including gestational hypertension and pre-eclampsia as separate disorders and based primarily on clinical criteria is proposed. A diastolic blood pressure (point IV) of 90 mmHg or more is proposed as the sole criterion for diagnosis of hypertension, and the occurrence of proteinuria (in the absence of chronic renal disease) as the sole clinical criterion for the diagnosis of pre-eclampsia. In the treatment of hypertension with anti-hypertensive agents more attention should be given to their effect on cardiac output and on renal and uterine blood flow and less on blood pressure *per se*. More attention should also be paid to the effect of anti-hypertensive drugs on salt and water excretion. If salt excretion and mean circulatory filling pressure are major determinants of blood pressure, then the use of diuretics in combination with vasodilator drugs may have to be reconsidered particularly in the long-term treatment of hypertension in pregnancy.

REFERENCES

Adams E M, MacGillivray I 1961 Long term effect of pre-eclampsia on blood pressure. Lancet ii: 1373–1375

Altchek A 1964 Renal biopsy and its clinical correlation in toxaemia of pregnancy. Circulation 29, 30 (Suppl II): 43–51

Blaustein M P 1977 Sodium ions, calcium ions, blood pressure regulation and hypertension: a reassessment and a hypothesis. American Journal of Physiology 232 (3): C 165–173

Breckenridge A 1966 Hypertension and hyperuricaemia. Lancet i: 15–18

Chesley L C 1971 Hypertensive Disorders of Pregnancy. In Hellmann L M, Pritchard J A (eds) Williams Obstetrics, p. 685. Appleton-Century-Crofts, New York

Chesley L C 1978a Hypertensive Disorders of Pregnancy, p. 40. Appleton-Century-Crofts, New York

Chesley L C 1978b Hypertensive Disorders of Pregnancy, p. 484. Appleton-Century-Crofts, New York

Chesley L C 1980 Hypertension in pregnancy: definitions familial factor and remote prognosis. Kidney International 18: 234–246

Chesley L C, Valenti C 1958 Evaluation of tests to differentiate pre-eclampsia from hypertensive disease. American Journal of Obstetrics and Gynecology 75: 1165–1173

Davison J M, Dunlop W, Ezimokhai M 1980 24-Hour creatinine clearance during the third trimester of normal pregnancy. British Journal of Obstetrics and Gynaecology 87: 106–109

Dustan H P, Tarazi R C, Bravo E L 1972 Dependence of arterial pressure on intra-vascular volume in treated hypertensive patients. New England Journal of Medicine 286: 861–866

Ferris T F, Veruto R C, Bay W H 1976 Studies of the uterine circulation in the pregnant rabbit. In: Lindheimer M D, Katz A I, Zuspan F P (eds) Hypertension in Pregnancy pp 351–361. John Wiley, New York

Fishberg A M 1939 Hypertension and Nephritis, 4th edn, p. 746. Lea and Febiger, Philadelphia

Friedman E A 1976 Progress in Clinical and Biological Research, Vol. 7. Blood Pressure, Edema and Proteinuria in Pregnancy, Ch 19, p. 279. Alan R Liss, New York

Friedman E A, Neff R K 1977a Pregnancy Hypertension, p. 238. PSG Littleton, Massachusetts

Friedman E A, Neff R K 1977b Pregnancy Hypertension, p. 46. PSG Littleton, Massachusetts

Friedman E A, Neff R K 1977c Pregnancy Hypertension, p. 169. PSG Littleton, Massachusetts

Friedman E A, Neff R K 1977d Pregnancy Hypertension, p. 170. PSG Littleton, Massachusetts

Gant N F, Worley R J 1980 Hypertension in Pregnancy, p. 1. Appleton-Century-Crofts, New York

Guyton A C 1980a Arterial Pressure and Hypertension, p. 497. W. B. Saunders, Philadelphia

Guyton A C 1980b Arterial Pressure and Hypertension, p. 7. W. B. Saunders, Philadelphia

Guyton A C 1980c Arterial Pressure and Hypertension, p. 495. W. B. Saunders, Philadelphia

Herrick W W, Tillman A J B 1936 The mild toxaemias of late pregnancy: their relation to cardiovascular and renal disease. American Journal of Obstetrics and Gynecology 41: 751–764

Ikedife D 1980 Eclampsia in multipara. British Medical Journal 1: 985–986

Kaplan N M 1982a Clinical Hypertension, p. 56. Williams and Wilkins, Baltimore

Kaplan N M 1982b Clinical Hypertension, p. 124. Williams and Wilkins, Baltimore

McCartney C P 1964 Pathological anatomy of acute hypertension of pregnancy Circulation 30 (Suppl 11): 37–42

MacGillivray I 1961 Hypertension in pregnancy and its consequences. Journal of Obstetrics and Gynaecology of the British Commonwealth 68: 557–569

MacGillivray I, Rose G A, Rowe B 1969 Blood pressure survey in pregnancy. Clinical Science 37: 395–407

Messerli F H, Frohlich E D, Dreslinski G R, Suarez D H, Aristimuno G G 1980 Serum uric acid in essential hypertension: an indicator of renal vascular involvement. Annals of Internal Medicine 93: 817–821

Nelson T R 1955 A clinical study of pre-eclampsia. Journal of Obstetrics and Gynaecology of the British Commonwealth 62: 48–57

O'Brien E T, O'Malley K 1979 ABC of blood pressure measurements. British Medical Journal 2: 775, 851, 920, 982, 1048, 1124, 1201

Page E W 1976 The impact of mean arterial pressure in the middle trimester upon the outcome of pregnancy. American Journal of Obstetrics and Gynecology 125: 740–746

Petrucco O 1981 Aetiology of pre-eclampsia. In: Studd J (ed) Progress in Obstetrics and Gynecology, Vol 1, pp 51–69. Churchill Livingstone, Edinburgh

Pollak V E, Nettles J B 1960 The kidney in toxaemia of pregnancy: a clinical and pathological study based on renal biopsies. Medicine 39: 469–526

Redman C W G, Beilin C J, Bonnar J, Wilkinson R H 1976 Plasma urate measurement in predicting fetal death in hypertensive pregnancy. Lancet i: 1370–1373

Reid D E, Teel H M 1939 Nonconvulsive pregnancy toxaemias; their relationship to chronic vascular and renal disease. American Journal of Obstetrics and Gynecology 37: 886–896

Rippmann E T 1969 Pra-eklampsie. Oder Schwangerschafts-Spatgestose? Gynaecology 167: 478

Robertson E G 1971 The natural history of oedema during pregnancy. Journal of Obstetrics and Gynaecology of the British Commonwealth 78: 520–529

Sheehan H L, Lynch J B 1973a Pathology of Toxaemia of Pregnancy, pp 211–215. Churchill Livingstone, Edinburgh

Sheehan H L, Lynch J B 1973b Pathology of Toxaemia of Pregnancy, p. 281. Churchill Livingstone, Edinburgh

Wood S M 1977 Assessment of renal functions in hypertensive pregnancies. Clinics in Obstetrics and Gynaecology 4 (3): 747–758

APPENDIX

RECOMMENDED METHOD FOR TAKING THE BLOOD PRESSURE IN PREGNANCY BY STANDARD MERCURY SPHYGMOMANOMETER

1. Procedure and position of patient

(a) Remove any tight clothing from R arm so that there is no constriction and the sphygmomanometer cuff can be applied easily.

(b) Arrange that patient lies comfortably on R side with approximately 30° of tilt towards observer and that R arm is well supported with upper arm at same level as heart, horizontal with the sternum at the 4th intercostal space and apply sphygmomanometer cuff.

(c) Ensure that patient rests comfortably lying undisturbed on R side for 2–3 min before blood pressure (BP) is taken.

2. Application of cuff

(a) Place sphygmomanometer cuff over inside of upper arm with connecting tubes to sphygmomanometer pointing headwards and with centre of bladder in cuff directly over the brachial artery leaving ante-cubical fossa free.

(b) Apply cuff evenly and firmly, but not tightly, around arm.

(c) Whenever possible use cuff with the acceptable range of arm circumference marked on cuff. If arm is too large, use larger cuff. If no large cuff is available, note that BP reading is suspect.

3. Taking the blood pressure

(a) Feel brachial artery in front of elbow and place stethoscope directly over artery and hold in place without undue pressure.

(b) Pump up cuff rapidly to 20–30 mmHg above point at which Korotkoff sounds disappear and take BP without delay.

(c) Let air out slowly so that mercury falls steadily at 2–3 mm/s;

(d) Take systolic blood pressure (SBP) as point where first clear tapping sound is heard, read top of mercury meniscus and record to nearest 2 or 5 mmHg.

(e) Take diastolic blood pressure (DBP) in pregnancy as point where sounds first become muffled (Point IV), read top of mercury meniscus and record to nearest 2 or 5 mmHg. If no clear point of muffling, take point of disappearance of Korotkoff sounds (Point V) and record.

(f) Let down cuff completely as soon as BP taken.

4. Choice of arm

(a) The BP should normally be taken in the R arm as this is the most convenient for the majority of observers.

(b) At first visit take BP in both arms. First take BP in R arm as described above and then turn patient on L side approximately 30° tilt with L arm well supported at level of heart; ensure patient rests comfortably on L side for 2–3 min and then take BP in L arm in same way as in R arm and record both measurements.

(c) If BP is 10 mmHg or more higher in L arm than R arm make special note in records and use L arm for all future measurements.

5. Repeat measurements if blood pressure high or unsure

(a) If BP unsure always repeat measurement but let cuff down completely and wait 2–3 min before repeating.

(b) If BP high, ensure patient is resting comfortably and at ease and wait 5 min before repeating measurements; also take and record pulse rate and note any signs of anxiety.

(c) Record all measurements, both initial and repeat, but only act on lowest BP unless there is reason to think it is a falsely low measurement.

6. Repeat by second observer

If action is indicated (e.g. admission to hospital, anti-hypertensive therapy) it is advisable that BP measurement should be repeated by second independent trained observer and reading confirmed.

Abruptio placenta

The purpose of this chapter is to present succinctly our concepts of abruptio placenta with emphasis on some of the newer aspects of diagnosis and management. Emphasis will be placed upon some of the newer techniques including ultrasound as it relates to initiating early diagnosis of the patient with abruptio placenta and the need to maintain an effective circulation to prevent serious complications.

The separation of the normally implanted placenta before the delivery of the fetus has been termed placental abruption, ablatio placenta, and premature separation of the placenta. We will utilise the terms abruptio placenta or placental abruption.

INCIDENCE AND IMPACT

Although the incidence of abruptio placenta appears to be decreasing along with a parallel decrease in severity (Blair 1973), abruptio placenta still occurs in 0.5–3.5% of pregnancies. The wide range in reported incidence occurs because the criteria for diagnosis vary with some studies including mild and dubious cases while others include only patients who are symptomatic. Modern diagnostic techniques and early and intensive management has decreased maternal mortality from 8.7% only 60 years ago (Harrar 1917) to less than 1% today. However, the perinatal mortality rate of 4/1000 births makes abruptio placenta the second most common cause of perinatal death in the Collaborative Perinatal Project (Naeye 1980), and it is responsible for 15–20% of all perinatal mortality in the United States. Despite our technological advances there remains a 25–50% chance of perinatal death in all abruption cases.

While symptomatic abruptio placenta appears to be a disease of the second half of pregnancy, there is controversy regarding the gestational age at which the peak frequency of abruptio placenta occurs. The occurrence rate has been reported by some to be widely distributed over the last trimester with a peak at 36–37 weeks (Nilsen 1958, Hibbard & Hibbard 1963), while others have found the occurrence to peak between 20 and 29 weeks and after 38 weeks (Naeye et al 1977). Still others have noted the peak frequency to be truly cyclic with peaks at 32, 36 and 40 weeks (Page et al 1954).

AETIOLOGY

In the vast majority of cases, no clear aetiology for the abruption is found. In a minority, an apparent association (sudden uterine decompression, trauma, inferior vena cava compression) is present. There is a controversial relationship between abruption and maternal age, parity, folate deficiency, and socioeconomic status. In addition to the above, there may be relationship between abruption and cigarette smoking, uterine anomalies, previous premature labor, and an unexplained second trimester elevated maternal serum alpha-fetoprotein level.

Several cases of abruptio placenta due to sudden uterine decompression at the time of spontaneous or induced rupture of the membranes in patients with hydramnios have been reported (Hibbard & Hibbard 1963, Pritchard 1970). Abruption secondary to external trauma has been reported. The most common traumatic events have been motor accidents with and without the use of 'lap' seat belts (Crosby & Costiloe 1971) and during attempted external cephalic version (Hibbard & Hibbard 1963). Of the abruption cases in the Collaborative Perinatal Project, none were felt to be due to trauma.

While inferior vena cava compression in laboratory animals and in humans just prior to opening the uterus at Caesarean delivery has been associated with abruption (Mengert 1953), this is probably not a common cause of abruptio placenta. Several women who have had inferior vena cava ligation for pulmonary emboli have gone through pregnancy without suffering abruption (Pritchard 1970). Angiographic studies (Kerr 1965) have clearly shown that in a significant percentage of women in late pregnancy, the interior vena cava may normally be completely occluded in the supine position without any evidence of abruption.

While most authorities agree that there is a relationship between abruptio placenta and chronic hypertension or acute pregnancy induced hypertension, controversy still exists regarding hypertension as the *aetiology* of the abruption. The bulk of the recent clinical and pathologic evidence suggest the abruption occurs before the hypertension (Naeye et al 1977) and that hypertension is not an important factor in the genesis of placental abruption.

The evidence regarding the relationship between abruptio placenta and maternal age and parity is conflicting. Hibbard & Hibbard (1963) and Pritchard (1970) found age not to be a factor while others have found a relationship between abruption and maternal age greater than 40 (Golditch & Boyce 1970, Paterson 1979). Paintin (1962), on the other hand, suggested that there is a higher incidence of abruption in primagravidas under the age of 20. Most authorities agree that there is a relationship between parity and abruption, particularly when parity is five or greater (Hibbard & Hibbard 1963, Golditch et al 1970).

Maternal folate deficiency was once thought to be important in the genesis of placental abruption (Hibbard & Hibbard 1963). However, recent studies have not confirmed this (Pritchard 1970, Naeye 1980). Furthermore, routine folate supplementation during pregnancy does not seem to reduce the risk of abruption (Golditch & Boyce 1970). It may be that the folate needs to be administered prior to conception and during the first trimester before any beneficial effect is seen.

The conditions for abruptio placenta may be in place much earlier in pregnancy than has previously been thought. Preliminary evidence from our laboratory indicates that patients who have an unexplained elevation of the maternal serum alpha-fetoprotein (above two multiples of the median) in the second trimester of pregnancy have an increased risk of placental abruption. The elevation of the maternal serum alpha-fetoprotein, unrelated to any fetal structural or amniotic fluid abnormality, may be related to abnormal placentation and subsequent leakage of the alpha-fetoprotein into the maternal serum. These data may further explain the theories linking abruption to a chronic process which may be further aggravated by cigarette smoking or hypertension.

It has become clear that cigarette smoking is a most important aetiologic factor in abruptio placenta. The two most common lesions associated with abruption are necrosis of the decidua basalis at the margin of the placenta and large, recent placental infarcts. The frequency of these lesions increases with the number of cigarettes smoked per day (Naeye et al 1977). It appears that smoking may have a vasoconstrictive effect on the uteroplacental circulation. Release of this spasm causes a surge of blood which in turn causes arterial rupture (Goujard et al 1975). The decidua at the edge of the placenta appears to be predisposed to the subsequent necrosis (Naeye 1980). Women who smoke have a six-fold higher risk of stillbirth from abruption than women who do not smoke. This effect of smoking is independent of parity (Goujard et al 1975, Naeye et al 1977). Women who stop smoking during pregnancy have a 23% lower incidence of abruption and a 50% decrease in fetal and neonatal deaths due to abruption than women who continue smoking and, in fact, they lower their risk of fetal death due to abruption to the level of women who have never smoked (Naeye 1980). This effect of smoking is probably an effect of nicotine (Barry 1963, Naeye et al 1977), or it may be related to a relative deficiency of folic acid or other vitamins. It has been reported that maternal serum alpha-fetoprotein is elevated in mothers who smoke (Thomsen et al 1983).

There is a controversial relationship between uterine anomalies and the risk of abruption. Two studies found a relationship between uterine anomalies and abruption (Lunan 1973, Naeye et al 1977), while a third study found that uterine anomalies were rare among abruption cases (Pritchard 1970). While an unusually short umbilical cord has been held responsible for occasional cases of abruption, large studies have found no such relationship (Pritchard 1970, Naeye 1980).

PATHOLOGY AND MECHANISM

The initiating event in abruption is uterine vasospasm and subsequent relaxation of the circulation causing vascular engorgement followed by arteriolar rupture into the decidua basalis which in turn leads to decidual haematoma formation and eventual decidual necrosis at the edge of the placenta. This is the most common pathological lesion seen with abruption. The decidua basalis is the layer that normally separates at delivery with most of the decidua remaining attached to the myometrium and a smaller portion attached to the maternal side of the placenta. The difference with normal separation at delivery is that the myometrium of the empty uterus contracts around the maternal sinuses to cause hemostasis.

The blood escaping under the decidua basalis can then pursue one of four courses: (1) dissect under the membranes (a large volume of blood may be concealed here) eventually leading to vaginal bleeding; (2) break through the membranes into the amniotic cavity (indeed, bloody amniotic fluid is often seen when the membranes rupture); (3) dissect under the placenta, separating it from the maternal surface; and (4) infiltrate the myometrium causing the uterus to contract and take on a purplish colour ('Couvelaire uterus') (Naeye et al 1977, Knab 1978).

The diapedesis of blood from the decidua into the myometrium acts like an ecbolic agent and is associated with a contraction that may be well-localised or diffuse and tetanic. If uterine relaxation does not occur, the uteroplacental circulation may be compromised leading to fetal hypoxaemia, acidosis and possible fetal death. In addition, the increased intra-amniotic fluid pressure secondary to the tetanic contraction may further jeopardise the uteroplacental circulation and fetal health.

The decidua is rich in thromboplastin (Pritchard 1968). As the decidua degenerates, it may release thromboplastin into the maternal circulation and start the process that may lead to disseminated intravascular coagulation (d.i.c.).

SIGNS AND SYMPTOMS

The onset of symptoms occurs before labour in slightly more than half the cases, after the onset of labour in 35% and simultaneously with the onset of labour in 7% of cases. Clinically, the patient with severe abruption presents with vaginal bleeding, a tonically-contracted uterus, absent fetal heart tones, and uterine tenderness. Even if the amount of vaginal bleeding is minimal the patient may present in shock with a rapid and weak pulse, hypotension, cold moist skin, and stupor. The majority of patients are asymptomatic until they experience sudden onset abdominal pain, vaginal bleeding, or both, but 11% of patients have experienced previous vaginal bleeding 1 to 49 days earlier (Paintin 1962).

Vaginal bleeding is the most common symptom (Hurd et al 1983), but there is little relationship between the amount of visible bleeding prior to delivery and the amount of placental separation, the amount of maternal haemorrhage, or the degree of hypofibrinogenemia. The amount of visible vaginal bleeding may be minimal even though the fetus is dead, the placenta is completely separated from the uterus, the mother is in shock, and severe d.i.c. exists (Pritchard 1968).

Abdominal pain is the second most common symptom, occurring in 35% of cases (Hurd et al 1983). The cause of the pain is unknown but is most likely due to disruption of myometrial fibres and intravasation of blood from the site of the abruption (Notelovitz 1974). Several cases of 'silent' abruption severe enough to be associated with fetal demise have been reported. In these cases the placental site was the posterior wall of the uterus, and persistent low back pain was the only feature (Notelovitz 1974). Usually the pain is constant, acute, and differs from labour pains (Nilsen 1958). Though epidural anaesthesia will relieve labour pain, the pain associated with abruption continues in spite of epidural anaesthesia (Paterson 1979). Epidural anaesthesia should not be used, however, as a test to differentiate between abruption and labour. Though the pain is variable, particularly with lesser degrees of abruption, uterine tenderness is almost always present (Notelovitz 1974).

On physical examination, uterine hypertonus is present in 17% of cases (Hurd et al 1983), and the uterus is nearly always tender. The uterine tension often makes it impossible to palpate the fetus or hear the fetal heart tones with a fetoscope (Lunan 1973). It is thus imperative that a sonogram be performed before a diagnosis of fetal death is made, because many of these fetuses with inaudible heart tones are alive.

In severe abruption, disseminated intravascular coagulation and shock are common features. In addition, intense systemic vasospasm commonly occurs, and this may in turn cause the patient to become hypertensive or normotensive in spite of marked hypovolemia.

DIAGNOSIS AND DIFFERENTIAL DIAGNOSIS

If pain, tenderness, and a tetanically contracted uterus are present, abruption is easily distinguished from placenta previa or local causes of vaginal bleeding. If bleeding is the only symptom, then a careful speculum exam should be performed to rule out local causes of vaginal bleeding and a careful sonogram should be performed to rule out placenta previa.

Though we still feel that the diagnosis of abruptio placenta is a clinical diagnosis, we have recently diagnosed abruptio placenta with real-time sonography (Fig. 7.1) in a patient with a confusing clinical presentation. A retroplacental haematoma is visualised sonographically as an anechoic collection between the placenta and the uterine wall. As the haematoma becomes organised, its echogenicity may increase presenting internal echos that may be difficult to distinguish from a degenerating leiomyoma.

If the cause of the bleeding still hasn't been found after the above procedures, the physician is faced with a diagnostic and management dilemma. The presence of albuminuria, hypertension, thrombocytopaenia, or hypofibrinogenaemia certainly should heighten clinical suspicion of abruption as should hypotension out of proportion to observed blood loss. Even in the

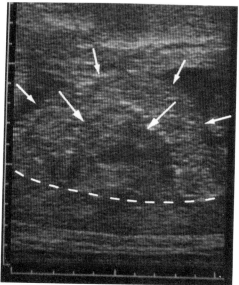 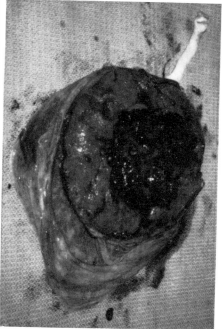

Fig. 7.1 Ultrasonographic appearance of abruptio placenta. The retroplacental haematoma was visualised sonographically (left) as an anechoic collection between the placenta and uterine wall. After delivery, the haematoma remained attached to the maternal side of the placenta (right) (courtesy of Dr John Seeds)

absence of any of these, the diagnosis of abruptio placenta cannot be excluded. But because a diagnosis cannot be made, there is often a delay in aggressive management, especially if the gestation is less than 36 weeks and symptoms are so minimal that prolongation of pregnancy in hopes of improving the chance of neonatal survival is important (Golditch et al 1970). It is in these cases that the visualisation of a retroplacental haematoma by sonography may be helpful.

COMPLICATIONS

The major complications of abruptio placenta are *postpartum haemorrhage, renal failure, d.i.c.,* and *hypertension with or without proteinuria.*

Renal failure is a major cause of maternal death in abruptio placenta. More than half the women who die from abruptio placenta are found at autopsy to have bilateral cortical necrosis (Nilsen 1958) while others are found to have lower nephron necrosis. The renal failure is related to prolonged maternal hypovolaemia (Porter 1960, O'Driscoll & McCarthy 1966, Golditch & Boyce 1970, Pritchard & Brekken 1967) and is largely preventable by appropriate fluid replacement (Pritchard & Brekken 1967, Golditch & Boyce 1970) and by the use of central venous pressure monitoring (O'Driscoll & McCarthy 1966).

In 1901 DeLee described a haemophilia-like syndrome associated with abruption, and in 1936 Dieckman found low levels of fibrinogen in these cases. In 1948, Kellog proposed that thromboplastin enters the maternal circulation from the decidua in abruption cases and causes d.i.c. (Page et al 1954).

In general, the greater the degree of placental separation, the more likely the development of a serious coagulation defect. However, dangerous *hypofibrinogenaemia* can even develop in cases of mild abruption. Overall hypofibrinogenaemia below 100 mg/dl occurs in 4–10% of abruption cases (Porter 1960, Sher 1977), but it occurs in about 30% of cases of abruption severe enough to cause fetal death (Pritchard 1968). Thrombocytopaenia below 100,000/mm³ often accompanies hypofibrinogenaemia. Factor VII and VIII levels, while reduced, may be in the low normal range since these clotting factors normally increase during pregnancy.

Evidence for d.i.c. should be sought in any patient with abruptio placenta. Prolonged bleeding from venapuncture sites indicates serious hypofibrinogenaemia. A serum fibrinogen level below 100 mg/dl or fibrin degradation products above 10 μg/ml confirms the diagnosis. A prolonged thrombin time indicates either hypofibrinogenaemia or increased levels of fibrin degradation products. While awaiting the results of these tests, a quick method of evaluating the patient for the presence of d.i.c. is to observe her freshly-drawn blood in a test tube. Failure of the blood to clot within 8 minutes indicates hypofibrinogenaemia. By the end of 1 hour the clot should retract from the sides of the tube; if not, thrombocytopaenia should be suspected. Furthermore, if the clot dissolves within 1 hour, it is likely that the patient has excessive fibrinolysis.

Of all obstetrical complications, the combination of d.i.c. and abruption tends to be the most lethal with nearly uniform perinatal mortality and very high maternal mortality (Sher 1977).

When d.i.c. does develop, it usually develops quite rapidly, nearly always within 8 hours of the onset of clinical symptoms of abruption. Conversely, when the fibrinogen concentration is above 150 mg/dl 6–8 hours after clinical onset of abruption, serious hypofibrinogenaemia usually does not develop even if delivery is delayed for several more hours (Pritchard 1968).

It is believed that the d.i.c. is initiated by release of thromboplastin from the decidua at the separation site (Pritchard 1968). This decidua is extremely rich in thromboplastin (Schneider 1950). At the same time, a fibrinolytic mechanism lyses much of the fibrin generated in the maternal circulation. It has become clear that the fibrinolysis is a secondary event to the intravascular coagulation in that all patients showing increased fibrinolytic activity have hypofibrinogenaemia while fibrinolysis (increased fibrin degradation products) occurs in only a small number of cases (Pritchard 1968).

After delivery the contracted myometrium normally compresses the maternal vascular sinuses, but approximately 27% of patients with the combination of abruption and d.i.c. may develop *postpartum haemorrhage* (Basu

1969). The occurrence of postpartum uterine bleeding is not related to the degree of hypofibrinogenaemia, but it is associated with an increase in fibrin degradation products. The presence of early products of fibrinogen proteolysis (fragments X or Y) is almost invariably associated with postpartum haemorrhage, whereas the presence of late products (fragments D or E) alone is not strongly associated with postpartum haemorrhage. *In vitro* contractility of myometrial strips removed from patients in labour is completely inhibited when exposed to fibrin degradation products.

Hypertension with or without albuminuria is present in up to two-thirds of cases of abruption, and the hypertension is severe (diastolic b.p.$\geqslant$110 mmHg) in up to one-third of cases (Porter 1960). While there may be some debate over which comes first, the abruption or the rise in blood pressure, the bulk of the evidence points to the abruption preceding the rise in blood pressure (Paintin 1962, Hibbard & Hibbard 1963). The intense vasospasm may be a response to maternal hypovolaemia and is likely responsible for some cases of renal failure. Unfortunately, the hypertension may mislead the obstetrician into an undertreatment of the underlying maternal hypovolaemia.

TREATMENT

Prompt diagnosis and treatment are the mainstays of management of abruption. The longer the interval from recognition to treatment, the worse the fetal prognosis and the greater the maternal hazard. The main goals of treatment are restoration of effective circulation, delivery of a non-acidotic fetus, and continued surveillance of the coagulation status of the mother.

Hypovolaemia is a major factor in the genesis of renal failure associated with abruption (Pritchard 1968). There is a tendency to grossly undertransfuse. A normal pulse rate and blood pressure may often be found with blood loss of up to 35% of the maternal blood volume, and tachycardia and pallor indicate that 40–50% of maternal blood volume has been lost (Barry 1963). External bleeding may be minimal while retroplacental bleeding is extensive. An indwelling urinary catheter should be placed so that the urinary output can be accurately monitored. The urine output should be at least 30 ml/hour and preferably greater than 60 ml/hour. If the urine output is less than 30 ml/hour, monitoring with a pulmonary artery catheter or central venous line is recommended. The central venous pressure may not reflect early pulmonary congestion; thus, it is important to observe the patient for rales and dyspnoea if a pulmonary artery catheter is not used. The central venous pressure is used to monitor the ability of the cardiovascular system to handle the intravenous infusion. Blood and lactated Ringers solution should then be infused in such proportions to keep the haematocrit above 30% and the urinary output above 30 ml/hour. Though undertransfusion is quite common, overtransfusion is rare. It has been shown that the amount of blood transfused is more adequate if the central venous pressure is monitored than if it is not (O'Driscoll & McCarthy 1966).

If d.i.c. accompanies abruptio placenta the therapeutic goals are to avoid trauma to the genital tract through spontaneous vaginal delivery. An episiotomy, if necessary, should be in the midline and should be carefully repaired. After delivery, intravenous oxytocin should be administered. Once hypofibrinogenaemia develops, it is unlikely that it will correct spontaneously prior to delivery. However, treatment is rarely required, though it is best to administer fresh blood if transfusion is required. After delivery, the plasma concentration of fibrinogen increases by approximately 100 mg/dl over the first 12–16 hours with a similar increase in other coagulation factors, though it may take several days for the platelet count to reach normal (Pritchard 1968). A well-contracted myometrium contributes more to haemostasis after delivery than does the coagulation mechanism. If excessive bleeding persists after delivery and is unresponsive to oxytocin administration and uterine massage, cryoprecipitate may be needed. Infusion of 10 units of cryoprecipitate increases the plasma fibrinogen concentration by 100 mg/dl, and in addition it will increase the factor VIII level. Fresh frozen plasma may occasionally be required to replace factor V.

If a Caesarean section is necessary in the face of obvious bleeding and hypofibrinogenaemia, the amount of bleeding can be greatly reduced when enough cryoprecipitate is given prior to Caesarean section to increase the plasma fibrinogen concentration to 150 mg/dl or greater.

About 3% of patients with abruption develop postpartum uterine atony unresponsive to oxytocin and uterine massage. This occurs because a high concentration of fibrin degradation products inhibits myometrial contractility. In these cases the protease inhibitor aprotinin may improve contractility (Basu 1969) as may intramyometrial injection of prostaglandin $F_2\alpha$.

When the diagnosis of abruption is made, immediate amniotomy should be performed to (1) allow for internal monitoring of the fetal heart, (2) hasten delivery, (3) decrease intervillous space pressure, and (4) possibly prevent thromboplastin from escaping into the maternal circulation.

In the presence of fetal death, vaginal delivery is preferable unless there is persistent haemorrhage in which case Caesarean delivery should be performed after administration of blood or blood component therapy to correct the hypovolaemia and coagulopathy. If the fetus is alive on admission, there is a close association between diagnosis to delivery time and perinatal mortality rate (Pritchard & Brekken 1967, Knab 1978). In the days before electronic fetal heart monitoring, there was a clear advantage in performing an immediate Caesarean section in all cases of moderate or severe abruption once hypofibrinogenaemia had been corrected. However, with internal monitoring of the fetal heart combined with liberal use of fetal scalp blood sampling, an equally good perinatal outcome can be obtained with a Caesarean rate of approximately 50% (Hurd et al 1983). Once the scalp electrode has been placed, an intravenous oxytocin infusion should be started to induce labour. Epidural anaesthesia should be avoided because of the maternal hypovolaemia that so often accompanies abruption.

PROGNOSIS

The maternal mortality has fallen from nearly 10% early in this century (Harrar 1917) to well under 1% today (Paterson 1979). Much of this reduction in maternal mortality has resulted from more liberal use of intravenous fluid therapy and transfusion of blood and blood components. Major causes of maternal death are bilateral renal cortical necrosis, lower nephron necrosis, and liver necrosis, all of which may be preventable through maintenance of an effective maternal blood volume. Other causes of death are subarachnoid haemorrhage and shock (Nilsen 1958, Porter 1960). Maternal mortality tends to be higher among women age 30 or greater, particularly if they are hypertensive and have evidence of a coagulopathy.

If a patient suffers an abruption in one pregnancy, she then stands an approximately 6 per cent chance of suffering a recurrence in each subsequent pregnancy (Hibbard & Hibbard 1963, Paterson 1979). Further, the recurrent abruption tends to be more severe than the initial episode (Golditch & Boyce 1970, Paintin 1962).

Abruptio placenta continues to be a major cause of perinatal mortality, accounting for 4 deaths per 1000 births. It was the second most common cause of perinatal mortality in the Collaborative Perinatal Project (Naeye et al 1977). Abruptio placenta accounts for 15% of all perinatal mortality in the United States and the overall perinatal mortality associated with abruption is 30%. With cases of severe abruption, the perinatal mortality is 70%, while with milder cases it is 12%. Perinatal mortality correlates with severity of the abruption, gestation at which the separation occurs, birth weight, the amount of concealed haemorrhage, and with maternal hypertension.

Premature survival correlates with the gestation at which the abruption occurs and with the birthweight of the infant. Survival at 28–32 weeks is only 23%, rising to a peak survival of 87% at 37–40 weeks, then falling to 67% after 40 weeks (Paterson 1979). Of those fetuses who are alive on admission and weighing more than 2500 g, the survival rate is more than 98% (Edson et al 1968, Lunan 1973). Thus it becomes clear that the vast majority of the mortality is accounted for by two factors: a large number of the fetuses are already dead on admission and a large number die from extreme prematurity.

In addition, the newborn is at risk for malformation, neonatal anaemia, d.i.c., respiratory distress syndrome, hyperbilirubinaemia, patent ductus arteriosus, and central nervous system depression from hypoxia. The risk of a major fetal anomaly is 4.4%, and the risk of a major central nervous system anomaly is three to five times higher than in the general population (Lunan 1973, Paterson 1979, Hurd 1983). Neonatal anaemia is diagnosed in 4–20% of cases (Golditch & Boyce 1970, Hurd et al 1983). This may be due to fetal to maternal transfusion that occurs in up to two-thirds of abruption cases (Haynes 1966). Cases of neonatal d.i.c. occurring in the face of maternal d.i.c. have been reported (Edson et al 1968).

Respiratory distress syndrome occurs in about half the live-born abruption cases, and hyperbilirubinaemia in about 25% (Hurd et al 1983). Newborns of abruption cases are significantly more depressed at 5 minutes of life, and these have a small chance of being normal on later exam (Niswander et al 1966).

PREVENTION

Patients at risk for abruptio placenta (those who have suffered a previous abruption, those of high parity, those of age 40 or greater, and those who smoke cigarettes) should receive preconceptional counselling. In addition, any patient with an unexplained elevation in a second trimester maternal serum alpha-fetoprotein should be considered at risk for developing a placental abruption.

The most significant impact the physician can make in prevention of abruption occurs when he persuades his patient to stop smoking. Mothers who stop smoking have a 23% lower frequency of abruption, and only one-half as many fetal and neonatal deaths due to abruption as those who continue smoking. In fact, when the mother stops smoking by the time of her first prenatal visit the risk of perinatal mortality secondary to abruption is almost as low as if she has never smoked (Naeye 1980).

Though the relationship between chronic hypertension and abruptio placenta remains uncertain, if a mother with chronic hypertension has suffered a previous abruption, consideration should be given to the use of antihypertensive agents starting early in pregnancy to prevent the vasospasm and subsequent relaxation of arterioles in the decidua basalis. Chronic hypertensive patients with a history of abruption should be maintained on antihypertensive medication unless specifically contraindicated in pregnancy.

Folate administration *during* pregnancy has not been shown to prevent abruptio placenta. It may be that the folate has to be administered during early placentation to be effective. The patient at risk for abruptio placenta should be offered folate supplementation *preconceptually* and throughout pregnancy.

Perinatal survival in abruptio placenta primarily depends upon two factors: gestational age at the time of the abruption and having a live fetus upon admission to the hospital. Sonography should be used early in the pregnancy accurately to assess gestational age. Furthermore, the patient should be made aware of the symptoms of abruptio placenta so that she can report these promptly. Any patient who is at risk for abruptio placenta and has vaginal bleeding during the last trimester of pregnancy should be hospitalised until delivery.

Consideration should be given to decreasing stress during pregnancy, and if the patient has an especially high risk for abruptio placenta, bed rest is prescribed. Finally, if anaemia is present, it should be corrected with iron and folic acid.

REFERENCES

Barry A 1963 Accidental haemorrhage or abruptio placentae clinical features. Journal of Obstetrics and Gynaecology of the British Commonwealth 70: 708–710

Basu H K 1969 Fibrinolysis and abruptio placentae. Journal of Obstetrics and Gynaecology
   15: 690–697
Blair R G 1973 Abruption of the placenta. Journal of Obstetrics and Gynaecology of the
   British Commonwealth 80: 242–245
Brame R G, Harbert G M, McGaugher H S, et al 1968 Maternal risk in abruption.
   Obstetrics and Gynecology 31: 224–227
Carter B 1967 Premature separation of the normally implanted placenta. Obstetrics and
   Gynecology 29: 30–33
Coopland A T, Israels E D, Zipursky A, et al 1968 American Journal of Obstetrics and
   Gynecology 100: 311–318
Crosby W M, Costiloe J P 1971 Safety of lap belt restraint for pregnant victims of automobile
   collisions. New England Journal of Medicine 284: 632–636
Douglas R G, Buchman M I 1955 Premature separation of the normally implanted placenta.
   Journal of Obstetrics and Gynaecology of the British Commonwealth 62: 710–714
Edson J R, Blaese R M, White J G, et al 1968 Defibrination syndrome in an infant born after
   abruptio placentae. Journal of Pediatrics 72: 342–346
Golditch I M, Boyce N E 1970 Management of abruptio placentae. Journal of the American
   Medical Association 212: 288–293
Goujard J, Rumeau C, Schwartz D 1975 Smoking during pregnancy, stillbirth and abruptio
   placentae. Biomedicine 23: 20–22
Harrar J A 1917 Abruptio placentae. Bulletin Lying-in hospital 11: 151–153
Haynes D M 1966 Premature separation of the placenta. American Journal of Obstetrics and
   Gynecology 96: 660–669
Hibbard B M, Hibbard E D 1963 Aetiological factors in abruptio placentae. British Medical
   Journal 2: 1430–1436
Hurd W W, Miodovnik M, Hertzbert V, et al 1983 Selective management of abruptio
   placentae: a prospective study. Obstetrics and Gynecology 61: 467–473
Kerr M G 1965 The mechanical effects of the gravid uterus in late pregnancy. Journal of
   Obstetrics and Gynaecology of the British Commonwealth 72: 513–519
Knab D R 1978 Abruptio placentae. Obstetrics and Gynecology 52: 625–629
Lunan C B 1973 The management of abruptio placentae. Journal of Obstetrics and
   Gynaecology 97: 681–700
Mengert W F 1953 Observations on the pathogenesis of premature separation of the normally
   implanted placenta. American Journal of Obstetrics and Gynecology 66: 1104–1110
Naeye R L 1980 Abruptio placentae and placenta previa: Frequency, perinatal mortality, and
   cigarette smoking. Obstetrics and Gynecology 55: 701–704
Naeye R L, Harkness W L, Utts J 1977 Abruptio placentae and perinatal death: A
   prospective study. American Journal of Obstetrics and Gynecology 128: 740–746
Nilsen P A 1958 Premature separation of the normally implanted placenta. Acta Obstetrica et
   Gynecologica Scandinavica 37: 195–260
Niswander K R, Friedman E A, Hoover D B, et al 1966 Fetal morbidity following potentially
   anoxigenic obstetric conditions. American Journal of Obstetrics and Gynecology 95:
   838–845
Notelovitz M 1974 Silent abruption of the posteriorly inserted placenta. South African
   Medical Journal 48: 93–95
O'Driscoll K, McCarthy J R 1966 Abruptio placentae and central venous pressures. Journal
   of Obstetrics and Gynaecology of the British Commonwealth 73: 932–929
Page E W, Fulton L D, Glendening M B 1951 The cause of the blood coagulation defect
   following abruptio placentae. American Journal of Obstetrics and Gynecology 61:
   1116–1122
Page E W, King E B, Merril J A 1954 Abruptio placentae. Obstetrics and Gynecology 3:
   385–393
Paintin D B 1962 The epidemiology of ante-partum haemorrhage. Journal of Obstetrics and
   Gynaecology 69: 614–624
Paterson M 1979 The aetiology and outcome of abruptio placentae. Acta Obstetrica
   Gynecologica Scandinavica 58: 31–35
Porter J 1960 conservative treatment of abruptio placenta. Obstetrics and Gynecology 15:
   690–697
Pritchard J A 1968 Treatment of the defibrination syndromes of pregnancy. Modern
   Treatment 5: 401–418

Pritchard J A 1970 Genesis of severe placental abruption. American Journal of Obstetrics and Gynecology 108: 22–27

Pritchard J A, Brekken A L 1967 Clinical and laboratory studies on severe abruptio placentae. American Journal of Obstetrics and Gynecology 97: 681–700

Schneider C L 1954 Obstetric shuck. Some interdependent problems of coagulation. Obstetrics and Gynecology 4: 273–279

Sher G 1977 Pathogenesis and management of uterine inertia complicating abruptio placentae with consumption coagulopathy. American Journal of Obstetrics and Gynecology 129: 164–170

Smith K, Fields H 1958 The supine hypotensive syndrome — a factor in the etiology of abruptio placentae. Obstetrics and Gynecology 12: 369–372

Thomsen S G, Isager-Sally L, Lange A P, et al 1983 Smoking habits and maternal serum alpha-fetoprotein levels during the second trimester of pregnancy. British Journal of Obstetrics and Gynaecology 90: 716–717

Post-term pregnancy

The editor wanted a discussion of postmaturity, but we settled on post-term pregnancy. In clinical jargon the two expressions are used more or less synonymously, one by paediatricians and the other by obstetricians. This makes sense as long as a child born post-term is defined as postmature, but difficulties start when we look for a postmaturity syndrome. Post-term is easier to define, but definitions can be equivocal, as will be shown below. Ironically, the American compilation of obstetric-gynaecological terms (Hughes 1972) defines prolonged pregnancy as one which goes beyond 294 days, but a post-term infant as one born after day 287.

Post-term pregnancy is an everyday problem for the obstetrician, who in each case must decide on a course of action. Such decisions vary widely. Induction policy often follows local tradition, based on evidence which may no longer be valid. A questionnaire survey of European countries in 1980 revealed a large variation in induction frequency between those few countries and regions which had information on local practice (Bergsjø et al 1983). Chalmers & Richards (1977) have commented upon the difference between England and Wales, and Norway, the induction frequencies in 1974 being 38.9% and 14.2% respectively.

It seems fitting to start the discussion with a historical outline.

THE CHANGING CONCEPT OF POSTMATURITY

The clinical aspect

It began as an obstetrical problem. Discussing postmaturity, Ballantyne (1902) set prolonged pregnancy and a larger-than-normal fetus as prerequisites for the diagnosis. Returning to the subject 20 years later, he emphasised that a high degree of ossification was also a part of the syndrome, but the authors (Ballantyne & Browne 1922) acknowledged that it was difficult to describe the condition accurately. Bøe (1950) presented the 1930–41 material from the National Hospital in Oslo and restricted his cases to children with birth weight over 4500 g and length over 54 cm, who were born later than day 290. Of these

9% died, and the maternal mortality was 1.1%, primiparae running the far greatest risk.

In those days, when the Caesarean operation was the ultimate resort, the indications were far stricter than today. Ballantyne & Browne (1922) advocated induction of labour before the fetus became too big and immoldable, while Bøe (1950) realised that a fair number of children's lives could have been saved by Caesarean section before, rather than after, rupture of the membranes.

Clifford (1954) described the postmaturity syndrome, changing the emphasis from the disproportionately big to the undernourished fetus, suffering because of placental ageing and dysfunction. He saw three stages of the syndrome, the peak prevalence shifting towards longer pregnancy with each succeeding stage. The theory of placental ageing was hard to verify, and Clifford admitted that attempts to demonstrate degenerative changes by histology had been disappointing. Be that as it may, malnutrition may clearly cause fetal growth retardation and intrauterine death.

This, however, is a chronic condition not restricted to the post-term period. Kloosterman (1979), who analysed almost 30 000 single births in Amsterdam, widened the definition of so-called clinical postmaturity to include 'every fetus that dies before or during labour or shows signs of severe fetal distress during a normal labour; whereas its development and degree of maturity would have guaranteed survival as a healthy individual if it had been brought into the outer world at a slightly earlier date'. Counting all cases of stillbirth by unknown causes past 28 weeks of pregnancy in the years 1958 to 1976, he found an incidence of 6.9 per 1000 pregnancies, 72% of them occurring before 40 weeks. The gestational age-specific rates rose slightly past term but were still as low as 6.3 and 8.2 per 1000 for nulliparae and multiparae, respectively, for births beyond 290 days.

In other words, the concept of postmaturity started with the big post-term baby and ended with the starving, small-for-dates fetus, which need not be post-term at all. For clinical purposes Kloosterman's definition makes sense, but the label does not.

The role of the placenta

It stands to reason that the placenta has a limited lifespan, the senescent phase of which will be a threat to the fetus, through diminishing nutritional supply. However, serious attempts to pinpoint features characteristic of ageing have failed, as Clifford (vide supra) had to admit. Neither Clayton (1941) nor Naeye (1978) were able to distinguish special changes as being particularly prevalent in the post-term period. Fox (1983) discussed ageing of the placenta in a previous volume of the present series. He explained the slowing of placental growth in the later stages of pregnancy as a process of maturation, following which supply meets demand without the need for further expansion, but there is still considerable reserve capacity.

It remains to be seen whether the postmaturity syndrome, as broadly applied to most of the nutrition-deprived fetuses, has a common denominator in a placental syndrome yet to be described.

Quite recently, umbilical cord blood flow measurements by pulsed Doppler ultrasound technique have been of help in picking out fetuses with poor placental circulation (W. Giles, lecture communication in Bergen, 1984). This may become a useful discriminator in addition to real-time-scanning and biochemical tests. If characteristic pathological changes can be found, placental biopsy may become another diagnostic tool.

POST-TERM PREGNANCY

Term dating

The mother expects to give birth on the promised day and grows increasingly anxious with further passage of time. Term is defined as day 280, counting from the start of bleeding of the last menstrual period. Pregnancies going beyond 2 weeks from that day are labelled post-term. Biologically these limits are fraught with pitfalls, as the exact times of ovulation and fertilisation are seldom if ever known (excepting *in vitro* fertilisation). A meticulous study of menstruation to ovulation intervals in pregnancies with reliable information reduced the rate of 'true postmature births' according to menstrual dating from 10.7% to 4.7% when based on ovulation (Boyce et al 1976).

The percentage of women with unreliable menstrual dates will vary with, among other things, contraceptive pill use. Kloosterman (1979) found that the percentage of mothers with uncertain dates in Amsterdam rose from about 5 in 1952–6 to about 13 in 1974–6, in all likelihood due to the advent of oral contraceptives, which in 1976 were used by 46% of the fertile female population in the Netherlands. Other reported figures for uncertain dates vary from 12 to 18% (McKiddie 1949, Schildbach 1953, Magram & Cavanagh 1960, Timonen et al 1965, Bergsjø et al 1982). The Swedish birth registry, which asks specifically for reliability of term assessment in the notification forms, reported 9.8% with uncertain dates among 1981 singleton births. How these influenced the post-term fraction is described below. Suffice it here to say that the average gestational age for singleton births with certain dates was 281.0 and for those with uncertain dates 284.6 days.

Post-term — definition and incidence

The most recent international definition of post-term comes from the International Federation of Obstetrics and Gynaecology (FIGO 1982), which, quoting WHO recommendations from 1967 and 1976, says it should be pregnancies lasting 'forty-two completed weeks or more (294 days or more)'. This contradicts another recent FIGO statement, defining post-term as 'pregnancy that is calculated to have proceeded beyond the end of the 42nd week (i.e. more than 294 days from onset of the last menstrual period)' (FIGO 1980). Whether this difference of 1 day is intentional or not, it shows that definitions can be tricky. The one day has little importance in the clinical situation but may count in statistical comparison. In addition, other variables such as induction policy, will weigh when differences in reported figures are encountered. A literature review, covering periods from the early 1920s to 1982 and including national, regional and hospital data from many countries, revealed that incidence rates for post-term pregnancy varied from 4.4% to 14.9% (material available on request). The fraction of pregnancies passing 43 completed weeks ranged from 2.1% to 7.3% in eight studies. While hospital materials are notoriously unreliable as epidemiological evidence, a few instances of population-based statistics will be mentioned, as they are better indicators.

In a study from the Hawaiian island Kauai almost every pregnancy was recorded from the onset, and there was little interference with the biological process. In this (epidemiological) paradise 14% of 3000 pregnancies went beyond 42 weeks and 6% beyond 43 weeks (Bierman et al 1965). All of the Nordic countries except Finland have national data on gestational age and birthweight. Table 8.1 shows the situation in 1979 (NOMESKO 1982), with between 8.1% (Denmark) and 18.6% (Iceland) going beyond term. Note, however, that Denmark lacked information about menstrual dates in 26.2% while Iceland had total coverage. As Sweden had the additional information about certainty of dates, a correction for this factor can be made. Using 1981 data for singleton births, the total post-term rate was 13.7%, but as much as 33.5% of those with uncertain dates passed the post term limit. Excluding those, the corrected post term rate was 11.6%, as seen in Table 8.2.

Consequently, the fraction of pregnancies proceeding beyond 42 completed weeks seems to be slightly over 10% when strict criteria for menstrual dating are used, given that the induction activity before this time limit is moderate. When all pregnancies are counted, the post-term fraction will be in the order of 15%.

Table 8.1 Frequency of pregnancies going beyond 42 weeks in four Nordic countries in 1979. National data including birthweights of 1000 g or more. Gestational age based on menstrual dates (NOMESKO 1982)

Country	Total no. of births	No. with gest. age known	<42 weeks ≤293 days	42–43 294–307	≥44 ≥308
Denmark	59347	43773	91.9	8.1	—
Iceland	4462	4462	81.4	18.0	0.6
Norway	51591	49390	85.0	12.8	2.2
Sweden	95696	94261	85.3	14.4	0.3

Table 8.2 Distribution of gestational age based on all singleton births in Sweden 1981 by reliability of term assessment

Term assessment		Total	Gestational age at birth, based on last menstrual period							
			<36 ≤251	36–37 252–265	38–39 266–279	40–41 280–293	42–43 294–307	44–45 308–321	≥46 >322+	Unknown
Certain	No.	82889	2417	5205	26526	39070	8461	784	356	70
	%		2.9	6.3	32.0	47.1	10.2	0.9	0.4	0.1
Uncertain	No.	9058	628	813	1800	2764	2069	631	323	30
	%		6.9	9.0	19.9	30.5	22.8	7.0	3.6	0.3
Total	No.	91974	3045	6018	28326	41834	10530	1415	679	100
	%		3.3	6.5	30.8	45.5	11.4	1.5	0.7	0.1

Post-term perinatal mortality

Post-term would be no problem were it not for the fear of perinatal death. Early reports found this primarily to be a risk for the nulliparous (Clifford et al 1951, Lindell 1956). In contrast, Timonen et al (1965) found no parity differences in post-term perinatal mortality rates. Kloosterman (1979), studying time trends between 1955–6 and 1976, found the rates dropping from 19.2 to 2.8 per 1000 for primiparae, while remaining almost constant at about 10 per 1000 for multiparae. Another statistical oddity which remains to be explained, is a preponderance of boys in some materials on post-term death (Butler & Bonham 1963, Bjerkedal & Bakketeig 1972, Kloosterman 1956).

Table 8.3 is a compilation of perinatal term and post-term mortality data from the four Nordic countries which have national coverage, for 1979, 1980 and 1981, derived from NOMESKO (1982) and unpublished data from the same source. It is seen that the rates for weeks 42 and 43 are almost as low as for weeks 40 and 41, and considerably below those for weeks 37 through 39. For pregnancies going beyond 43 weeks, that is, lasting 308 days or more, the rates for the four countries combined, although rising, are still slightly lower than in weeks 37–39. Recalling that those with uncertain dates make up a relatively large proportion of post-term pregnancies, it is tempting to hypothesise that these may also take a considerable share of the perinatal deaths in that period. Wenner & Young (1974) showed that women with non-specific menstrual

Table 8.3 Term and post-term gestational age-specific perinatal mortality in the four Nordic countries 1979–81, excluding birthweight of less than 1000 grams (NOMESKO 1982 and unpublished data from the same source)

Country		Perinatal mortality numbers and rates			
		37–39 weeks 259–279 days	40–41 weeks 280–293 days	42–43 weeks 294–307 days	≥44 weeks ≥308 days
Denmark	1979	95 (8.6)	72 (2.7)	10 (2.8)	0 (0)
	1980	81 (6.5)	62 (2.3)	8 (2.3)	0 (0)
	1981	95 (8.0)	53 (1.9)	15 (3.6)	1 (28.6)
Iceland	1979	9 (11.4)	6 (2.2)	3 (3.7)	0 (0)
	1980	9 (9.8)	6 (2.1)	1 (1.5)	0 (0)
	1981	7 (7.8)	6 (2.3)	3 (4.5)	1 (7.1)
Norway	1979	122 (8.2)	96 (3.9)	21 (3.3)	6 (5.5)
	1980	106 (7.0)	74 (3.1)	27 (4.3)	7 (8.1)
	1981	91 (6.2)	59 (2.5)	24 (3.8)	9 (9.2)
Sweden	1979	147 (5.0)	113 (2.4)	36 (2.7)	2 (8.1)
	1980	162 (4.8)	107 (2.5)	39 (3.4)	11 (4.8)
	1981	140 (4.2)	88 (2.1)	25 (2.3)	6 (2.9)
Total	1979	373 (6.7)	287 (2.8)	70 (2.9)	8 (5.7)
	1980	358 (5.8)	249 (2.6)	75 (3.4)	18 (5.6)
	1981	333 (5.4)	206 (2.1)	67 (3.1)	17 (5.4)

dating had poor reproductive outcome in general. This question could be resolved through a detailed case analysis.

What are the causes of post-term perinatal death? Few large-scale investigations have been done. In a US collaborative study, Naeye (1978) found that the excess mortality post-term compared to term was due to severe congenital anomalies in 26%, amniotic fluid infections in 19%, abruptio placentae in 10%, Rh erythroblastosis in 8%, large placental infarcts in 8%, growth-retarded placentas in 8%, and the rest a variety of other disorders. These results were largely substantiated by another US multicentre study (Lucas et al 1965), in which various anoxic conditions, congenital anomalies and neonatal infections were the main causes. Zwerdling (1967) found that excess post-term mortality was not related to birthweight, and that significantly increased mortality rates persisted into the second year of life for children born after 43 completed weeks.

ALTERNATIVES TO MENSTRUAL DATING

Because of the errors inherent in menstrual dating, auxiliary or alternative methods are employed, to ensure optimal assessment of true gestational age. The time of the first quickening is unreliable, but HCG assays can be helpful if employed early. Needless to say, the mother may give additional information which must not be ignored.

Ultrasound dating is very much in vogue, and in some centres adjustment of term based on fetal body measurements in the presumed 16th–18th week is done routinely. When the biparietal diameter was used on 1000 pregnancies in Malmø, in 1976–8, the readjusted dates resulted in only 1.5% spontaneous births after the end of the 42nd week, as compared to 11.6% in the same group when menstrual dates were used for prediction. However, 152 cases were excluded from the comparison, 148 of them because of induction (Grennert et al 1978). A similar study from King's College Hospital in London gave corresponding figures of 6.3% and 11%, respectively (Warsof et al 1983). The latter authors also showed that the real clinical gain was in the group with unsatisfactory menstrual history, that the biparietal diameter is a better predictor than the crown-rump length and that measurements after the 24th week have no predictive value.

Such figures, showing that births following spontaneous labour cluster nicely around the ultrasonically adjusted term, are used to warrant ultrasound screening of all pregnant women. However, expert results may deceive because they derive from experts. With widespread use the likelihood of errors increases and should not be taken lightly. Furthermore, with too much reliance on ultrasound, other important criteria for term assessment may be neglected. Let us therefore discuss the clinical implications in perspective.

CLINICAL IMPLICATIONS

To pick up the thread from the introduction, those who go beyond 42 weeks of pregnancy are customarily examined with a view to specific action, the issue being whether to induce labour or not. This is a noble intention, but nowhere do indication rates differ more widely than for this problem.

Some require a high Bishop score as condition for induction. This is a gateway to success, as spontaneous labour is just around the corner anyway. However, it is the mother who benefits. It is hard to envisage the cervix and the fetus always maturing in unison. The ripeness argument can therefore, with good reason (see for example Harris et al 1983) be turned upside down. Social considerations often weigh heavier than medical ones, and elective post-term induction is intervention for convenience.

If a definite gain, whether in medical or more general terms, can be demonstrated in favour of post-term induction, then the practice is probably justified. So far, the arguments have not been too convincing. Numerous articles comparing different modes of induction with oxytocin, prostaglandin or artificial rupture of membranes, enthusiastically attest to the safety of such procedures. Most of these studies compare relatively small and carefully selected groups. One point which is often neglected is that many induction attempts remain just that. In a study of post-term oxytocin induction from a Norwegian hospital in 1974–7 only 70% of first induction attempts were successful. The rest of the mothers experienced up to three more attempts, some resulting in delivery while others had spontaneous labour and birth between courses (Bergsjø et al 1982). The intensity and duration of oxytocin medication are important for the success rate, other things being equal (Bergsjø & Jenssen 1969). Going to extremes, 100% success can be achieved by prolonging an oxytocin course indefinitely and resorting to Caesarean section when necessary. With a debatable indication for elective delivery this is clearly too aggressive. With cautious use of oxytocin one important question is whether the rates of operative delivery in post-term cases will be altered. Table 8.4 shows that this appeared to be the case in Akershus Central hospital in Norway. A similar conclusion was reached by Gibb et al (1982), who compared labour and outcome in two post-term groups randomly assigned to two consultant units with different induction policy. The Caesarean section rates in the group of 'certain postmature' patients were 9.8% among the non-induced and 26.7% among the induced cases. Chalmers et al (1976) studying two teams with different approaches to obstetric care in Cardiff, recorded a significantly higher incidence of Caesarean section in labour in patients managed by the more liberal induction practice. Smith et al (1984) also found that elective term and post-term inductions resulted in more Caesarean sections because of failure to progress than birth of spontaneous onset.

None of the quoted studies satisfy strict criteria for randomisation. In fact, few prospective, controlled studies have been published. One, from Glasgow, compared induction in weeks 39 and 40 to induction at 41 weeks, in those who

Table 8.4 Operative delivery during induced labour past 40 completed weeks of pregnancy, compared with a group in spontaneous labour, matched for gestational age (from Bergsjø et al 1982) (in percentages)

Parity	Group	Total number	No intervention	Forceps	Vacuum extraction	Caesarean section	Two or more interventions	Not stated
0	Induction	302	69.9	2.6	16.9	7.6	0.3	2.6
	Control	302	79.8	2.6	13.2	2.0	0.3	2.0
1+	Induction	419	89.7	0.7	5.5	2.9	0.5	0.1
	Control	419	94.5	0.2	1.7	1.2	0.5	1.9

did not go into spontaneous labour (Cole et al 1975). This 'term versus almost post-term' induction revealed no significant differences in operative delivery rates among the 228 pregnancies studied. A similar protocol for randomisation of non-risk cases was employed by Breart et al (1982) in Paris, who compared induction at 40 weeks to induction at 42 weeks. There were significantly more forceps deliveries among those in the early induction group and more with low Apgar scores in the newborns induced at 42 weeks. A third study with almost the same design was performed in Belfast (Martin et al 1978). There were 92 in each group completing the study. Those in the planned delivery group received more pethidine while the control group had more meconium-stained amniotic fluid. These three well-designed studies weighed the alternatives of whether to start artificial labour at term or 1 to 2 weeks later, both of which I consider too aggressive. I am not insensitive to the idea that modern obstetrics may have contributed to the low term and post-term perinatal mortality rates, but consider large-scale term induction a shot far above the target. O'Driscoll & Meagher (1980), outlining the active management of labour at the National Maternity Hospital in Dublin, go as far as to say that as it is not practical to prohibit all induction, it 'should be accepted as a necessary burden limited to a small number of cases in which conditions are favourable'.

More randomised studies on post-term policy are clearly needed, but the emphasis should be on induction versus continued clinical surveillance in order to detect those in need of acute delivery.

CONCLUSION

Going past term is not as dangerous as it was once thought. Perinatal mortality is at its lowest from week 40 up to 44 completed weeks. Placental ageing of abrupt post-term onset has not been demonstrated as a common phenomenon. The so-called postmaturity syndrome of the newborn is an expression of chronic malnutrition, a process which is not confined to the post-term period. It has never been convincingly shown that elective induction of labour at or past term is of benefit, except perhaps socially to the mother. On the other hand, inductions may result in more operative deliveries than would otherwise be necessary.

By introducing routine intervention we tend to dismiss our clinical watchfulness. The real task is to try to discover those few fetuses which suffer from a poor supply line and to save them before they are permanently damaged or dead, a task not confined to the post-term period only. This is truly difficult, but application of a set of simple rules is essential, otherwise all sophisticated measures will fail.

1.   Detailed information on menstrual rhythm and the last menstrual period, use of contraceptive pills, abortion or lactation immediately preceding the pregnancy, and date of first positive HCG-assay should be

obtained as early as possible. This will be the basis for deciding whether term is 'certain' or 'uncertain'.
2. Previous birth experience. Post-term tends to repeat itself as a normal phenomenon.
3. Assessment of uterine size as early as possible. This is unreliable, so do not be too confident in your own judgement. However, there may be twins.
4. Symphysis to fundus distance all through pregnancy. This was found to be a better discriminator of fetal growth retardation than both the biparietal diameter and serum oestriol, by an Uppsala group (Cnattingius et al 1983).
5. Ultrasound examination for term prediction in week 16–18 of those with uncertain dates, and in cases where the uterus appears to be too small or big.
6. Post-term examinations should be supplied with electronic fetal non-stress tests at intervals of one week or less. Amnioscopy may be useful. Decreasing girdle circumference is a warning sign.

Of course, any clinical suspicion of pathology must be explored further with clinical biochemical, ultrasonic or other tests as indicated. Shime et al (1984) found a 'biophysical profile', a scoring system of nonstress test results, amniotic fluid pocket depth, fetal movements and fetal breathing helpful in finding the dysmature post term fetuses in need of elective delivery.

It may seem naive to produce this list of trivia. However, 'carefully obtained historical and physical examination remains a cornerstone of appropriate obstetric care' (Hertz et al 1978). Our most common sin is that we do not pay attention to clinical detail, and I believe that more is to be gained here than in routine application of expensive machines and biochemical assays.

Acknowledgement

I wish to thank director Anders Ericson, Medical Birth Registry of Sweden, The National Board of Health and Welfare, for providing the Swedish figures for 1981 used in Table 8.2.

REFERENCES

Ballantyne J W 1902 The problem of the postmature infant. The Journal of Obstetrics and Gynaecology of the British Empire 2: 521–554
Ballantyne J W, Browne F J 1922 The problems of fetal post-maturity and prolongation of pregnancy. Journal of Obstetrics and Gynaecology of the British Empire 29: 177–238
Bergsjø P, Jenssen H 1969 Nasal and buccal oxytocin for the induction of labour: a clinical trial. Journal of Obstetrics and Gynaecology of the British Commonwealth 76: 131–136
Bergsjø P, Bakketeig L S, Nome Eikhom S 1982 Case-control analysis of post-term induction of labor. Acta Obstetricia et Gynecologica Scandinavica 61: 317–324
Bergsjø P, Schmidt E, Pusch D 1983 Differences in the reported frequencies of some obstetrical interventions in Europe. British Journal of Obstetrics and Gynaecology 90: 628–632

Bierman J M, Siegel E, French F E, Simonian K 1965 Analysis of the outcome of all
    pregnancies in a community. American Journal of Obstetrics and Gynecology 91: 37–45
Bjerkedal T, Bakketeig L 1972 Medical Registration of Births in Norway, 1967–68. Some
    Descriptive and Analytical Aspects, p. 144. University of Bergen, Institute of Hygiene and
    Social Medicine, Medical Birth Registry of Norway, Bergen, Norway
Bøe F 1950 Hypermature pregnancy. Acta Obstetricia et Gynecologica Scandinavica 30:
    (Suppl 1): 31
Boyce A, Mayaux M J, Schwartz D 1976 Classical and 'true' gestational postmaturity.
    American Journal of Obstetrics and Gynecology 125: 911–914
Breart G, Goujard J, Maillard F, Chavigny C, Rumeau-Rouquette C, Sureau C 1982
    Comparison de deux attitudes obstetricales vis-a-vis du declenchement artificiel du travail a
    terme. Journal de Gynecologie, Obstetrique et Biologie de la Reproduction 11: 107–112
Butler N R, Bonham D G 1963 Perinatal Mortality. The first report of the 1958 British
    Perinatal Mortality Survey under the auspices of The National Birthday Trust Fund,
    p. 304. E & S Livingstone, Edinburgh
Chalmers I, Lawson J G, Turnbull A C 1976 Evaluation of different approaches to obstetric
    care Part I. British Journal of Obstetrics and Gynaecology 83: 921–929
Chalmers I, Richards M 1977 Intervention and Causal Inference in Obstetric Practice. In:
    Chard T, Richards M (eds) Benefits and Hazards of the New Obstetrics, Ch 3, pp 34–61.
    Spastics International Medical Publications, London
Clayton S G 1941 Foetal Mortality in Post-maturity. Journal of Obstetrics and Gynaecology
    of the British Empire 48: 450–460
Clifford S H 1954 Postmaturity — with placental dysfunction. Clinical syndrome and
    pathologic findings. Journal of Pediatrics 44: 1–13
Clifford S H, Reid D E, Worcester J 1951 Postmaturity. American Journal of Diseases of
    Children 82: 232–235
Cnattingius S, Axelsson O, Lindmark G 1983 Diagnosis of Intra-uterine Growth Retardation
    in Late Pregnancy. Acta Obstetricia et Gynecologica Scandinavica Suppl 116, Abstract no.
    17, p. 17
Cole R A, Howie P W, Macnaughton M C 1975 Elective Induction of Labour. A
    Randomised Prospective Trial. Lancet i, 767
FIGO 1980 International Classification of Diseases: Update. International Journal of
    Gynaecology and Obstetrics 17: 634–640
FIGO 1982 Report of the Committee following a workshop on Monitoring and Reporting
    Perinatal Mortality and Morbidity. Figo Standing Committee on Perinatal Mortality and
    Morbidity, International Federation of Gynecology and Obstetrics, p. 78. The Chameleon
    Press, London
Fox H 1983 Placental pathology. In: Studd J (ed) Progress in Obstetrics and Gynaecology,
    Vol. 3, pp 47–56. Churchill Livingstone, Edinburgh
Gibb D M F, Cardozo L D, Studd J W W, Cooper D J 1982 Prolonged pregnancy: is
    induction of labour indicated? A prospective study. British Journal of Obstetrics and
    Gynaecology 89: 292–295
Grennert L, Persson P-H, Gennser G 1978 Benefits of ultrasonic screening of a pregnant
    population. Acta Obstetricia et Gynecologica Scandinavica (Suppl) 78: 5–14
Harris B A, Huddleston J F, Sutliff G, Perlis H W 1983 The Unfavorable Cervix in
    Prolonged Pregnancy. Obstetrics and Gynecology 62: 171–174
Hertz R H, Sokol R J, Knoke J D, Rosen M G, Chik L, Hirsch V J 1978 Clinical estimation
    of gestational age: Rules for avoiding preterm delivery. American Journal of Obstetrics and
    Gynecology 131: 395–402
Hughes E C 1972 Neonatology. In: Obstetric-Gynecologic Terminology, Section 8,
    pp 459–523. F. A. Davis Company, Philadelphia
Kloosterman G J 1956 Prolonged pregnancy. Gynaecologia 142: 373–388
Kloosterman G J 1979 Epidemiology of postmaturity. In: Keirse M J N C et al (eds) Human
    Parturition, pp 247–261. Martinus Nijhoff Publishers, The Hague
Lindell A 1956 Prolonged Pregnancy. Acta Obstetrica et Gynecologica Scandinavica 35:
    136–162
Lucas W E, Anctil A O, Callagan D A 1965 The problem of postterm pregnancy. American
    Journal of Obstetrics and Gynecology 91: 241–250
Magram H M, Cavanagh W V 1960 The problem of postmaturity. American Journal of
    Obstetrics and Gynecology 79: 216–223

Martin D H, Thompson W, Pinkerton J H M, Watson J D 1978 A randomized controlled trial of selective planned delivery. British Journal of Obstetrics and Gynaecology 85: 109–113

McKiddie J M 1949 Foetal Mortality in Postmaturity. Journal of Obstetrics and Gynaecology of the British Commonwealth 56: 386–392

Naeye R L 1978 Causes of perinatal mortality excess in prolonged gestations. American Journal of Epidemiology 108: 429–433

NOMESKO 1982 Fødsler i Norden. Medicinsk fødselsregistrering. Births in the Nordic Countries. Registration of the Outcome of Pregnancy 1979. Nordisk Medicinal-Statistisk Kommitte, nr. 17, p. 80. Offsetmundir hf, Reykjavik

O'Driscoll K, Meagher D 1980 Active Management of Labour, p. 192. W. B. Saunders, Philadelphia

Schildbach H R 1953 Neue Erkentnisse über die Dauer der Schwangerschaft beim Menschen mit Hilfe der Basaltemperaturmessung. Klinische Wochenschrift 31: 654–656

Shime J, Douglas J G, Andrews J, Bertrand M, Salgado J, Whillans G 1984 Prolonged pregnancy: Surveillance of the fetus and the neonate and the course of labor and delivery. American Journal of Obstetrics and Gynecology 148: 547–552

Smith L P, Nagourney B A, McLean F H, Usher R H 1984 Hazards and benefits of elective induction of labor. American Journal of Obstetrics and Gynecology 148: 579–585

Timonen S, Vara P, Lokki O, Hirvonen E 1965 Duration of pregnancy. Annales Chirurgiae et Gynaecologiae Fenniae 54 (Suppl 141): 33

Warsof S L, Pearce J M, Campbell S 1983 The Present Place of Routine Ultrasound Screening. In: Ultrasound in Obstetrics and Gynaecology: Recent Advances. Clinics in Obstetrics and Gynaecology, Vol. 10, No. 3, pp 445–458. W. B. Saunders, Philadelphia

Wenner W H, Young E B 1974 Nonspecific data of last menstrual period. American Journal of Obstetrics and Gynaecology 120: 1071–1079

Zwerdling M A 1967 Factors pertaining to prolonged pregnancy and its outcome. Pediatrics 40: 202–212

Note

Part of this work was done when the author was Visiting Scientist at the Biometry Branch, Epidemiology and Biometry Research Program, National Institute of Child Health and Human Development, National Institutes of Health, Bethesda, Maryland, USA.

The psychological response to stillbirth and neonatal death

In 1967 I could find no textbook account or journal article on the grief reactions of women who had delivered stillborn babies or whose babies had died in the neonatal period. For this reason I studied, during 1968 and 1969, the reactions of 40 women to the loss of their babies in the perinatal period (Giles 1970). There is still (early 1983) no account of this subject in any obstetric textbook.

What are the bereaved mother's reactions? Those of her partner and children? Does she need help? Is the doctor's help needed, and adequate? What are the doctor's own reactions? What are the nurses' reactions? Should help be offered, and, if so, how should it be given? These and a consideration of the importance of mourning are some of the questions reviewed in this article.

THE MOTHER'S REACTION TO PERINATAL DEATH

In 1970 the first descriptions by doctors of a mother's reaction to the death of her baby in the perinatal period were published. That year there were papers by Giles, by Kennell et al, and by Wolff et al.

Giles, of the University of Western Australia, analysed the reactions of 40 women who had had perinatal deaths. Nineteen women said they would have liked to have been told of their baby's death when it occurred and not, as had happened, at a time judged more suitable by medical or nursing staff. Eighteen women believed that they would have been helped to bear the loss if a doctor had explained why their babies had died. Five women were disappointed that no senior doctor had visited them especially when junior doctors had intimated that a senior doctor would call. Each of the 40 women showed the classical physical and psychological features of grief reaction: emptiness, restlessness, numbness, sadness, fatigue, self-blame and questioning. Some felt that they had failed their husbands, others doubted whether they would ever be able to have a baby. Giles suggested ways of helping these women and concluded that they could have been helped much more if their own doctors had appreciated their need for explanation, reassurance and support.

Kennell et al (1970), of the Case Western Reserve School of Medicine, Cleveland, Ohio, described the mourning responses of 20 parents to the death of a newborn infant. Their three main conclusions were: that a classical grief

134

reaction occurred irrespective of the baby's gestational age or age at death; that parents were not prepared for their own mourning responses; and that a disturbed husband–wife relationship was not uncommon. They suggested that parents should be advised of the mutual benefit of talking freely to each other about their feelings and should be told of the reactions they may experience.

The third study in 1970 was by Wolff et al of the University of Illinois. They studied the reactions of 50 women who had lost their babies at or shortly after birth. These 50 women were first seen in the immediate post-partum period and 40 women were followed up for 3 years. All the women showed a typical grief reaction. None developed significant psychiatric disturbances. The group was almost equally divided in intending to have more children, and time showed that each mother seemed to abide by her decision.

Two years later, Cullberg (1972) published his findings of the mental reactions of 56 women, as assessed 1 or 2 years after perinatal death. Nine said that they had had no reaction to the death, but the remaining 47 said they had suffered grief, emptiness, apathy and inadequacy for 2 to 3 months. He reported a feature not noted in previous studies — the presence, in 19 of the 56 women, of psychiatric symptoms: delusions, phobias, anxiety attacks, depressive thoughts or deep depression.

Zahourek & Jensen's (1973) study of 25 mothers who had lost babies in the last trimester of pregnancy drew attention to the reactions of shock and disbelief experienced by many of the mothers. In most cases there had been no warning during the pregnancy that the baby might die. Many mothers had been anaesthetised or heavily sedated at delivery, so had not seen or touched their baby. Lewis (1976) drew attention to the special problems of the mother of a stillborn baby. Because of society's 'abhorrence' of a stillbirth she was likely to feel avoided by her doctor, her husband and her friends. She tended to isolate herself, too, because of her own feelings of failure, and because of shame and guilt that her thoughts or actions might have caused the death.

Grief scores were used by Benfield et al (1978) to quantify the grief response of 50 couples to neonatal death. They found that parents' grief was not related significantly to their babies' birth weight, duration of life, extent of parent–infant contact, parental age or previous perinatal loss. However the attitudes of family, friends and hospital attendants often had an adverse effect on parental grieving.

Clarke & Williams (1979), of the University of Leicester, studied post-partum depression with the Beck inventory in two groups of over 300 women. They found that the difference in prevalence of depression between women who had had live births and women whose babies had died in the perinatal period was influenced by age. In women aged under 24 years post-partum depression at 6 months was just as common in those whose babies had lived as in those whose babies had died. A 2-year follow up was advised by Lockwood & Lewis (1980), of Tasmania; this was because, in their study of the grief reaction of 26 women (and 11 of their husbands), they had found that grief lasting longer than 18 months required special help.

Cooper (1980), a social worker, found that shock and anger were the predominant emotional reactions of 17 couples to stillbirth. She also observed how little sympathy and support doctors and nurses appeared to give these couples. Standish (1982), a psychiatric social worker, interviewed 32 women 6 months and 14 months after stillbirth or neonatal death. She found that those who had held their babies were glad that they had done so, particularly when it had dispelled frightening fantasies. Many parents, in retrospect, had wished that they had been told the truth of their babies' deaths at the time they had occurred in pregnancy. Nicol et al (1982a), of Perth, Western Australia, used a structured questionnaire to study the reactions of 110 women for 6–36 months after stillbirth or neonatal death. Twenty-one per cent showed a marked deterioration in health, as assessed by the general health inventory of Maddison & Walker (1967). The investigators found that mothers who had had a crisis during their pregnancy, who did not consider their husbands or family to be supportive, or who saw but did not hold their baby were more likely to experience a marked deterioration in health. Nicol et al (1982b) suggested that these women, who ought to be easily identifiable in the early puerperium, should be given additional support by hospital staff in the hope of preventing pathological grief reactions.

Wilson et al (1982), of the South Dakota School of Medicine, studied eight families who lost both newborn twins and eight families who lost one of twins. They found that the presence of a live baby did not lessen the grieving process. However, friends and hospital staff tended to assume that the grief of parents would be lessened because of the surviving twin; for this reason they saw less need to support such families or to allow the parent an opportunity to mourn. (Incidentally, it is my impression that hospital staff treat people such as health professionals, who lose a baby, similarly; they mistakenly assume that such people can handle their loss unaided.)

THE FATHER'S REACTION TO PERINATAL DEATH

Self-blame, anger and a feeling of helplessness in knowing how to support his wife are common reactions for the dead baby's father (Seitz & Warrick 1974). The father's grief reaction to perinatal death seems to be less intense and prolonged than that of his wife (Wilson et al 1982). Assuming that the doctor's help is needed, each parent should be prepared for the probable mourning reactions, told that there are likely to be differences between their reactions and that this can place stress on the husband–wife relationship (Kennell et al 1970). Ways of improving communication and supportiveness between the parents is an area which needs further study.

THE OTHER CHILDREN'S REACTION TO PERINATAL DEATH

Perinatal death will affect the surviving children, at least to some degree.

If the bereaved parents are depressed, preoccupied and irritable, the children may feel abandoned and unloved (Cain et al 1964). If the children cannot talk freely they may conceal their emotions and later suffer guilt reactions. If explanations such as 'taken by God', 'asleep' are used by the parents to account for the baby's death, the other children may develop distorted ideas about illness, death and doctors (Hardgrove & Warrick 1974). The children need to be allowed to grieve, to have their questions answered, yet still to feel loved. How to help parents help their children is an area that warrants much more attention (Parkes 1977, Drotar & Irvin 1979).

Occasionally a surviving sibling may be chosen as a 'scapegoat', a displacement object for a mother's sense of guilt and self hatred; mothers' long continued harsh treatment of these children has eventually led to the children being taken into protective legal custody (Tooley 1975).

THE BEREAVED MOTHER'S NEEDS

The woman who has lost a baby in the perinatal period needs help. She is likely to be haunted by thoughts that she is to blame and that she may never have a live baby. As a result of the loss of her baby she may feel empty and physically exhausted. If there was a complication in late pregnancy she may have been referred to a major hospital and admitted under the care of an unfamiliar specialist. Naturally she cannot speak to him as freely as to her own doctor and this adds to her feelings of strangeness.

Doctors and the bereaved mothers

Doctors in my study (Giles 1970) treated the bereaved mother's physical symptoms and prescribed sedatives liberally but in half the cases they avoided discussing the baby's death with the mother. This may have been due, as Williams (1963) observed about doctors in a children's hospital, to the youth and inexperience of the doctors or to their inability to provide support when they themselves were feeling defeated or perhaps responsible for the death.

In our society, it has traditionally been the doctor or the priest to whom the bereaved looks for reassurance and explanation (Elkinton 1967, Knapp & Peppers 1979). However, the patients studied by Nicol et al (1982a) rated the obstetrician and the chaplain as less supportive than their own partners, the hospital's paediatricians or senior labour ward sisters.

Stillbirth can cause a marked deterioration in the doctor-patient relationship (Bourne 1968). Cullberg (1972) and Lewis (1972) both found that doctors tended to avoid contact with the bereaved mothers and to discharge them from hospital prematurely.

In cases where a doctor is blaming himself for the death he should remember that the parents are certainly more distressed than he is. Not uncommonly, aggression and hostility are part of the parents' bereavement reactions and are not directed against the doctor personally.

Perinatal death may affect the doctor in ways other than those described above. Savage (1978) observed that doctors also respond to perinatal death by shock (a physically sickening sense of unreality), by denial (re-checking the fetal heart, resuscitation continued far too long); by sadness, by anger and hostility (to others concerned with the patient's care); and by guilt and shame. Savage recalls that she felt helpless and useless at her first stillbirth.

A perinatal death may make even an obstetrician over-cautious in managing other antenatal patients. He may perform an excessive number of tests or resort to Caesarean section unnecessarily. On the other hand, if the fetus is dead or grossly abnormal, the doctor may go to such lengths to obtain a vaginal delivery that he puts the mother's life at risk.

The nurse and perinatal death

The first articles published on the psychological reactions to stillbirth and neonatal death were by nurses (Bruce 1962, McLenahan 1962).

McLenahan, Assistant Professor of Obstetric Nursing at the University of Pittsburg School of Nursing, discussed the nurse's and mother's reactions to perinatal death in the light of Freud's (1917) work on grief and Lindemann's (1944) work on the importance of mourning.

Bruce, Head Nurse at the Boston Lying-In Hospital, made two important points. Firstly, that the nurse must recognise and resolve her own feelings of failure, guilt, helplessness and anger, which result from the perinatal death, before she can help the bereaved parents. Secondly, that the mother wants from the nurse care and sympathy rather than scientific reasons for the baby's death. The nurse can show her sympathy and understanding by being a willing listener, by avoiding platitudes, by respecting the way each mother expresses her grief, by being willing to talk about the baby, and by demonstrating to the bereaved mother that she is being cared for.

Nurses should be taught how to deal with the mother who has an intra-uterine fetal death. They should be able to ask parents calmly and compassionately whether they would like to see and to hold their dead baby, and should be able to show them the baby.

Nurses should be prepared for the stress that perinatal death may cause in themselves and in their colleagues, and should themselves be able to be given care and support when needed.

GRIEF AND THE IMPORTANCE OF MOURNING

According to Freud (1917), grief is the self-limited normal reaction to the loss of a beloved person. He emphasised that it is not a pathological condition nor one that calls for medical treatment. Lindemann (1944) observed that grief is a specific psychological process which cushions the impact of the loss and enables the bereaved to readjust to an environment in which the deceased is missing, and later to form new relationships.

Freud and Lindemann's studies show that grief has psychological and physical features. Initially there is numbness, shock and disbelief. Later there comes a gradually increasing acute awareness of the loss with sadness, self-blame, hopelessness, guilt and anger, and preoccupation with the image of the deceased. These reactions are usually accompanied by physical symptoms such as insomnia, epigastric emptiness, weariness and loss of appetite (Lindemann 1944, Hinton 1967). Family and friends respond to the bereaved's grief by providing support. The funeral rites help by emphasising the reality of the loss (Engel 1964). Sooner or later, family and friends withdraw their sympathy and support (Gauthier & Marshall 1977) and in time the bereaved becomes increasingly able to establish new interests and relationships.

Maddison & Walker (1967) found that inadequate mourning and suppression of grief hinders psychological recovery, especially for those who have no social support. In such a case it would help the bereaved to externalise her suppressed sadness, anger or guilt by talking with a willing listener about her memories of her lost loved one.

The evidence that loss of a spouse affects both mental and physical health is very strong. Parkes (1975), in his review of the subject, reports that in the first year after bereavement there is an increased death rate (due to heart disease especially) and an increase in psychiatric admissions (because of reactive and neurotic depression).

Is grief after perinatal death comparable with grief after the death of an older person?

The only opinion which I could find on this question before my study in the late 1960s was that of Helene Deutsch (1945) who held that grief following stillbirth or early neonatal death was not the same as that following the death of a loved person but was rather the non-fulfillment of a wish fantasy. My own impression in 1970 was that there was no qualitative difference between the reactions following early and late neonatal deaths, and that the grief reactions in mothers with a perinatal death were similar to those described in recently bereaved widows (Clayton et al 1968). One can, however, appreciate Deutsch's viewpoint: that there is a marked difference in grieving for the elderly who have lived their lives and for babies who die in the perinatal period, for their potential can never be realised.

Peppers & Knapp (1980) used a grief score to measure the grief responses of mothers to miscarriages, stillbirth and neonatal death. The grief scores for each of these events, at the time of the loss, and later, were remarkably similar. From their results they concluded that affectional ties develop very early in pregnancy.

On the other hand, Furman (1978) came to a conclusion which I see as close to that of Helene Deutsch's. Furman argues that the fetus is not regarded by the mother as a separate person but as part of the mother's body for some time after birth. The mother's reaction to the loss of her baby, therefore, is not to the loss of a separate person but is more like that to the loss of a limb. Accordingly, the mother has to readjust to think of herself as an incomplete human being, deprived of fulfillment. She experiences emptiness, loss of self-esteem, and depression. People tend to shun her, as they tend to shun an amputee or so it seems to her.

Peppers & Knapp (1980) found that grief scores of women after miscarriage were comparable with those of women bereaved by stillbirth and neonatal death. This is surprising, at least to me. If the grief score used is a reliable index of grief then we should be devoting considerably more attention to the psychological needs of the woman who aborts or who chooses to be aborted.

SPECIAL PROBLEMS IN MOURNING FOR A STILLBORN CHILD

The parents' memories of their stillborn child will facilitate the process of mourning. The mother of a stillborn baby may not have seen her child and thus have no actual person to mourn. In hospital, a conspiracy of silence may have surrounded her. Then after her discharge from hospital, she finds that people tend to avoid her. She avoids people because of shame and guilt she associates with the stillbirth.

Lewis (1976), who drew attention to this special problem, points out that we can do a lot to help mothers and fathers in this position. They should be encouraged to see, hold and touch their dead baby (provided, of course, that they consider it fitting) so that they will have memories to help in the mourning process. Giving the baby a name, taking a photograph of the baby and holding a funeral can also help (Lewis & Page 1978).

What is the place of bereavement counselling?

Does bereavement counselling work? Parkes (1980) reviewed the evidence and concluded that professional help, and professionally supported voluntary help can reduce the risk of the psychiatric and psychosomatic disorders which can result from bereavement.

Counselling seemed to be of most benefit for those who considered that their families were unsupportive. This was shown in a controlled study by Raphael (1977) who attempted to lower post-bereavement morbidity in widows by supporting them in their grief and encouraging mourning for 3 months. She was able to show most reduction in morbidity (as assessed by a health questionnaire 13 months later) in a high risk group of women who considered that their social network was very unsupportive.

The only study of the effectiveness of support and counselling after perinatal bereavement is that of Forrest et al (1982) of Oxford. Fifty families were studied; they were allocated randomly either to the group which received support and counselling or to the control group who were left to their own devices. At 6 months and 14 months the members of each group were assessed by semistructured interviews and by two self-rating scales (the General Health Questionnaire and the Leeds scales). At 6 months, only 2 of 16 mothers of the supported group, but 10 of 19 mothers of the non-supported group, showed psychiatric disability. At 14 months there was no difference between the groups. Forrest et al (1982) found that it was the women who could not name a single person who had been supportive or the women who had very poor communication with her husband who had a higher incidence of psychiatric symptoms at 6 months.

CARE OF THE BEREAVED PARENTS

The doctor's contribution

Telling the parents about their child's death should not be postponed. It should be done by the doctor himself in a place where the parents will feel quite free to weep. This is not the time for detailed explanation but for sympathy and for privacy.

The initial shock may be so great that the parents may have difficulty in grasping anything else than the fact of the death. Later a simple explanation of why the child died may help to relieve guilt, and it may allay their fears about the future.

The doctor can help the couple to accept the reality of the death. He can help to create memories for them of their child by encouraging them to see, touch and hold the baby — a more rewarding task than treating their grief with sedatives.

The parents need time to talk; their repeated questions should be answered patiently and they should be reassured that nothing they did (or failed to do) was the cause of the death. Subjects that could be discussed at this time are suppression of lactation, accommodation in a single room, early discharge and the use of a hypnotic to ensure a night's sleep. Decisions can be made with the parents about a postmortem examination, about burial and death certification.

The parents should be told what reactions are likely and should be reassured that restlessness, anger, sadness, and exhaustion are natural and expected responses to shock and grief. Some may even fear that they may be going mad, and they need reassurance that this also is a response to grief. They should be warned that this time could be a time of stress between husband and wife, and that other children need special consideration (see above).

It is generally accepted that prescribing drugs for the parents is less helpful than spending time with them, for a compassionate listener can offer lasting support, explanation and reassurance.

The parents should be seen by the doctor at least two or three times while the mother is in hospital. They should feel free to contact the hospital doctor or their family doctor as often as they wish after discharge and should certainly return 4–6 weeks later for the usual postnatal visit when the postmortem findings should be available. This is the time to review the whole case and to discuss any plans for future pregnancy with the parents. Generally it is advisable to wait until grief is waning before embarking on another pregnancy; Forrest et al (1982) found that pregnancy within 6 months of perinatal bereavement was associated with a higher incidence of psychiatric symptoms in women who had no support for their grief.

The now well recognised 'replacement child syndrome' (Poznanski 1972) should be mentioned to the parents.

Of course, the patient's family doctor should be told of his patient's loss as soon as practicable. Naturally, many parents find it easier to ask questions of their family doctors and this is especially so if they feel that the hospital staff could have done more to prevent the death. The family doctor is also in a better position than hospital staff to assess marital stresses, to detect depression in the bereaved parents, and to help with the anxieties which may arise in the next pregnancy.

Fetal death in utero and gross fetal abnormalities

Ultrasonography has simplified the diagnosis in pregnancy of fetal death *in utero* and of fetal abnormalities incompatible with life. In general it is advisable to be completely honest with both parents about the findings, and to outline for them the methods of management of such complications. The mother with a dead fetus *in utero* should be reassured that it will do her no harm and that the delivery will not be complicated because of it. She should be prepared for any disturbing psychological reactions and should be warned of the possible attitudes of family and friends.

Organised care in hospital

Perinatal mortality bereavement clinics have been established in some hospitals in North America and England (Morris 1976, Cohen et al 1978, Kellner et al 1981). Besides providing organised support for parents they also provide education for the hospital staff and influence the practice of the hospital in general. It is important that the bereaved are not overwhelmed by numerous well-meaning advisers, and that each member of the team is flexible and knows what other members have told the parents (Hildebrand & Schreiner 1980).

If a staff member appears to be unaware that a baby has died the parents can feel very hurt. On the other hand, there are simple ways of helping the parents in hospital, e.g. by providing a bed in the patient's room for her husband and ensuring that the same doctor is available to talk with the parents. Knowing the answers to questions about funeral arrangements or registration of the death provides a good entrée for establishing rapport with the parents (Forrest et al 1981).

Booklets on parental reactions to perinatal death cannot replace the compassionate case of another person but they do provide information for the bereaved parents and they can be instructive for the general community. One excellent booklet is 'The Loss of your Baby', produced by the Health Education Council of Great Britain (Beard et al 1978) — it is simply and compassionately written, giving sensible answers to questions which the parents may not have been able to ask.

Education of junior medical staff

Young medical officers receive little organised training in this field. They should at least observe how a colleague treats bereaved parents. Discussion groups may make them more aware of their own and of their colleagues' reactions to perinatal deaths. By attending bereaved parents' self-help support groups (Wilson & Soule 1981) they might learn more of the bereaved parents' reactions and of any deficiencies of care in hospital.

CONCLUSION

The reactions of a woman whose baby is stillborn or dies in the neonatal period have been little mentioned in the obstetric literature. Perinatal death causes psychological and physical reactions in the mother and father, in the family and in the attendant medical and nursing staff. Before they can help bereaved couples, doctors and nurses must be aware of all these reactions, of the psychological needs of the bereaved and of the importance of mourning.

Further research is needed to identify those most in need of help and to evaluate the effectiveness of help. There is also a need to train young doctors in this field. A sympathetic doctor who is prepared to spend time with parents who have lost their baby can relieve feelings of inadequacy and guilt and can do much to help them face the future with hope and confidence.

REFERENCES

Beard R W et al 1978 Help for parents after stillbirth. British Medical Journal 1: 172–173

Benfield D G, Leib S A, Vollman J H 1978 Grief response of parents to neonatal death and parent participation in deciding care. Pediatrics 62: 171–177

Bourne S 1968 The psychological effects of stillbirths on women and their doctors. Journal of the Royal College of General Practitioners 16: 103–112

Bruce S J 1962 Reactions of nurses and mothers to stillbirths. Nursing Outlook 10: 88–91

Cain A C, Fast I, Erickson M E 1964 Children's disturbed reactions to the death of a sibling. American Journal of Orthopsychiatry 34: 741–752

Clarke M, Williams A J 1979 Depression in women after perinatal death. Lancet i: 916–917

Clayton P, Desmaris L, Winokur G 1968 A study of normal bereavement. American Journal of Psychiatry 125: 168–178

Cohen L, Zilkha S, Middleton J, O'Donnohue N 1978 Perinatal mortality: assisting parental affirmation. American Journal of Orthopsychiatry 48: 727–731

Cooper J D 1980 Parental reactions to stillbirths. British Journal of Social Work 10: 55–69

Cullberg J 1972 Mental reactions of women to perinatal death. In: Morris N (ed) Psychosomatic Medicine in Obstetrics and Gynaecology, 3rd International Congress, London, 1971, pp 326–329. Karger, Basel

Deutsch H 1945 The psychology of women: a psychoanalytic interpretation, Vol 2, Motherhood, p. 263. Grune & Stratton, New York

Drotar D, Irvin N 1979 Disturbed maternal bereavement following infant death. Child: Care, Health & Development 5: 239–247

Elkinton J R 1967 Life and death and the physician. Annals of Internal Medicine 67: 669

Engel G L 1964 Grief and grieving. American Journal of Nursing 64: 93–98

Forrest G C, Claridge R S, Baum J D 1981 Practical management of perinatal death. British Medical Journal 282: 31–32

Forrest G C, Standish E, Baum J D 1982 Support after perinatal death: a study of support and counselling after perinatal bereavement. British Medical Journal 285: 1475–1479

Freud S 1917 Mourning and Melancholia. Standard Edition, Hogarth Press, London 14: 243–258

Furman E P 1978 The death of a newborn: care of the parents. Birth and the Family Journal 5: 214–218

Gauthier J, Marshall W L 1977 Grief: a cognitive-behavioral analysis. Cognitive Therapy & Research 1: 39–44

Giles P F H 1970 Reactions of women to perinatal death. Australian and New Zealand Journal of Obstetrics & Gynaecology 10: 207–210

Hardgrove C, Warrick L H 1974 How shall we tell the children? American Journal of Nursing 74: 448–450

Hilderbrand W L, Schreiner R L 1980 Helping parents cope with perinatal death. American Family Physician 22: 121–125

Hinton J 1967 Dying, pp 167–182. Penguin Books, Middlesex

Kellner K R, Best E K, Chesborough S, Donnelly W, Green M 1981 Perinatal mortality counselling program for families who experience a stillbirth. Death Education 5: 29–35

Kennell J H, Slyter H, Klaus M H 1970 The mourning response of parents to the death of a newborn infant. New England Journal of Medicine 283: 344–349

Knapp R J, Peppers L G 1979 Doctor-patient relationships in fetal/infant death encounters. Journal of Medical Education 54: 775–780

Lewis E 1972 Reactions to stillbirth. In: Morris N (ed) Psychosomatic Medicine in Obstetrics & Gynaecology, 3rd International Congress, London, 1971, pp 323–325. Karger, Basel

Lewis E 1976 The management of stillbirth: coping with an unreality. Lancet ii: 619–620

Lewis E, Page A 1978 Failure to mourn a stillbirth: an overlooked catastrophe. British Journal of Medical Psychology 51: 237–241

Lindemann E 1944 Symptomatology and management of acute grief. American Journal of Psychiatry 101: 141–148

Lockwood S, Lewis I C 1980 Management of grieving after stillbirth. The Medical Journal of Australia 2: 308–311

Maddison D, Walker W L 1967 Factors affecting the outcome of conjugal bereavement. British Journal of Psychiatry 113: 1057–1067

McLenahan I G 1962 Helping the mother who has no baby to take home. American Journal of Nursing 62: 70–71

Morris D 1976 Parental reactions to perinatal death. Proceedings of the Royal Society of Medicine 69: 837–838

Nicol M T, Tompkins J R, Campbell N A 1982a Mothers' views of perinatal death: implications for care. Australian Paediatric Journal 18: 141

Nicol M T, Tompkins J R, Campbell N A 1982b Maternal bereavement: factors affecting mothers' responses to perinatal death. Australian Paediatric Journal 18: 142

Parkes C M 1975 The broken heart. In: Bereavement, Ch 2, pp 29–45. Penguin Books, Middlesex

Parkes C M 1977 Family reactions to child bereavement. Proceedings of the Royal Society of Medicine 70: 54–55

Parkes C M 1980 Bereavement counselling: does it work? British Medical Journal 281: 3–6

Peppers L G, Knapp R J 1980 Maternal reactions to involuntary fetal/infant death. Psychiatry 43: 155–159

Poznanski E O 1972 The 'replacement child': a saga of unresolved parental grief. Journal of Pediatrics 81: 1190–1193

Raphael B 1977 Preventive intervention with the recently bereaved. Archives of General Psychiatry 34: 1450–1454

Savage W 1978 Perinatal loss and the medical team. Midwife, Health Visitor and Community Nurse. Part 1, 14: 292–295, Part 2, 14: 348–351

Seitz P, Warrick L 1974 Perinatal death: the grieving mother. American Journal of Nursing 74: 2028–2033

Standish L 1982 The loss of a baby. Lancet i: 611–612

Tooley K 1975 The choice of a surviving sibling as 'scapegoat' in some cases of maternal bereavement — a case report. Journal of Child Psychology & Psychiatry 16: 331–339

Williams H 1963 On a teaching hospital's responsibility to counsel parents concerning their child's death. Medical Journal of Australia 2: 643–645

Wilson A L, Soule D J 1981 The role of a self-help group in working with parents of a stillborn baby. Death Education 5: 175–186

Wilson A L, Fenton L J, Stevens D C, Soule D J 1982 The death of a newborn twin: an analysis of parental bereavement. Pediatrics 70: 587–591

Wolff J R, Nielson P E, Schiller P 1970 The emotional reaction to a stillbirth. American Journal of Obstetrics & Gynaecology 108: 73–77

Zahourek R, Jensen J S 1973 Grieving and the loss of the newborn. American Journal of Nursing 73: 836–839

Pregnancy, childbirth and mental illness

Mental illness can adversely affect obstetric outcome and childbearing can cause or exacerbate mental illness. This review examines some of the more important points of contact between obstetrics and psychiatry and it emphasises the need for obstetricians to pay careful attention to the psychological welfare of their clients. The word 'client' is used advisedly instead of 'patient' because, in fact, most of the consumers of the obstetric services are relatively healthy individuals, but they are receiving 'treatment' from doctors and nurses in an 'illness' setting. This ambiguity of the doctor-patient relationship may partly explain the continuing concern that is felt about the *unnecessary* medicalisation of childbirth and about the indifference to the emotional aspects of childbearing that is characteristic of some aspects of the maternity services (Chard & Richards 1977, MacIntyre 1977, Cartwright 1979, Oakley 1980, Social Services Committee: Short Report 1980, Kumar 1982). Changes in the maternity services will not be brought about by planting a psychiatrist in every antenatal clinic, nor will they be achieved by exhortations to the staff to do better and to be more sympathetic (Social Services Committee: Short Report 1980). The answer lies in demonstrating that early recognition and appropriate responses to psychiatric problems, whether they are noted in pregnancy or in the puerperium, can bring about tangible benefits to the mother, to her baby and to her family. In addition to considering measures of prevention and treatment, it is also important to recognise that the circumstances surrounding pregnancy, delivery and the puerperium can have a profound and lasting significance for *every* mother. This generalisation reflects echoes of the growing chorus (predominantly middle-class and articulate) of a demand for a more personalised and psychologically oriented approach to childbearing (Oakley 1980, Boyd & Sellars 1982); the fact that there are no 'good varicose vein guides' (c.f. Kitzinger 1979) indicates by contrast the special importance that is assigned to obstetricians and to the service that they supply.

The Social Services Committee: Short Report (1980) underlined the contribution of social and psychological factors to disturbing regional variations in perinatal and maternal survival rates. Similarly, it is now accepted that the ways in which babies are nurtured in special care units can interact with maternal personal and social characteristics and so affect the attachment process and, consequently, the risk of child abuse (e.g. Lynch & Roberts 1977). This review contains many similar examples, drawn from a variety of obstetric settings and, therefore, it repeatedly underlines the need for awareness in obstetricians of problems that are traditionally seen as belonging to the domain of psychiatrists and social workers. The article is divided into two broad sections, the first of which examines some of the ways in which psychological and social factors can influence pregnancy and childbirth and the baby's health. The second section is concerned with the psychiatric disorders which follow childbirth.

The topic of psychopathology in pregnancy is a particularly fascinating one and the reader is referred elsewhere to reviews and discussions (Deutsch 1945, Chertok 1969, Pines 1972, Breen 1975, Rapoport et al 1977, Chodorow 1978, Raphael-Leff 1980, Brockington & Kumar 1982a). Hyperemesis may indicate a symbolic rejection of the fetus or it may reflect some sort of metabolic disorder; but together with other more esoteric conditions such as pica and pseudocyesis it pales into insignificance against the fact that about one in every six pregnancies in residents of England and Wales is terminated each year, mostly on social and psychological grounds. In numerical terms alone, this is one of the most important determinants of the outcome of conception.

PSYCHOLOGICAL AND SOCIAL FACTORS AND OBSTETRIC OUTCOME

Termination of pregnancy

Since the introduction of the Abortion Act 1967, it is no longer necessary for doctors to assert that to continue with a given pregnancy would almost certainly result in the mother becoming a 'physical or mental wreck' (BMJ 1938). Almost annual attempts are made to amend or reverse this Act and they are based upon religious, moral and ethical arguments. Questions about the viability of the fetus, distinctions between contraception and abortion, concerns about the timing of abortion, are now somewhat overshadowed by the ethical implications of developments in *in vitro* fertilisation, the maintenance and preservation of embryos and the use of surrogate mothers. Increasing emancipation of women from continuous childbearing between menarche and the menopause has occurred as one consequence of medical progress and it is a change with profound social and perhaps political implications. Questions about who has the right to decide whether or not a pregnancy shall go to term, although intrinsically the same, are nowadays posed in a very different social and medical context to that which pertained a generation ago.

The psychiatric evidence in relation to the abortion debate is fairly clear — quite apart from the attendant risks of criminal abortion for those women who are determined not to have a baby, there is evidence following refusal, of an increased risk of suicide (Whitlock & Edwards 1968, Visram 1972) of depression (Höök 1963, Pare & Raven 1970), and of more conduct problems in the children (Forssmann & Thuwe 1966, Dytrych et al 1975). Studies of refused abortion have, however, to be interpreted with caution (see Illseley & Hall 1976).

The incidence of psychiatric disorder following therapeutic abortion is substantially less than that seen after childbirth and the manifest pathology is less severe. For example, post-abortion psychosis is virtually unknown (Brewer 1977) and handicapping depressive reactions are also relatively uncommon (Osofsky & Osofsky 1972, Greer et al 1976). Feelings of guilt can persist for several months and, indeed, may remain dormant until they are uncovered by a subsequent pregnancy (Kumar & Robson 1978). Women who repeatedly seek terminations and those whose pregnancies are aborted because of suspected fetal abnormalities (Donnai et al 1981) may be at greater risk of becoming depressed. More work is needed to characterise those who are most 'at risk' from the psychiatric point of view in order that counselling can be more effectively directed to them.

Spontaneous abortion

There is a small and somewhat dated literature on the possible psychological antecedents of spontaneous abortion. It has been suggested that repeated miscarriage is connected with maternal immaturity and dependency, hostility towards the spouse and with deep-seated conflicts (Deutsch 1945, Mann 1959, Weil & Tupper 1960, Grimm 1962). As Grimm (1967) observes, such studies do not demonstrate a causal link and, furthermore, they do not exclude the possibility that it is the miscarriage which brings about the psychological disturbance. The relatively small samples, the possibility of retrospective bias, the lack of reliable methods of measurement and the absence of adequate controls are deficiencies which must be overcome in any future investigations of psychological mechanisms in habitual abortion.

Anxiety, life stress and pregnancy complications

Links have been made between anxiety and stress and pre-eclamptic toxaemia (Coppen 1958, Hetzel et al 1961), abnormalities of parturition and infant health (McDonald & Christiakos 1963, Gorsuch & Key 1974) and the onset of premature labour (Newton et al 1979). Others (e.g. McDonald 1968, Nuckolls et al 1972, Chalmers 1982) have failed to come up with positive findings. Kumar & Robson (1984) have recently illustrated an indirect route through which psychological factors might influence fetal development. Women who were depressed in early pregnancy were more likely to describe past and present conflicts about wanting to go through to term with their pregnancies, they were also significantly more likely to be still smoking cigarettes in the third trimester. This is just one small example of the ways in which drug use and abuse in pregnancy may be linked with physical and behavioural teratogenicity or developmental problems (see reviews by Coyle et al 1976, Goldberg & Di Mascio 1978, Proc Symp B A P 1981, Brockington & Kumar 1982b).

Psychiatric disorder and failure to attend ante-natal clinics

Failure to attend ante-natal clinics is linked with a sharp increase in perinatal mortality (Butler & Bonham 1963, Ryan et al 1980), but there is no simple relationship between frequency of attendance and pregnancy outcome (c.f. DHSS 1978). For example, socio-economic status can independently influence attendance as well as being linked with differing maternal and fetal morbidity and mortality rates (Adelstein et al 1980, MacFarlane et al 1980). Whatever the mechanisms, there is little doubt, however, that 'women who are most likely to attend late are those most at risk' (Hall & Chng 1982). The existing major surveys of late or poor attenders (Butler & Bonham 1963, Robertson & Carr 1970, McKinlay & McKinlay 1972, Scott-Samuel 1979, Law 1980, Lewis 1982) point to associations between indices such as perinatal mortality and birthweight, and factors such as parity, ethnic group, social class, unplanned pregnancy, illegitimacy, negative attitudes and low motivation towards the pregnancy, unstable homes and insecurity in the areas of housing, finance and marital relationships. Some of these correlates of late attendance closely resemble the factors that were picked out by Brown & Harris (1978) in their important study of depression in women in an urban environment.

There is, therefore, a strong possibility that the prevalence of psychiatric problems may be substantially higher in women who do not attend ante-natal clinics. The types of disturbance one might expect to see would include depressive and anxiety neuroses, phobic disorders, drug dependence (Stauber et al 1982) (including alcohol), severe personality disorder and, finally, certain kinds of psychotic illness. Such patients are likely to require special attention when they return home after delivery.

PSYCHIATRIC DISORDERS IN THE PUERPERIUM

Maternity blues

More than half of recently delivered women experience transient episodes of tearfulness, emotional vulnerability and mild depression 4 or 5 days after the birth of their babies (Yalom et al 1968, Kendell et al 1981a). They may also manifest some mild impairments of attention and concentration and of memory (Pitt 1973). The immediate puerperium is a time of very considerable physiological change but, as yet, no particular metabolic or endocrinological disturbances have been specifically implicated as being responsible for the blues syndrome (Stein 1982). Research interest in this condition springs mainly from the hope that investigation of such disturbances may shed light on biological mechanisms underlying more serious mental disorders such as post-natal depression or puerperal psychotic illnesses. Other factors, e.g.

hospitalisation, effects of drugs, lack of sleep, pain and soreness, adaptation to the demands of the baby may all play some part in bringing about the blues.

Post-natal depression

The incidence of depression is raised in the first 3 months after delivery. The clinical picture of depression is typical of depression in other situations, and is characterised by some or several of the following features: lowered mood and self-esteem, tearfulness, hopelessness, guilt and self-reproach, tiredness, loss of energy, appetite and libido, insomnia, irritability, inability to cope, isolation and social withdrawal. The borderline between neurotic and psychotic depression remains a matter of controversy in general psychiatry and the distinction is based upon assessments of severity, suicidal intent, prominent somatic symptoms and sometimes the presence of delusions. The typical and common post-natal depressions are of moderate severity and are found to occur in 10–15% of mothers between 6 and 12 weeks after delivery (Pitt 1968). The incidence and prevalence of this condition is therefore very high bearing in mind that about half a million babies are born each year in England and Wales. Recent studies (reviewed by Kumar 1982) suggest that the rate of occurrence is not greatly influenced by race or culture or by social class. Individual risk factors in one study of primiparae (Kumar & Robson 1984) were found to include maternal age (over 30 years), sub-fertility (trying to conceive for 2 or more years), a history of marital conflict, early severe doubts about going through with the pregnancy and evidence of difficulties in the mother's relationships with her own parents. Other important factors are likely to be an accumulation of recent life-events in the context of inadequate domestic and family support (Paykel et al 1980) and a previous history of psychiatric problems. The impact of a depressive disorder at a potentially critical time for the mother and her developing baby is one further reason why it is worth paying more attention to recognition, treatment and prevention of such disturbances. Some mothers who are depressed are more likely to respond aggressively towards their babies, others may over-protect and yet others may not be able to cope with the demands of their infants in addition to those of the rest of their families (Weissman et al 1972).

Quite simple measures of support and practical help may be of great benefit once the problem is recognised. In cases where the depression is severe and persistent, tricyclic anti-depressant drugs can be prescribed in the knowledge that they do not enter the breast-milk in sufficient quantities to affect the infant. Benzodiazepines and phenothiazine drugs do, however, appear in breast-milk (Brockington & Kumar 1982b).

Puerperal psychosis

A severe mental illness can manifest itself, usually within a month of delivery in about one in 500 to a 1000 mothers, often with catastrophic impact on the mother, her baby and her family. Such illnesses are often unexpected in the sense that there may be no prior history of similar disorder in the patient or her family. The early days after delivery are often unremarkable and many observers have commented on the presence of a 'lucid' interval. Within a week or so, the mother may experience symptoms such as irritability, lability of mood, insomnia, restlessness, all of which may be difficult to distinguish from the blues. Of more sinister significance, there may be signs of suspiciousness, irrational ideas and unusual reactions to the baby.

The full clinical picture of puerperal mental illness usually takes the form of an affective psychosis, manic or depressive in type, or it may take a mixed or schizo-affective form (Hamilton 1962, Kendell et al 1976, 1981b, Dean & Kendell 1981, Brockington et al 1982). It has been noted, in addition, that there may be some clouding of consciousness, perplexity and confusion, but not actual disorientation. The majority of women who become ill in this way are primiparae and a few may develop symptoms during pregnancy (Dean & Kendell 1981), but most become ill within a fortnight of delivery. Weak associations have been found by some workers but not by others with obstetric variables such as dystocia (Paffenbarger 1964) and with Caesarian section (Kendell et al 1981b). The biological antecedents of puerperal psychosis remain unknown and the nosological status of this condition is controversial (Granville-Grossman 1971, Brockington et al 1982, Hamilton 1982). It is argued that as there is no coherence to the clinical syndrome, what is being seen is merely a latent predisposition to an affective or a schizophrenic condition which is then precipitated by the metabolic and psychological trauma of delivery. However, many women who experience a first psychotic breakdown after childbirth have neither any constitutional (genetic) predisposition nor any significant premorbid personality trait.

As puerperal psychosis is a relatively rare condition and 'mother and baby' units are expensive to staff and maintain, many mothers are nursed apart from their babies who may be cared for at home by relatives or other helpers. In some cases where there is concern about infanticidal impulses such separation may be temporarily necessary but, as far as possible, the aim should be to provide opportunities in a therapeutic setting for the mother to care for her baby with nursing supervision and help (Margison & Brockington 1982). The choice of physical treatment for puerperal illnesses depends upon the clinical picture which predominates and it is the same as that for similar types of psychotic disorders in other clinical settings.

The immediate prognosis is fair and the majority of mothers are able to leave hospital within 2 or 3 months of admission (Protheroe 1969), but careful out-patient follow-up is essential. The chances of recurrence after a subsequent pregnancy rise a hundredfold to about one in five or ten (Paffenbarger 1964). The risk of psychotic breakdown outside pregnancy is also raised. Epidemiological surveys suggest that once having had a mental hospital admission for a puerperal illness, at some time later in their lives about a third of such mothers may require one or more admissions to a mental hospital that are unrelated to childbirth. Women with a previous history of mania or hypomania are especially prone to recurrence in the puerperium. Such patients, as well as any with a previous history of puerperal mental illness are therefore particularly vulnerable in the days and weeks following delivery.

There is much room for improvement in the detection and treatment of psychological disturbances in pregnant and parturient women and the initial burden is on those who are likely to be in the closest contact with the patient; viz the midwife, the health visitor, the general practitioner and the obstetrician.

CASE HISTORIES

Case 1. Maternity blues

The subject was a healthy, twenty-six year old, first-time mother. She had had one miscarriage 2 years previously. She was happily married and the pregnancy was planned and wanted. She had felt tired and uncomfortable in the last month of pregnancy. Labour and delivery had been uncomplicated and the baby was healthy. She had felt immediate affection for her child and had put him to the breast very soon after delivery. Her husband was present at the birth. Three to 4 days after the birth she began to experience an exacerbation of perineal soreness and also found that her sleep was disturbed by noises in the ward. On the fifth day she felt unaccountably miserable and was upset when a midwife snapped at her for not getting on with changing her baby. Her husband was not reassuring when he visited, and they had an argument. She felt unreasonably irritable and demanding and cried on and off for several hours. She was still weepy the next day. At one point she had felt unable to concentrate and people had seemed 'distant', but she was never confused. By the time of her discharge on the 7th day she was once again her normal cheerful and confident self.

Case 2. Puerperal Psychosis

Background.

The patient was a 19-year-old primigravida who had no previous significant medical or psychiatric history. Her mother had suffered from depression for many years and had received anti-depressant treatment from her GP and from psychiatric out-patients; there was no other history of illness in the family. The patient had become married a year before to a 24-year-old man who had a prison record for theft and drug abuse. The marriage was described as 'stormy'; the baby was unplanned but wanted. The pregnancy was uneventful and delivery of a healthy male baby was normal, though about a week overdue.

Psychiatric history.

About 2 days after delivery she was said to have been tearful and 'things had seemed unreal'. There had been a row with her husband around the same time.

She was discharged home after 6 days and on the 7th day began to behave oddly. She was initially agitated and unable to cope with the baby's feeds (she had given up breast-feeding). She then described feeling persistently sad and became withdrawn and isolated. She was unable to concentrate and felt perplexed, but she knew where she was, who she was and what time it was. Her husband took over the baby's care after 2 days at home, by which time she had begun to feel that the child might not be her own. She suffered severe insomnia, waking in the early hours, and her appetite and energy were depressed. She was brought to a psychiatric clinic on the 12th day post-partum and was admitted together with her baby. At this time she was also noted to be hearing voices; her auditory hallucinations were religious in content and lasted for several days. Simultaneously, she began to assert that her baby was Jesus, and although she could be convinced otherwise for a time the thoughts soon recurred.

She was treated with an anti-depressant drug together with a phenothiazine. ECT was considered but she recovered gradually during the course of the next 6 weeks and was discharged home after 8 weeks. She remained well on follow-up and the anti-depressant medication was maintained for 6 months, the phenothiazine having been stopped after 1 month. She required considerable support from her social worker and from doctors in the year that followed. She separated from her husband and was rehoused in a flat nearby her parents. Contact was lost about 18 months after the birth of her baby. Her notes do not indicate whether she had received counselling about the risks of relapse in future pregnancies, nor whether she was taking adequate contraceptive precautions as she formed new relationships.

Case 3. Puerperal Psychosis

Background.

She was an illegitimate child who had been brought up by her mother and maternal grandmother; she had had a generally happy childhood, but in adolescence had experimented with drugs — LSD and cannabis regularly, and amphetamines occasionally. At the age of 18 she had had a termination of pregnancy, prior to which she was seen by a psychiatrist. She was described as a lively and cheerful person, with no history of affective disturbance other than a tendency to be irritable before periods. There was no relevant family history of illness.

Pregnancy 1.

Aged 25 years — this was planned and, aside from threatened miscarriage at 5 months, uneventful. She had, however, been intermittently miserable and weepy, upset about stopping her work and about her cramped accommodation. Labour was induced because she was 2 weeks overdue and she was delivered normally of a healthy male infant. On the 5th day post-partum she was noted to be distressed and weepy and on the 7th day she became unaccountably excitable, overactive and disinhibited. She thought she had special powers (extrasensory perception), was preoccupied with religious ideas and with her illegitimacy. She wanted to leave hospital in order to find her father. There was also a suggestion that she was experiencing auditory hallucinations. She was transferred to a psychiatric ward (with her baby), treated with chlorpromazine and recovered rapidly over a period of 4–6 weeks.

Pregnancy 2.

Aged 28 years — this was again planned and uneventful and was followed by normal labour and delivery of a healthy girl. Nothing untoward was recorded until the 4th day post-partum when she was seen to be writing continuously and noted to be expressing religiose ideas. On the 9th day she began to suffer from insomnia, was overtalkative, restless and overactive. Her behaviour was bizarre, e.g. she wrapped her baby in wet towels. She was transferred to a psychiatric ward and treated with haloperidol and chlorpromazine. Recovery was a little slower this time and she was discharged home after 9 weeks.

Pregnancy 3.

Aged 30 years — this pregnancy was unplanned and was due to contraceptive failure; the baby was nevertheless wanted as soon as she discovered she had conceived. A formal assessment of her mental state 1 month prior to delivery revealed no abnormality. Four days before delivery she fell down some stairs with her daughter, avoided injury to herself, but the daughter aged 2 sustained a fractured tibia and fibula. On the next day her son developed chicken pox. Labour and delivery were again normal and for the first 2 days she was her usual self. On the third day, the only abnormality on interview was slight disinhibition and mild euphoria. By day 7 she was elated, laughing infectiously, beginning to sleep poorly and was moved to a psychiatric ward. Her condition worsened perceptibly on the 10th day when, simultaneously, she came out in a chicken pox rash. She was overactive, somewhat promiscuous and disinhibited in an amicable sort of way. She showed pressure of speech, flight of ideas and punning. There were no abnormal experiences and she was well-oriented. Treatment with chlorpromazine and haloperidol was started and there was rapid improvement over the next 2 weeks. She was discharged home after 8 weeks.

On the first occasion a provisional diagnosis of a schizophrenic illness was entertained, but with hindsight the clinical picture on all three admissions was consistent with that of a manic depressive psychosis — manic type.

Case 4. Postnatal depression

The patient was a 32-year-old married woman with two children, aged 2½ years and 4 months. She was referred to psychiatric outpatients by her GP for persistent depression which had not responded to pharmacotherapy. She had had a normal pregnancy and delivery and there had been no post-partum complications.

Psychiatric history.

She had been tearful for a day or so at home a week after the birth. Her symptoms of depression had begun a month later and had progressively worsened. By 4 months she was persistently low spirited, with diurnal variation of her mood, she was irritable and had frequent tiffs with her husband, she often shouted at the toddler but had never hit her, even though she sometimes felt like it. She was very guilty about her inability to cope and about her aggressive feelings. At times she thought she would be better dead and phantasised about taking an overdose. She never acted on her impulses, however. She avoided social contact to the extent that going out shopping alone had become impossible and, in the last month, she had begun to drink to the point of sedation, a bottle of wine or sherry every evening. Her concentration and memory were affected. She suffered from early morning waking, loss of energy and her libido was non-existent. Three months after the delivery, her GP had prescribed imipramine 75 mg at night but she had not been helped by the drug and had stopped it.

There was no significant family history of mental illness but the patient herself had briefly attended psychiatric out-patients some years before, following the break-up of her first marriage. She had been prescribed anti-depressants then, but had taken them erratically. She had had one termination of pregnancy at a private clinic, at the time she was single and the pregnancy was unplanned and unwanted. This baby was wanted, but she sometimes regretted having had her, especially in view of her deteriorating relationship with her husband. He was an academic who worked long hours away from home.

She was again prescribed a tricyclic anti-depressant (imipramine) and the dose was increased to 150 mg at night, at which level adequate plasma concentrations were maintained. She agreed to try and reduce her alcohol intake and she and her husband were seen conjointly on two occasions to try and negotiate mutually satisfactory ways of reorganising their domestic lives. After 4 weeks she described herself as much improved, this had begun about 2 weeks after starting the anti-depressant. She was optimistic, more relaxed, she and her husband were enjoying social occasions for the first time in months and had also resumed sexual intercourse. She was unable to reach orgasm, however. She felt physically better. She had cut her alcohol consumption to about a bottle of wine a week. At the time of writing (6½ months post-partum) she was continuing to improve gradually and further discussions were planned with her husband. It was agreed that she would remain on anti-depressants for at least 6 months.

COMMENTARY

These four case histories illustrate some important clinical features of post-partum psychiatric syndromes. The two patients with psychotic illnesses show that signs of impending severe mental disturbance occur early, often before the patient has left the obstetric ward, or at least while she is still under the daily surveillance of the midwife. There is still much room for improvement in methods of early detection and in the distinction of prodromal psychotic disturbances from the blues. But there is a simple lesson to be learned from the patient with the recurrent illness. Liaison with psychiatric services is advisable whenever there is a previous history of severe puerperal mental illness and, indeed, in all cases of pregnancy where the mother has had a past functional psychotic illness; she will probably have received in-patient psychiatric treatment for this. Liaison is much more likely to be effective if the process is begun in pregnancy. The personal lives and social relationships of mothers with puerperal psychotic illnesses can be drastically affected and physical treatment in hospital is only one of several potential therapeutic measures that may be required in the process of rehabilitation.

The fourth patient with the insidious onset, postnatal depressive condition is typical of many who attend for post-natal checks or who take their babies to clinics (sometimes unnecessarily often), but whose depressive disorders are not always picked up by doctors, midwives or health visitors for some considerable time. Many post-natal depressions remit after about 3 months, but in a significant sub-group of women they persist and may become severe, as in this patient. Anti-depressants in therapeutic doses are usually beneficial, but drug treatment should always be combined with psychological support and counselling. As yet, there are no reliable methods of early detection, e.g. at 3 to 4 weeks postnatally, of those women who are likely to become severely and chronically depressed. Anti-depressant therapy, if started early, might prevent or abort the illness in such cases. Most women with postnatal depression do not require anti-depressants, but all may benefit from counselling aimed at specific areas, such as their marital and sexual relationships, or at the ways in which their daily routines and care of the baby are affected.

As a general conclusion, it seems clear that there is still much room for improvement in the services that are available to meet psychological and social needs of pregnant and parturient women. One consequence of improvements in this direction may be a significant amelioration in the physical health of both mothers and babies.

REFERENCES

Adelstein A M, Macdonald Davies I M 1980 Perinatal and infant mortality: social and biological factors 1975–77. Studies on medical and population subjects, No 41 (O P C S) HMSO, London
Boyd C, Sellars L 1982 The British Way of Birth. Pan Books, London

Breen D 1975 The Birth of a First Child. Tavistock, London

Brewer 1977 Incidence of post abortion psychosis: a prospective study. British Medical Journal 1: 476–477

British Medical Journal 1938 Charge of procuring abortion: Mr Bourne acquitted. 2: 199–205

Brockington I F, Kumar R (eds) 1982a Motherhood and Mental Illness. Academic Press, London

Brockington I F, Kumar R 1982b Drug addiction and drug treatment during pregnancy. In: Brockington I F, Kumar R (eds) Motherhood and Mental Illness, pp 239–255. Academic Press, London

Brockington I F, Winokur G, Dean Christine 1982 Puerperal psychosis. In: Brockington I F, Kumar R (eds) Motherhood and Mental Illness, pp 37–69. Academic Press, London

Brown G, Harris T 1978 Social Origins of Depression. Tavistock, London

Butler N R, Bonham D G 1963 Perinatal Mortality. Livingstone, Edinburgh

Cartwright A 1979 The Dignity of Labour. Tavistock, London

Chalmers B 1982 Psychological aspects of pregnancy: some thoughts for the eighties. Social Science and Medicine 16: 323–331

Chard T, Richards M (eds) 1977 Benefits and Hazards of the New Obstetrics. Spastics International Medical Publications. Heinemann, London

Chertok L 1969 Motherhood and Personality. Tavistock, London

Chodorow, N 1978 The Reproduction of Mothering. University of California Press, Berkeley and Los Angeles

Coppen A 1958 Psychosomatic aspects of pre-eclamptic toxaemia. Journal of Psychosomatic Research 2: 241–265

Coyle I, Wayner M J, Singer G 1976 Behavioral terato-genesis: a critical review. Pharmacology, Biochemistry & Behavior 4: 191–200

Dean C, Kendell R E 1981 The symptomatology of puerperal illnesses. British Journal of Psychiatry 139: 128–133

Deutsch H 1945 The Psychology of Women, Vol II. Grune and Stratton, New York

DHSS 1978 Reaching the consumer in the antenatal and child health services. HMSO, London

Donnai P, Charles N, Harris R 1981 Attitudes of patients after 'genetic' termination of pregnancy. British Medical Journal 1: 621–622

Dytrych Z, Matejcek Z, Schuller V, David H, Friedmann H 1975 Children born to women denied abortion. Family Planning Perspectives 7: 165–171

Forssman H, Thuwe I 1966 One hundred and twenty children born after application for therapeutic abortion refused. Their mental health social adjustment and education level up to the age of 21. Acta Psychiatrica Scandinavica 42: 71–88

Goldberg H L, Di Mascio A 1978 Psychotropic drugs in pregnancy. In: Lipton M A, Di Mascio A, Killam K F (eds) Psychopharmacology: A Generation of Progress, pp 1047–1055. Raven Press, New York

Gorsuch R L, Kay M K 1974 Abnormalities of pregnancy as a function of anxiety and life stress. Psychosomatic Medicine 36: 352–362

Granville Grossman K 1971 Psychiatric aspects of pregnancy and the puerperium. In: Recent Advances in Clinical Psychiatry Vol 1, pp 266–310. Churchill Livingstone, Edinburgh

Greer H S, Lal S, Lewis S C, Belsey E M, Beard R W 1976 Psychosocial consequences of therapeutic abortion. King's termination study. III British Journal of Psychiatry 128: 74–79

Grimm E R 1962 Psychological investigation of habitual abortion. Psychosomatic Medicine 24: 369

Grimm E R 1967 Psychological and social factors in pregnancy, delivery and outcome. In: Richardson S A, Guttmacher A F (eds) Childbearing — Its Social and Psychological Aspects, pp 1–52. Williams and Wilkins, New York

Hall M, Chng P 1982 Antenatal care in practice. In: Enkin M and Chalmers I (eds) Effectiveness and Satisfaction in Antenatal Care, pp 60–68. Heinemann, London

Hamilton J A 1962 Postpartum Psychiatric Problems. C V Mosby, St Louis

Hamilton J A 1982 The Identity of Postpartum Psychosis. In: Brockington I F, Kumar R (eds) Motherhood and Mental Illness, pp 1–17. Academic Press, London

Hetzel B S, Bruer B, Poidevin L O S 1961 A survey of the relation between certain common antenatal complications in primiparae and stressful life situations during pregnancy. Journal of Psychosomatic Research 5: 175–182

Höök K 1963 Refused abortion: a follow-up study of 249 women whose applications were refused by the National Board of Health in Sweden. Acta Psychiatrica Neurologica Scandinavica Suppl 168

Illsley R, Hall M H 1976 Psychological aspects of abortion. A review of issues and needed research. Bulletin of the World Health Organisation 53: 83–106

Kendell R E, Wainwright S, Hailey A, Shannon B 1976 The influence of childbirth on psychiatric morbidity. Psychological Medicine 6: 297–302

Kendell R E, McGuire R J, Connor Y, Cox J L 1981a Mood changes in the first three weeks after childbirth. Journal of Affective Disorders 3: 317–326

Kendell R E, Rennie D, Clarke J A, Dean C 1981b The social and obstetric correlates of psychiatric admission in the puerperium. Psychological Medicine 11: 341–350

Kitzinger S 1979 The Good Birth Guide. Fontana Paperbacks, William Collins, Glasgow

Kitzinger S, David J A (eds) 1978 The Place of Birth. Oxford University Press, London

Kumar R 1982 Neurotic disorders in childbearing women. In: Brockington I F, Kumar R (eds) Motherhood and Mental Illness, pp 71–118. Academic Press, London

Kumar R, Robson K 1978 Previous induced abortion and antenatal depression in primiparae: preliminary report of a survey of mental health in pregnancy. Psychological Medicine 8: 711–715

Kumar R, Robson K M 1984 A prospective study of emotional disorders in childbearing women. British Journal of Psychiatry 144: 35–47

Law E H 1980 Memorandum — Social work with antenatal defaulters. Appendix 5. Paper 663 pp 40–41. House of Commons Social Services Committee: Chairman Mrs Short

Lewis E 1982 Attendance for antenatal care. British Medical Journal 1: 788

Lynch M, Roberts J 1977 Predicting child abuse: signs of bonding failure in the maternity hospital. British Medical Journal 1: 624–626

MacFarlane A, Chalmers I, Adelstein A M 1980 The role of standardization in the interpretation of perinatal mortality rates. Health Trends 12: 45–50

MacIntyre S 1977 The management of childbirth: a review of sociological research issues. Social Science Medicine 11: 477–484

Mann E C 1959 Habitual abortion: a report in two parts, on 160 patients. American Journal of Obstetrics and Gynecology 77: 706–718

Margison F, Brockington I F 1982 Psychiatric Mother and Baby Units. In: Brockington I F, Kumar R (eds) Motherhood and Mental Illness, pp 223–238. Academic Press, London

McDonald R L 1968 The role of emotional factors in obstetric complications: a review. Psychosomatic Medicine 15: 222–237

McDonald R L, Christiakos A C 1963 Relationship of emotional adjustment during pregnancy to obstetric complications. American Journal of Obstetrics and Gynecology 86: 341–348

McKinlay J B, McKinlay S M 1972 Some social characteristics of lower working class utilisers and under-utilisers of maternity care services. Journal of Health and Social Behaviour 13: 369–382

Newton R W, Webster P A C, Binu P S, Maskrey N, Phillips A B 1979 Psychosocial stress in pregnancy and its relation to the onset of premature labour. British Medical Journal 2: 411–413

Nuckolls K B, Cassel J, Kaplan B H 1972 Psychosocial assets, life crises and the prognosis of pregnancy. American Journal of Epidemiology 95: 431–441

Oakley A 1980 Women Confined — Towards a Sociology of Childbirth. Martin Robertson, Oxford

Osofsky J D, Osofsky H J 1972 The psychological reaction of patients of legalised abortion. American Journal of Orthopsychiatry 42: 48–60

Paffenbarger R S 1964 Epidemiological aspects of post-partum mental illness. British Journal of Social Preventive Medicine 18: 189–195

Pare C M B, Raven H 1970 Follow-up of patients referred for termination. Lancet i: 653–658

Paykel E S, Emms E M, Fletcher J, Rassaby E S 1980 Life events and social support in puerperal depression. British Journal of Psychiatry 136: 339–346

Pines D 1972 Pregnancy and motherhood: interaction between fantasy and reality. British Journal of Medical Psychology 45: 333–343

Pitt B 1968 Atypical depression following childbirth. British Journal of Psychiatry 114: 1325–1335

Pitt B 1973 Maternity blues. British Journal of Psychiatry 122: 431–435

Proceedings of the Symposium of the British Association for Psychopharmacology 1981 Behavioural Teratology. Neuropharmacology 20: 1237–1269

Protheroe C 1969 Puerperal psychoses: a long term study 1927–1961. British Journal of Psychiatry 115: 9–30

Raphael-Leff J 1980 Psychotherapy with pregnant women. In: Blum B L (ed) Psychological Aspects of Pregnancy, Birthing and Bonding, pp 174–205. Human Sciences Press, New York

Rapoport R, Rapoport R N, Strelitz Z, Kew S 1977 Fathers, Mothers and Others. Routledge & Kegan Paul, London

Robertson J S, Carr G 1970 Late bookers for antenatal care. In: MacLachan G, Shegog R (eds) Studies of Maternity Services: In the Beginning, pp 81–102. Oxford University Press, Oxford

Ryan G, Sweeney P J, Solola A S 1980 Prenatal Care and pregnancy outcome. American Journal of Obstetrics and Gynecology 137: 876–881

Scott-Samuel A 1979 Delayed booking for antenatal care. Public Health London 93: 246–251

Social Services Committee 1980 Perinatal and neonatal mortality. Vol 1, Second report from the Social Services Committee Session 1979–1980. HMSO, London

Stauber M, Schwerdt M, Tylden E 1982 Pregnancy, birth and puerperium in women suffering from heroin addiction. Journal of Psychosomatic Obstetrics and Gynaecology 1: 128–138

Stein G 1982 The Maternity Blues. In: Brockington I F, Kumar R (eds) Motherhood and Mental Illness, pp 119–154. Academic Press, London

Visram S A 1972 A follow-up study of 95 women who were refused abortion on psychiatric grounds. In: Morris N (ed) Psychosomatic Medicine in Obstetrics and Gynaecology, pp 561–563. Karger S, Basel

Weil R J, Tupper C 1960 Personality, life situation and communication; a study of habitual abortion. Psychosomatic Medicine 22: 448

Weismann M M, Paykel E S, Klerman G L 1972 The depressed woman as a mother. Social Psychiatry 7: 98–108

Whitlock F A, Edwards J E 1968 Pregnancy and attempted suicide. Comprehensive Psychiatry 9: 1–12

Yalom I, Lunde D, Moos R, Hamburg D 1968 Post partum blues syndrome. Archives of General Psychiatry 18: 16–27

Post-pregnancy and post-abortion contraception

The methods of contraception suitable for use in the puerperium after miscarriage and termination of pregnancy are reviewed in this article. Often in the past, the choice of contraception and 'when to start' following a pregnancy, has been hampered by lack of information on side-effects and morbidity. Over the last 5 years this information has been collated through multicentre international studies. When taken with our present understanding of the physiological changes in the puerperium and the role of lactation, a logical choice of contraceptive method can be made.

THE PHYSIOLOGY OF THE PUERPERIUM AND POST-ABORTAL STATE

During pregnancy, virtually every organ system adapts to the metabolic and physical demands of the fetus. While some of these changes occur in the first few weeks, most become more pronounced with the duration of the pregnancy. Reversion to normal after delivery is rapid. Six to 8 weeks is conventionally taken as the time limit for the puerperium yet many of the cardiovascular adaptations have regressed within a few days and most of the anatomical changes have been accomplished by 2 weeks. By contrast return of endocrine normality is determined by the period of lactation which may last for months. As a result the conventional notion of the puerperium is inadequate and contraceptive use should be tailored to the individual's needs, based upon a knowledge of the physiological changes taking place.

Endocrine Changes

Lactation

During pregnancy raised levels of oestrogen and progesterone induce hyperplasia of the lactotrophs and increased synthesis of Prolactin (Kletzky et al 1980). After delivery the fall in progesterone and oestrogen remove the inhibition for lactation while prolactin secretion continues.

160

Hypothalamic-pituitary axis

It has been suggested that there is hypothalamic hypofunction post-partum, possibly induced by high pregnancy oestrogen levels (Morishita et al 1984) giving rise to low levels of GnRH. Also there is a pituitary refractoriness to GnRH in the immediate post-partum period resulting in low FSH and LH levels (Canales et al 1974, Nakano et al 1974, Canales et al 1981, Falsetti et al 1982).

During recovery of pituitary responsiveness to LRH it is FSH secretory response which is recovered before that of LH, a pattern seen during initiation of gonadotrophin secretion at the menarche.

Positive feedback of oestrogen to produce an LH surge is inoperative during lactation (Canales et al 1981) though a negative feedback to reduce FSH is demonstrable. In the absence of lactation recovery of the normal oestrogen feedback mechanisms can be demonstrated by the third week post-partum.

High prolactin levels render the ovary less sensitive to the already low gonadotrophin stimulation (Archer et al 1976) (see Falsetti et al 1982) resulting in ovarian inactivity, low oestrogen status and anovulation. Even when ovarian activity resumes, raised levels of prolactin give rise to short luteal phases and reduced fertility (Delvoye et al 1980).

Thus the picture of the first 3 weeks post-partum is one of hypopituitary hypothalamo ovarian inactivity which is prolonged by lactation under the influence of prolactin secretion.

Ovulation — influence of lactation

The return of ovulation and menstruation is variable and unpredictable. Two per cent of non-lactating women show evidence of ovulation before 28 days partum (Cronin 1968, Flynn 1981) and 33% ovulate before the first menstruation. In this group the mean duration of amenorrhoea was 58.9 days.

Prolonged lactation produced elevated levels of prolactin (Vemer & Rolland 1981). Cronin (1968) did not find evidence of ovulation during the first 10 weeks post-partum where full breast feeding was in progress. Pascall (1969) also suggested that one-third of lactating women have evidence of ovulation before their first menstruation.

Howie et al (1981) have shown that ovulation did not occur, provided 'full lactation' was maintained. It appears that suckling episodes of 6 or more in 24 hours, duration of suckling >60 min/24 hours and suckling during night hours, to reduce the intervals between feeds, are the important factors in delaying ovulation (Howie et al 1982). Once supplementary feeds are introduced and suckling episodes decline approximately 75% develop follicular development and 50% ovulate within the next 16 weeks even though lactation is maintained.

The number of patients in the above series was small. Perez et al (1972) in a larger series of 200 mothers reported 14 ovulating while fully lactating and two of them conceived though the definition of full lactation and frequency of suckling was not rigidly defined. He calculated that the probability of ovulation in the first 9–10 weeks to be only 1/1250 in lactating mothers.

Thus following delivery, ovulation can and does occur within 28 days when the mother is not lactating (after termination of pregnancy, or spontaneous abortion this interval is even shorter). Ovulation is deferred beyond 10 weeks and possibly for the duration of suckling in lactating mothers provided the criteria given by Howie et al (1982) for suckling frequency are noted. In both lactators and non-lactators, when ovulation occurs, this event will precede menstruation in one-third of women.

Uterine changes

Endometrium. After delivery only the basal portion of the endometrium remains. By the seventh day there is a definite surface epithelium and the stroma exhibits its normal non-pregnant characteristics (Sharman 1953). Proliferative activity is detectable by the sixteenth. Sharman in this series could not demonstrate secretory activity before day 44 — somewhat later than would be expected from the other means of inferring ovulation already described.

Involution of the placental site may take up to 6 weeks (Williams 1931) though more recent studies suggest that the placental site is restored to normal at the same rate as the rest of the endometrium (Anderson & Davis 1968).

Corpus. Reduction in weight from 1000–1200 g to 500 g occurs in the first week, it is not palpable abdominally by 2 weeks and reaches its non-pregnant size and weight by 6 weeks (Monheit et al 1980).

The cavity itself undergoes rapid reductions in size between days 1 and 3, and 5 and 8. No difference is found between primiparas and multiparas nor between breast feeders and artificial feeders (Rodeck & Newton 1976).

Cervix. During the first week the cervix regains its non-pregnant morphology with the cervical canal reducing to a 1 cm diameter or less (Pritchard & Macdonald 1976). Histological changes in the stroma can be seen for up to 4 months (McLaren 1952).

Clotting Mechanisms

The complex changes in the coagulation and fibrinolytic systems are beyond comprehensive review here. However, the risk of thromoembolism in the immediate post-delivery period is well recognised. Review of the data on coagulation factors indicates that return to non-pregnant values has occurred by the fifth day post-partum (Beller & Ebert 1982, Bonnar et al 1970).

CONTRACEPTION

Hormonal

The general considerations for the use of these agents must be the same as when used outside the immediate post delivery period. However, there are specific considerations which apply to the lactating woman regarding their effect on lactation and the penetration of the hormones into breast milk.

For non-lactating women it would appear that contraception should be started certainly within the first 4 weeks and since there is evidence for return of hypothalamic-pituitary activity in the first 3 weeks it would seem advisable to pre-empt this activity.

For fully lactating women there is no need to start contraception before 10 weeks but if full lactation is not achieved or supplementary feeding is instigated, this should be the signal for contraceptive use (see Table 11.1 for Hormonal preparations).

Monophasic combined oestrogen/progestogen pills

Their effect depends upon the suppression of gonadotrophins (Ryu & Hong 1983).

It has been noted that oestrogens tend to raise prolactin levels (Kochenour 1980) and prolactin secretion. However, it has been shown that low dose combined contraceptive preparations (ethinyl oestradiol 0.03 mg and levonorgestrel 0.15 mg) even when used in women with well established lactation, showed a higher incidence of subsequent supplemental feeding and lower infant weight increase than controls though no long term ill effects were noted (Paralta et al 1983, Diaz 1983, Croxatto et al 1983). Thus it must be accepted that a moderate inhibitory effect on lactation is produced, and this seems to be dose related (Drill 1966). The efficacy of this form of contraception and incidence of side-effects are no different from non-puerperal women.

Since oestrogens have an effect on clotting mechanisms particularly in reducing the effect of anti-thrombin III (Howie et al 1975), it would therefore seem reasonable to allow the pregnancy effects to subside before commencement of combined preparations. Thus non-breast feeders should start 'the pill' between the first and second weeks. For lactating mothers these preparations should be used with caution. While no significant effect on milk composition has been shown (Thompson et al 1975), the hormones do enter breast milk and their effect on the fetus is uncertain. No significant deleterious effect has been shown to date (Hull 1981).

The minor side-effects often seen in the first few cycles of pill taking — break through bleeding, occasional nausea and infrequent breast tenderness — can all occur when pills are started in the puerperium. However, these are often masked by the natural symptomatology of the puerperium, and hence combined oral contraception will have a higher patient acceptability rate.

Phasic preparations

Two types are currently available — biphasic (2 step dose regime) and triphasic (3 step dose regime). Table 11.1 lists the hormonal composition of these preparations.

Table 11.1 Hormonal preparations

COMBINED OESTROGEN / PROGESTOGEN PILLS

(A)   MONOPHASIC   (1) *Oestrogen: ethinyl oestradiol 30 μg*
       Progestogen: levonorgestrel 150 μg : Microgynon 30, Ovranette
                                   levonorgestrel 250 μg : Eugynon 30, Ovran 30
                                   desogestrel   150 μg : Marvelon
                        ethynodiol diacetate   2 mg : Conova 30

                                              (2) *Oestrogen: ethinyl oestradiol 35 μg*
       Progestogen: Norethisterone 0.5 mg : Brevinor, Ovysmen
                                   Norethisterone 1.0 mg : Norimin

                                              (3) *Oestrogen: ethinyl oestradiol 50 μg*
       Occasionally these are needed when drug interaction is present, e.g. with anti-
       convulsant drugs, see British National Formulary for list

(B)   PHASIC PREPARATIONS
       Binovum :   Oestrogen: ethinyl oestradiol 35 mg
       (biphasic)   Progestogen: norethisterone 0.5 mg for 7 days
                                                         1.0 mg for 14 days

       Trinordiol/Logynon:
       (triphasic)   Regime   6   5   10 Days
                            Oestrogen ethinyl oestradiol   30 μg   40 μg   30 μg
                            Progestogen levonorgestrel   50 μg   75 μg   125 μg

       Trinovum (triphasic)   Regime   7   7   7 Days
                            Oestrogen: ethinyl oestradiol   30 μg   35 μg   35 μg
                            Progestogen: Norethisterone   0.5 mg 0.75 mg 1.0 mg

       PROGESTOGEN ONLY PILLS
       Norethisterone   :   350 μg Micronor, Noriday
       Levonorgestrel   :   30 μg Microval, Norgeston
       Levonorgestrel   :   75 μg Neogest
       Ethynodiol diacetate   :   500 μg Femulen

       INJECTABLE PROGESTOGENS
       Medroxyprogesterone acetate   :   150 mg Depo-Provera
          given every 12 weeks.
       Norethisterone oenanthate   :   200 mg Noristerat
          given every 10–12 weeks.

The effect of these formulations is to reduce the total amount of steroid ingested per cycle of treatment (up to 40% reduction in progestogen dose when compared with monophasic preparations). This reduction in progestogen dose, however, has to be traded off against a slight increase in oestrogen daily dose for the levonorgestrel triphasic preparations — this is equivalent to an extra 42 μg per cycle.

By reducing the dose with the levonorgestrel pills the metabolic, clotting and other side-effects are reduced. However, there is in some women an increase in break through bleeding. This is more easily tolerated by women in the puerperium and post-abortal states. The norethisterone preparations do not have an increase in oestrogen and the dose of progestogen is midway between the monophasic 0.5 mg and 1.0 mg pills (see Table 11.1). Therefore the effects of these preparations are appropriate to the dose of steroid ingested.

Progestogen only formulations

1. Oral

Taken everyday, these preparations have been advocated, particularly for lactating mothers because they have little effect on milk production (Hull 1981). However, the hormone does enter the milk though the amount is small and considered insignificant (Melis et al 1981).

Side-effects such as menstrual irregularity seem no more common than in the general use and are more tolerated in the puerperium due to the patients acceptance of irregular bleeding at this time. The failure rate appears to be higher than combined contraceptive pills and this risk must be weighed against the patient's needs.

It would seen appropriate to use these agents for breast feeding mothers with the option to change to a combined preparation when menstruation returns if a safer form of contraception is required.

2. Injectable progestogens

These preparations may be appropriate where long-term contraception is required without the reliance on user reliability or for coverage of Rubella vaccination. Two preparations are available medroxyprogesterone acetate (Depo-Provera) and norethisterone oenanthate (Novistat).

Side-effects. Croxatto et al (1982 a, b) have used progesterone subdermal implants to reduce the possible effect on the fetus of synthetic progestogens. They have attested to the contraceptive efficacy, low incidence of side-effects and no diminution in lactation in those mothers who breast feed. The effects could be prolonged to 5 months depending upon implant dosage.

Melis (1981) has documented similar results for norethisterone oenanthate implants.

Hormonal contraception: general conclusions

It is safe to use hormonal contraception in the puerperium bearing in mind the normal contraindications to pill use. Contraception should be started in the non-lactating women within 3 weeks of birth, in the lactating women when full breast feeding ceases. Steroid contraceptives do pass into the breast milk and therefore it is wise to use the lowest suitable dose for any given women. For lactating women this will be a progestogen only pill, for non-lactators the same or combined pills of the low dose monophasic or phasic type. Alternatively, injectable progestogens can be used.

When lactation ceases, it may be necessary to change directly from a progestogen only pill to a combined preparation. If break through bleeding is a problem then a change to a higher dose pill will control it, i.e. phasic to monophasic pill, or increase the strength of the progestogen component in the combined pill.

The side-effects of the pill in the puerperium or post-abortal state are minimal and often more acceptable due to natural physiological changes masking the pill effect. Routine examinations of blood pressure, weight, pelvic examination and cervical smear (if not done within the last 5 years) is mandatory.

Barrier methods

Sexual activity may be resumed at any time in the puerperium. It has been suggested that this may occur 3–4 weeks post-partum and earlier post-abortion (Keith et al 1979), depending upon symptoms and degree of discomfort. By this time, the anatomic changes of pregnancy have regressed and the use of barrier or chemical methods of contraception should present no specific differences from their use generally. Since fertility in this period is somewhat reduced naturally, there is no evidence to suggest a higher pregnancy rate than when these methods are used at other times.

Intrauterine devices

Insertion of a intrauterine contraceptive device (IUCD) as an intermenstrual (interval) procedure is well established and is accepted by clinicians as being safe and simple (for reviews see Newton 1982, Mishell 1983). Post-partum insertion of an IUCD is not so readily accepted by clinicians and this concern stems mainly from review articles suggesting that post-partum uterine perforation is more likely to occur (Davis 1972, Tatum 1976, Gentile & Seigler 1977). The original basis for this idea comes from a single report in Singapore, where in one study using a Lippes loop, a perforation rate of 1.8% was found (Ratnam & Tow 1970). This has not been confirmed in other studies especially those using the modern copper bearing IUCDs (Newton et al 1977, Mishell & Roy 1982, Kamal et al 1980).

Other reasons for concern are the effects of post-partum insertion on menstrual bleeding, intermenstrual bleeding, lochia, infection and expulsion of the device. Recently, a considerable amount of data has been collected on these effects. (To reassure the clinician and make post-partum IUCD insertion a practical contraceptive method, especially for the high risk patient who may find clinic visits difficult, or who may default and for the breast feeding mother who does not want to use hormal contraception.)

Timing of insertion

IUCDs have been inserted at various times following delivery, these are: *Immediate post-placental insertion*, i.e. within 10 to 30 minutes of delivery

(Newton et al 1977, WHO 1980, Apelo et al 1976, Thiery 1980). *Early post-partum insertion*, i.e. before the patient is discharged from hospital, 2 to 8 days after delivery (Emens & Shah 1982, Banhaurisupawat & Rosenfield 1971, Emens et al 1978). *Late post-partum insertion*, i.e. 4 to 8 weeks following delivery (Mishell & Roy 1982, Tietze & Lewit 1970, Wathen et al 1978).

Results of clinical studies

Early studies reported by Tietze & Lewit (1970) with inert plastic devices in the co-operative statistical programme, showed higher rates for pregnancy and expulsion when IUCDs were inserted up to 12 weeks after delivery compared with later insertion. However, removals for pain and bleeding were less — presumably the natural occurrence of post delivery discharge and bleeding made any IUD related bleeding tolerated more easily.

Mishell & Roy (1982) compared insertion of copper bearing IUCDs between 4 and 8 weeks after delivery and compared these with IUCDs inserted after 8 weeks. The types of IUCD investigated were the copper 7 and several models of the copper T. Follow-up was for 2 years, no uterine perforation occurred and there was no significant difference in the termination rates (medical removals, expulsion and pregnancy) between the two groups. Many of the 'early insertions' in this group were carried out by house staff in training, compared with experienced family planning staff who inserted most of the 'later' group. They conclude the insertion of IUCDs before 8 weeks after delivery is safe, effective and not associated with an increased morbidity or decrease in effective IUCD use.

Wathen et al (1978) also confirm these results in their study of the Multiload. More recently IUCDs releasing hormones, e.g. levonorgestrel, have been developed (Nilsson & Luukkainen 1977) and this has been compared with the Nova T device by Heikkila (1982) for post-partum use. The levonorgestrel devices released either 10 μg or 30 μg per day, while bleeding and spotting was more common with these devices for the first 3 months, it was well tolerated. All devices were inserted at 6 weeks (range 29–56 days) and expulsion rates were low.

Many types of IUCDs have been studied in the puerperium (for review see Brenner 1983), in general early insertion of the IUCD in the puerperium gives a higher expulsion rate. This in part may be due to the involution of the uterus. Emens & Shah (1982) also found a higher expulsion rate with early post-partum insertion (days 2–8) using the Multiload IUCD. Other studies have reported expulsion rates as high as 68% (Diamond & Freeman 1973).

For this reason immediate post-partum or post-placental insertion of devices was developed. Initial studies concentrated on the design of an IUCD that would 'flex' as the uterus involuted — the LEM device (Apelo et al 1976) — but this had an unacceptable partial expulsion rate. Newton et al (1977) used conventional devices with special long inserters for correct fundal placement and found a low and acceptable expulsion rate. With conventional insertion tubes, however, the expulsion rate was higher (WHO 1980), and for this reason other methods have been tried to increase the retention rate of IUCDs by the use of biodegradable membranes attached to the device or biodegradable sutures attached to the top of the device: Brenner (1982) — Copper T, and Kamal et al (1980) — Lippes loop. The use of these sutures does improve retention rate but only if a fundal insertion is achieved by the use of a long 25 cm inserter. In addition the placing of the IUCD at the fundus with the 'pull' insertion technique rather than the old fashioned 'push out' technique reduced the chance of uterine perforation.

Brenner (1982) confirms a low expulsion rate with no uterine perforation and no increase in morbidity or infection when this modified copper T — the Delta T — is inserted up to 55 hours after delivery.

Heikkila & Luukkainen (1982) studied duration of breast feeding and infant development in two groups of women — those using a levonorgestrel releasing IUCD and those using a copper Nova T. There were no differences in the children. However, twice as many mothers (44%) at 75 days post-partum discontinued breast feeding with the levonorgestrel (30 μg/day) IUCD, than the control group (20%).

Heikkila et al (1982) also studied levonorgestrel concentrations in milk and plasma with the same devices. They found a levonorgestrel plasma to milk ratio initially of 100:15 and at 3 months 100:75. There was no difference between the two devices and they calculated the total excretion of levonorgestrel per day in 600 ml breast milk to be approximately 0.1% of the daily release dose of 30 μg.

General conclusions. Clinical studies of copper devices, devices modified with biodegradable suture material and hormone releasing IUCDs can safely be inserted immediately after delivery. The use of a long (25 cm) inserter is recommended together with fundal placement of the device. No increase in morbidity is seen, expulsion rates are low, bleeding problems, if they occur, are well tolerated and pregnancy rates are similar or lower than intermenstrual insertion studies.

The use of an IUCD in this situation is to be recommended especially for those high risk mothers who are unlikely to return to the clinic. It also has a special place in the family planning programme of the developing world.

Copper IUCDs are to be preferred because of their lower pregnancy rates and higher continuation rates.

STERILISATION

Voluntary sterilisation of either partner is the most frequently used method of permanent contraception. It is clear that significant increases in the use of this method have occurred over the last 10 years; Stepan et al (1981) estimate that of more than 260 million couples using contraception world wide, at least one-third chose sterilisation.

Methods. From the classical tubal ligation methods of Pomeroy, Madlener Irving & Uchida introduced since the 1930s, methods have now changed to those suitable for laparoscopy or mini laparotomy, namely diathermy, tubal rings (Falope) or clips (Hulka or Filshie), for a recent review see Newton (1983).

The trend in recent years has been to use a safe, simple method that destroys the least possible amount of tube, and yet provides effective sterilisation. Many centres employ local anaesthetics and so methods have to be adapted for its use. In many areas of the world the sophisticated equipment needed for laparoscopy is not readily available and so mini laparotomy (<7 cm abdominal incision) is the preferred method of exposing the tubes.

Figure 11.1 shows the rings and clips in common use; these can be used either with laparoscopy (single or double portal) or at mini laparotomy.

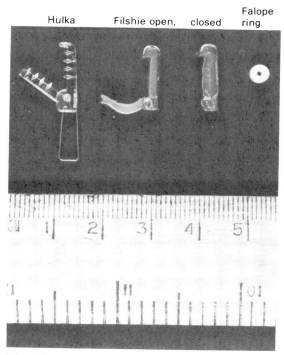

Fig. 11.1

Clinical studies

1. Falope ring

Mumford & Bhiwandiwala (1981) report on 10 086 post-partum cases in a multi-centre IFRP programme. The falope ring is made of silastic, has an outer diameter of 3.6 mm, an inner diameter of 1 mm and is 2.2 mm thick. When applied over a knuckle of tube it destroys approximately 3 cm of its length. At intervals sterilisation difficulties in application of the ring were experienced (Newton 1983) and these were also seen at puerperal sterilisation in 1.2% of cases. The difficulty was due in 60% of the cases to the patients characteristics, i.e. obesity, previous pelvic surgery, and in 40% of cases to instrument problems — the applicator or the rings. However, despite these difficulties it was possible in most cases to continue with the operation. Surgical complications (1.86%) did occur and were usually due to torn tubes; however, serious complications were rare. With the thick tubes found post-partum it is often best to employ the three stage grasping technique, gradually introducing the tube knuckle into the applicator milking the tube and so decreasing its diameter, thus preventing tearing of the tube.

The failure rate of this method at 1 year was 0.6 per 100 women and 0.86 per 100 women at 2 years — a low and acceptable rate, though it is higher than that reputed for interval sterilisation (Motashaw 1983).

2. Hulka Clips

The spring loaded clip developed by Hulka & Clemens (1972) has been widely used for sterilisation. However, some of its failures have been attributed to incomplete occlusion, a situation magnified by the thicker tube found in the puerperium. Bhiwandiwala et al (1982) compared different methods of sterilisation (diathermy, clip, rings) and found no method to have a distinct advantage. The failure rate is said by Leiberman (1983) to be less than 5/1000 cases. Surgical difficulty and complication rates are very similar to tubal rings being less than 2% (Bhiwandiwala et al 1982).

3. Filshie Clips

This, the newest of the clips to be used for sterilisation, is reviewed by Filshie (1983). The design of the Mark 5 clip allows the silicone rubber insert to accommodate for the different size of tube found in the puerperium. Failure rates vary between 0.9 and 4.9/1000 cases, and surgical complication rates were lower than with other clips or rings.

4. Diathermy

Conventional unipolar diathermy should now not be used for sterilisation due to the higher rate of serious complications (see RCOG Laparoscopy Survey 1978). Other electrical methods, unipolar diathermy and heat (thermal coagulation) have been used but destroy more tube than the methods mentioned above.

5. Mini laparotomy

This small abdominal incision (<7 cm) to expose the tubes, when coupled with uterine elevation is suitable for puerperal sterilisation. All of the methods (1 to

4) above can be used for tubal occlusion, but a common method is a modified Pomeroy tubal ligation. The WHO study (1982) reviewed a multicentre analysis of 1026 cases. Major complications only occurred in three subjects (0.3%) and minor complications in only 42 (4.2%). Local or general anaesthesia were used, and a modified Pomeroy technique applied to occlude the tubes. They concluded that mini laparotomy was a safe and effective method for puerperal sterilisation.

6. Culdotomy

An incision through the posterior vaginal fornix into the Pouch of Douglas is the standard method of approach to the Fallopian tubes in some countries (Wortman & Pistrow 1973). However, skilled vaginal surgeons are needed for this method, the overall complication rate is higher than the other methods mentioned above and the presence of pelvic disease and adhesions can cause technical failure in at least 2.1% of cases. This method is not recommended as a routine procedure.

Pregnancy following puerperal sterilisation

The failure rates of puerperal sterilisation are higher than for interval procedures (Chi et al 1981a for review). The methods reviewed were diathermy, tubal rings and clips, in 9399 cases. They were able to compare interval with post abortal and post delivery sterilisation and found a 2.4 fold increase in pregnancy rates after puerperal sterilisation. They comment on two reasons for this difference, first that gravid women may be more fecund and second mechanical problems with the equipment and the thicker post-partum tube (47.3% of cases) may play a part.

Ectopic pregnancy is known to occur after sterilisation (Chi et al 1981b for review). Factors known to increase the incidence of ectopics are prior pelvic or abdominal surgery or pelvic infection. Ectopics were also more common after diathermy sterilisation. It took longer to conceive ectopics, also the ratio of ectopics to intra-uterine pregnancies was 1:14 in the first year and 1:2 in the third and subsequent years post-sterilisation. Vessey et al (1983) confirmed a four times higher pregnancy rate in the first year post-sterilisation than subsequently. They also confirmed a higher ectopic rate in the second year when compared with the first year following sterilisation.

General conclusions

Sterilisation is safe when carried out in the puerperium. The increased failure rate has to be balanced against the need for the patient to be sterilised. Both mini laparotomy and laparoscopy can be used. For tubal occlusion a modified Pomeroy method or Filshie clips are recommended. Diathermy carries an increased risk of ectopic pregnancy while Hulka clips and Falope rings are at a disadvantage due to their design and the thickness of puerperal tubes. Male sterilisation (vasectomy) is a realistic and convenient alternative for many couples.

NATURAL FAMILY PLANNING (NFP)

The physiological changes in the puerperium, the influence of lactation or partial lactation all combine to make the recognition of ovulation difficult. As these changes are essential to the effective methods of natural family planning, the symptothermal method and the Billing's ovulation method (see Klause 1982 for review) confusion may occur. Both Billings et al (1980) and Kippley & Kippley (1977) make provision for this in their guides to these methods. Both presume that warnings will occur with changes in the cervical mucus, cervical os and the basal temperature. Harrison (1973) and Flynn et al (1983), both studying puerperal women, showed changes in the cervical mucus before temperature changes occurred, both studies also confirmed these changes with biochemical evidence of pre-ovulatory hormonal change and Flynn et al (1983) in addition carried out ultrasound scanning of ovarian follicles.

When NFP is to be used it is essential to have a properly trained teacher to teach these mucus and cervical os changes. It is helpful if the woman has been taught prior to pregnancy so that she can understand the normal cyclical changes and therefore be more able to recognise these changes in the puerperium and post-abortal state. Patients need to begin mucus observation following cessation of the lochia, regardless of their lactational state.

CONTRACEPTION POST-ABORTION (SPONTANEOUS AND INDUCED)

Ovulation occurs earlier than in the puerperium. The pregnancy changes are slighter due to the shorter length of gestation and therefore the normal state is resumed more quickly.

Hormal contraception

All methods can be used with safety. It is advisable to start 'the pill' the day after the miscarriage especially if the preceding pregnancy was unplanned or unwanted. It is logical to start with a combined formulation and not a progestogen only pill. Progestogen only pills should be restricted to those with medical indications for use, e.g. the older woman who smokes. Injectable contraception can also be used with safety.

Break-through bleeding often occurs during the first cycle of pill use, but again it can be disregarded and is often acceptable to the patient as she expects this after a miscarriage.

Intra-uterine contraception

In the past clinicians have been reluctant to insert an IUD immediately following termination of pregnancy or a miscarriage fearing an increased risk of uterine perforation, infection and expulsion of the IUD. However, there have now been several publications showing that this is safe and not associated with infection or uterine perforation (Andolsek 1972, Goldsmith et al 1972, Nygren & Johansson 1973, Timmen & Luukkainen 1974, Hue et al 1974).

Recently two multicentre studies by WHO looked at IUD insertion after spontaneous miscarriage (WHO 1983a), and termination of pregnancy (WHO 1983b). Both these studies confirmed the safety of immediate IUD insertion. Expulsion rates were not increased above intermenstrual rates when the pregnancy was less than 12 weeks. After termination no symptoms were reported by 90.9% of the subjects, and there were no perforations of the uterus. Of the three devices tested, the Lippes loop, Copper 7 and Copper T 220C, the Copper T performed best with the highest continuation rate at 390 and 750 days. However, all three devices had a higher expulsion rate ($\times 8$ to $\times 10$) when the pregnancy was more than 13 weeks and immediate IUD insertion is not recommended in this situation. There was no difference in the rate for medical removals (pain and bleeding).

Sterilisation

All methods and approaches are applicable but sterilisation does carry a higher morbidity and failure rate immediately after miscarriage or termination of pregnancy (see p. 00). However, this risk must be weighed against the risk of another unwanted pregnancy and failed contraception.

SUMMARY

Most of the anatomical changes in pregnancy have returned to normal by the end of the second week in the puerperium. The metabolic and endocrine changes take longer to regress.

Ovulation following pregnancy is variable and unpredictable in non-lactating women, this can be before 28 days, and at least one-third ovulate before the first period.

Full lactation will cause amenorrhoea and postpone ovulation but this requires 6 or more feeds totalling 60 or more minutes of suckling in each 24 hours.

Hormonal contraception is safe and effective. For lactating women, as the steroids cross into breast milk, a progestogen only pill is preferable. All other pill acceptors should have the lowest suitable dose and this may be a normophasic combined pill or a phasic preparation. These low dose pills have minimal side-effects and break-through bleeding, common in the first cycle, is masked by the post-pregnancy changes and more acceptable to the patient.

Injectable progestogens are a logical alternative for those who wish to use this method.

The immediate insertion of an IUD following pregnancy (post-placental) is safe and effective provided a long (25 cm) inserter is used. Insertion in the first week of the puerperium is associated with a higher expulsion rate. Insertion from 4 weeks onwards is safe and expulsion rates are low.

Post-abortal or post termination immediate insertion of an IUD is not associated with an increased risk of infection or other side-effects. Expulsion is low if the pregnancy is less than 12 weeks. For second trimester patients an IUD can be inserted with safety but there is a higher expulsion rate.

Natural family planning methods and barriers are effective for those who wish to use them, but both have problems in relation to failure rates and use.

Sterilisation is a very effective and safe method of permanent contraception. Laparoscopy or mini-laparotomy are both suitable methods to approach the Fallopian tubes. For tubal occlusion, the modified Pomeroy method or the newer type of clips (Filshie) are preferable. Other methods have a higher technical failure rate and an increased incidence of surgical difficulty. Pregnancy rates are higher following sterilisation post-partum and post-abortion but in the published studies at least half these failures are due to equipment malfunction or operator error. The newer methods avoid this. Diathermy is associated with an increased ectopic rate and is not to be recommended. Regret and guilt following sterilisation only occur if a hasty decision has been reached involving one partner; if in doubt it is best to use alternative methods and re-discuss sterilisation some months later.

Too often clinicians delay the start of contraception and ask the patient to await the first period. Immediate post-pregnancy contraception is safe and will avoid unnecessary unplanned pregnancy.

REFERENCES

Anderson W R, Davis J 1968 Placental site involution. American Journal of Obstetrics and Gynecology 102: 23–31

Andolsek L 1972 Immedate Post Abortion IUD insertion. In: Lewit S (ed) Abortion Techniques and Services, pp 63–67. Excerpta Medica, Amsterdam

Apelo R, Ramos R, Thomas M 1976 The LEM device in an immediate post partum contraceptive programme. Fertility and Sterility 27: 517–522

Archer D F, Josimovich J B 1976 Ovarian response to erogenous gonadotropins in women with elevated serum prolactin. Obstetrics and Gynecology 48: 155–159

Banharnsupawat L, Rosenfield A G 1971 Immediate post partum IUD insertion. Obstetrics and Gynecology 38: 276–285

Beller F K, Ebert C 1982 The coagulation and filirinolytic enzyme system in pregnancy and the puerperium. European Journal of Obstetrics, Gynaecology and Reproductive Biology 13: 177–197

Bhiwandiwala 1982 A comparison of different laparoscopic sterilization occlusion techniques in 24 439 procedures. American Journal of Obstetrics and Gynecology 144: 319–331

Billings E, Billings J J, Catarinich M 1980 Atlas of the Ovulation Method. Advocate Press, Australia

Bonnar J, McNicol G P, Douglas A S 1970 Coagulation and filirinolytie mechanisms during and after normal childbirth. British Medical Journal 2: 200–203

Brenner P 1983 A clinical trial of the Delta T IUD. Immediate post partum use. Contraception 28: 135–147

Canales E S, Zarate A, Garrido J et al 1974 Study of the recovery of pituitary FSH function during puerperium using synthetic LRH. Journal of Clinical and Endocrinological Metabolism 38: 1140–1144

Canales E S, Fonseca M E, Mason M, Zarate A 1981 Feedback effect of estradiol on Follicle-stimulating hormone and prolactin secretion during the puerperium. International Journal of Gynaecology and Obstetrics 19: 79–81

Chi I C, Mumford S D, Gardner S D 1981a Pregnancy risk following laparoscopic sterilization in non-gravid and gravid women. Journal of Reproductive Medicine 26: 289–294

Chi I C, Lauffe L E, Atwood R J 1981b Ectopic Pregnancy following female sterilisation procedures. Advances in Planned parenthood XVI 52–58

Cronin T J 1968 Influence of lactation upon ovulation. Lancet ii: 422

Croxatto H B, Diaz S, Peralta O, Juez G, Casado M E, Salvatierra A M, Duran E 1982a Comparative performance of progesterone implants versus placebo and copper T. American Journal of Obstetrics and Gynecology 144: 201–208

Croxatto H B, Diaz S, Peralta O, Salvatierra A M, Brandeis A 1982b Plasma progesterone levels following subdermal implantation of progesterone pellets in lactating women. Acta Endocrinologica 100: 630–6

Croxatto H B, Diaz S, Peralta O, Juez G, Herreros C, Casado M E, Salvatierra A M, Miranda P, Duran E 1983 Fertility regulation in nursing women: long term influence of a low dose combined oral contraceptive initiated at day 30 post partum upon lactation and infant growth. Contraception 27: 13–25

Davis H J 1972 Intrauterine contraceptive devices. American Journal of Obstetrics and Gynecology 114: 134

Delvoye P, Delogne-Desnoeck Robyn C, 1980 Hyperprolactinaemia during prolonged lactation: evidence for anovulatory cycles and inadequate corpus luteum. Clinical Endocrinology 13: 243–247

Diamond R A, Freeman D W 1973 Insertion of IUCDs in the early post partum period. Minnesota Medicine 56: 49–50

Diaz S, Peralta O, Juez G, Herreros C, Casado M E, Salvatierra A M, Miranda P, Duran E, Croxatto H B 1983 Fertility regulation in nursing women: short term influence of a low-dose combined oral contraceptive upon lactation and infant growth. Contraception 27: 1–11

Drill V A 1966 Oral Contraceptives. New York, McGraw-Hill

Emens J M, Shah S 1982 Early post partum insertion of the Multiload. British Journal of Obstetrics and Gynaecology (Suppl) 4: 43–45

Emens J M, Gustafson R C, Jordan J A 1978 The use of an IUD in the early post partum period. British Journal of Fertility and Contraception 2: 38–41

Falsetti L, Voltolini A M, Pollini C, Pontiroli A E 1982 A study of prolactin, follicle-stimulating hormone and luteinizing hormone in puerperium: spontaneous variations and effect of nutergoline. Fertility and Sterility 37: 397–401

Filshie G M 1983 The Filshie Clip. In: Van Lith D A F, Naith L G, Van Hall E V (eds) New Trends in Female Sterilization, pp 115–124. Year Book Medical, Chicago

Flynn A 1981 A survey of postpartum fertility studies with particular reference to the breastfeeding mother. International Journal of Fertility 26: 203–208

Flynn A M, Lynch S S, Docker M, Morris R 1983 Clinical Hormonal and Ultrasonic Indications of Returning Fertility. In: Harrison R F et al (eds) Fertility and Sterility Proceedings of XIth World Congress of Fertility and Sterility, pp 325–335. MTP Press, Lancaster

Gentile G P, Seigler A M 1977 The missing IUD. Obstetrics and Gynaecology Survey 32: 627

Goldsmith R, Goldberg H et al 1972 In: Snowdon R, Goldsmith R (eds) IUD Insertion Post Abortion. Family Planning Research Conference, pp 59–67. Excerpta Medica, Amsterdam

Harrison P E F 1973 Returning Fertility during Lactation. Ovulation Method Workshop. Catholic Family Life Centre, Australia

Heikkila M 1982 Puerperal Insertion of a copper releasing and a levonorgestrel releasing IUD. Contraception 25: 561–572

Heikkila M, Haukkamaa, Luukkainen T 1982 Levonorgestrel in milk plasma of breast feeding women with levonorgestrel releasing IUDs. Contraception 25: 41–49

Heikkila M, Luukkainen T 1982 Duration of breast feeding and development of children after levonorgestrel IUCDs. Contraception 25: 279–292

Hennart P, Delogne-Desnoeck J, Vis H, Robyn C 1981 Serum levels of prolactin and milk production in women during a lactation period of thirty minutes. Clinical Endocrinology 14: 349–353

Howie P W, Evans K, Forbes C D 1975 The effects of stilboestrol and quimestrol upon coagulation and filirinolysis during puerperium. British Journal of Obstetrics and Gynaecology 82: 968–974

Howie P W, McNeilly A S, Houston M J, Cook A, Boyle H 1981 Effect of supplementary food on suckling patterns and ovarian activity during lactation. British Medical Journal 283: 757–759

Howie P W, McNeilly A S, Houston M J, Cook A, Boyle H 1982 Fertility after childbirth: infant feeding patterns, basal PPL levels and post partum ovulation. Clinical Endocrinology 17: 315–322

Hue K, Kwan H Y et al 1974 Efficiency and safety of post abortal IUD insertion. American Journal of Obstetrics and Gynecology 118: 975–978

Hulka J F, Omran K F 1972 Comparative tubal occlusion rigid and spring loaded clips. Fertility and Sterility 23: 633

Hull V J 1981 The effects of hormonal contraceptives on lactation. Studies in Family Planning 12: 134–155

Husni E A, Pena L I, Lenhert A E 1967 Thrombophlebitis in pregnancy. American Journal of Obstetrics and Gynecology 97: 901–905

Inman W H W, Vessey M P, Westerholm B, Engelund A 1970 Thromboembolic disease and the steroidal content of oral contraceptives. A report of the Committee on the Safety of Drugs. British Medical Journal 2: 203–209

Kamal I, Ezzat R, Zaki S, Shaaban H, L'eisel E 1980 Immediate post partum insertion of a sutured lippa loop. International Journal of Obstetrics and Gynecology 18: 26–30

Keith L, Labbok M, Petty J, Berger G S 1979 Postpartum and Post Abortal Contraception, p. 4. Synapse Publications, Pennsylvania

Kippley J F, Kippley S 1977 The Art of Natural Family Planning. The Couple to Couple League International, USA

Klaus H 1982 Natural family planning, a review. Obstetrical and Gynaecological Survey 37: 128–150

Kletzky O A, Marrs R P, Howard W F, McCormick W, Mishell D R 1980 Prolactin synthesis and release during pregnancy and puerperium. American Journal of Obstetrics and Gynecology 136: 545–550

Kochonour N K 1980 Lactation Suppression. Clinical Obstetrics and Gynaecology 23: 1045–1059

Lieberman B A 1983 The Hulka Clemens Clip. In: Van Lith D A F, Naith L G, Van Hall E V (eds) New trends in Female Sterilization, pp 105–114. Year Book Medical, Chicago

McLaren H C 1952 The Involution of the Cervix. British Medical Journal 1: 347–350

Melis G B, Strigini F, Fruzzetti F, Paoletti A M, Rainer E, Dusterberg B, Fioretti P 1981 Norethisterone enanthate as an injectable contraceptive in puerperal and non puerperal women. Contraception 23: 77–88

Mishell D R Jr 1983 In: Newton J R (ed) Intrauterine Devices in Clinics in Obstetrics and Gynaecology. W. B. Saunders, Philadelphia

Mishell D R Jr, Roy S 1982 Copper IUCD event rates following insertion 4 to 8 weeks post partum. American Journal of Obstetrics and Gynecology 143: 29–35

Monheit A G, Cousins L, Resnik R 1980 The puerperium: anatomic and physiologic readjustments. Clinical Obstetrics and Gynaecology 23: 973–983

Morishita H, Higuchi K, Nakago K, Hashimoto T, Mitani H, Mori T, Oshima I 1984 Hypothalamic function in women during the first month post partum. Acta Endocrinologica 105: 145–148

Motashaw N D 1983 The Falope ring technique. In: Van Lith D A F, Naith L G, Van Hall E V (eds) New Trends in Female Sterilization, pp 97–104. Year Book Medical, Chicago

Mumford D S, Bhiwandiwala P P 1981 Tubal ring sterilization experience with 10 086 cases. Obstetrics and Gynaecology 57: 150–157

Nakano R, Kayashima F, Mori A, Kotsuti F 1974 Gonadotropin response to luteinising hormone releasing factor (LRF) in puerperal women. Acta et Obstetrica Gynaecologica Scandinavica 53: 303–309

Newton J R 1982 Copper intrauterine devices. British Journal of Obstetrics and Gynaecology (Suppl) 4: 20

Newton J R 1983 Sterilization. In: Newton J R (ed) Clinics in Obstetrics and Gynaecology. W. B. Saunders, Philadelphia

Newton J, Harper M, Chan K K 1977 Immediate post placental insertion of IUCDs. Lancet ii: 272–274

Nilson C G, Luukkainen T 1977 Improvement of a norgestrel releasing IUD. Contraception 15: 295–306

Nygren K G, Johansson E D B 1973 Insertion of T.Cu. 200 Immediately After Termination. Contraception 7: 299–306

Pascal J 1969 Some aspects of post partum physiology: contribution of the basal body temperature and its application to birth regulations. A statistical study of 750 cases. M.D. Thesis. University of Nancy, France

Peralta O, Diaz S, Juez G, Herreros C, Casado M E, Salvatierra A M, Miranda P, Duran E, Croxatto H B 1983 Fertility Regulation in nursing women: long term influence of low-dose combined oral contraceptive initiated at day 90 post partum upon lactation and infant growth. Contraception 27: 27–38

Perez A, Vela P, Masnick G S, Potter R G 1972 First ovulation after childbirth: the effect of breast feeding. American Journal of Obstetrics and Gynecology 114: 1041–1047

Pritchard J A, MacDonald P C 1976 Williams' Obstetrics, 15 edn, pp 374–375, 377. Appleton-Century-Crofts, New York

Ratnam S S, Tow S H 1970 In: Wolfer D D (ed) Translocation of the Loop in Post Partum Contraception. Excerpta Medica, Amsterdam

Rodeck C H, Newton J R 1976 Study of the uterine cavity by ultrasound in the early puerperium. British Journal of Obstetrics and Gynaecology 83: 795–801

RCOG 1978 In: Chamberlain G, Lawson Bourne J (eds) Laparoscopy Survey Publ: Royal College of Obstetrics & Gynaecologists. pp 105–139

Ryu K, Hong S S 1983 The effect of combined oral contraceptive steroids on the gonadotrophin response to LH-RH in lactating women with regular menstrual cycles resumed. Contraception 27: 605–617

Sharman A 1953 Postpartum regeneration of the human endometrium. Journal of Anatomy 87: 1–10

Stepan J, Kellog E H, Piotrow P T 1981 Legal Trends and Issues in Voluntary Sterilization. Population Report (E), No. 6

Tatum H J 1977 Clinical aspects of intrauterine contraception. Fertility and Sterility 28: 3

Thiery M 1980 Immediate post partum insertion of intrauterine devices. Contraceptive Delivery Systems 1: 228–230

Tietze C, Lewit S 1970 An evaluation of IUDs: Nuth progress Report to the C.S.S.P. Studies in Family Planning 55: 14

Thomson A M, Hytten F E, Black A E 1975 Lactation and Reproduction. Bulletin of the World Health Organisation 52: 337–349

Timmen H, Luukkainen T 1974 Immediate post abortion Insertion of the Copper T. Contraception 9: 153–160

Vemer H M, Rolland R 1981 The dynamics of prolactin secretion during the puerperium in women. Clinical Endocrinology 15: 155–163

Vessey M, Higgins G, Lawless M, Yeates D 1983 Tubal sterilization: findings in a large prospective study. British Journal of Obstetrics and Gynaecology 90: 203–209

Wathen N C, Sapire M E, Davey D A 1978 Post partum insertion of the multiload IUD. South African Medical Journal 54: 473–476

Williams J W 1931 Regeneration of the uterine mucosa after delivery, with special reference to the placental site. American Journal of Obstetrics and Gynecology 22: 664–669

WHO 1978 Annual report of the special programme in Human Reproduction

WHO 1980 Comparative multicentre trial of three IUDs inserted immediately following delivery of the placenta. Contraception 22: 9–18

WHO 1982 Mini incision for post partum sterilisation. Contraception 26: 495–503

WHO 1983a IUD insertion following termination of pregnancy. Studies in Family Planning 14: 99–107

WHO 1983b IUD Insertion following Spontaneous Abortion. Studies in Family Planning 14: 109–114

Wortman J, Pistrow P T 1973 Colpotomy the vaginal approach. Population Reports (c) No. 3

Confidential enquiry into maternal deaths

Dame Janet Campbell was not an obstetrician but did more for the maternity service than many clinicians who were working in the subject. Dame Janet joined the administrative Health Service soon after qualifying and when the new Ministry of Health was formed in 1918 Sir George Newcombe took her with him to this Department. Here she established herself rapidly in the field of maternal and child care and reviewed the subject of maternal mortality in a report published in 1924 (Campbell 1924); she came down hard on the inadequacies of the maternity services. During the 1920s the maternal mortality rate rose significantly (see Fig. 12.1). The Ministry of Health was concerned about this and a central committee was formed which asked Medical Officers of Health confidentially to investigate each maternal death occurring in their geographical area. This was done with varying degrees of completeness and reports were published in the early 1930s. Unfortunately, Dame Janet Campbell left the Ministry of Health in 1933 when she married and before the results of her penetrating questioning bore fruit.

Up until 1953, comments on the Ministry's assessment would appear in the Chief Medical Officer's Annual Reports but the fuller system of Confidential Reports on the Enquiries into Maternal Deaths for England and Wales started in 1952. The report of the Chief Medical Officer (CMO) for that year (1953) considered the old system of enquiries which were often incomplete and commended the new system. The new Enquiry would place a clinical assessment of the factors of each death in the hands of practising clinical obstetricians. The clinical assessors were also asked to examine the cases to tease out avoidable factors. From then on, the reports have been produced in triennia up to the latest published in 1982 which covered the years 1976–78 (DHSS 1982).

In parallel with this, Scottish reports have been produced examining the years 1965–75 and from Northern Ireland four reports have appeared assessing the years 1956–77. In both these Celtic Kingdoms, the populations were smaller and the numbers of maternal deaths were few compared with those of England and Wales which has a much larger number of births. However, these reports should be examined in conjunction for they give a complete picture of

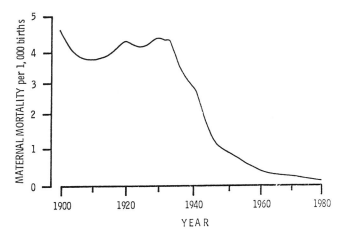

Fig. 12.1 The Maternal Mortality Rate this century. Note the rise in the 1920s

the United Kingdom, a single country under a reasonably unified Health Service, dealing with a varied population.

The usefulness of such complex enquiries depends greatly on the completeness of the reporting; among the missing cases are often the most important from which to learn. The first Report on the Confidential Enquiry into Maternal Deaths in England and Wales covered the years 1952–54 and examined 77% of all known registered true maternal deaths. The 1976–78 report covered 227 out of 228 known true maternal deaths — 99.6% of the total population and the one missing case was submitted, although too late for the published report.

MECHANISM OF THE ENQUIRY

The Confidential Enquiry into Maternal Deaths is voluntary, performed by the professionals without statutory obligations. It depends upon confidentiality. Only one copy of a report on a given maternal death is made and this is initiated by the District Medical Officer (England and Wales) or to the Chief Administrative Medical Officer (Scotland and Northern Ireland). Other cases are reported directly to the Department of Health by coroners. Details from medical and nursing staff about the care of the patient are obtained and, if performed, those of autopsy investigations are also included. The information collected is then examined by a senior appointed Regional Obstetrical Assessor. Where there are relevant aspects, Regional Anaesthetic or Pathology Assessors are also consulted. With the conjoint Assessors' comments and opinions, the papers are referred to the CMO where all patient identification is removed. The documents are dealt with at the DHSS by one medical officer on behalf of the CMO and considered by four Central Advisors. Once the Report for that triennium has been prepared, all documents are destroyed.

Essential to the confidentiality of the system is that no copies of the report or any related papers on the maternal death which are prepared for the enquiry are kept in the hospital notes or at any other stage. In the United Kingdom the Courts can empower lawyers or their nominated medical advisers to examine hospital notes in certain litigant circumstances; anything that is contained in the medical and nursing records must be made available. Hence no copy of the report sent to the District Medical Officer should be kept in the hospital records or by the Health Authority. Recently this precaution was not observed and in consequence there was a potential hazard to the whole Confidential Enquiry. The Enquiry mechanism was stopped by the Chief Medical Officer for 8 months but was restarted when it was clear that requests from a Court for the disclosure of documents related to the Enquiry could be resisted on public interest grounds. No attempt has yet been made to obtain a court order for disclosure of documents completed for the purposes of the Enquiry. Should this happen a claim for *public interest immunity* would be vigorously pressed before the Court by the Crown on the grounds that production of such documents would be against the public interest because not only this Enquiry, but also other similar types of confidential enquiry already being planned, would certainly have to be discontinued if absolute confidentiality was not observed. This has not been tested in the Courts but the assurances of the CMOs on this point have reassured the professionals and allowed this unique self-audit to continue.

The data are grouped and analysed by the Central Assessors and the chapters of the Report are discussed with the Regional Assessors, so that the final assessments have taken their views into account and these have been coordinated by the authors to produce a report which is generally acceptable to them all. A report on each Triennium is produced with the statistical assistance of OPCS (The Office of Population Censuses and Surveys) and published by HMSO.

CHANGE IN DEFINITIONS

With the altered definitions of maternal death and the changing denominator against which it is set, the rates are difficult to compare from one country to another and from one time to another in the same country. Generally speaking in Britain, the International Classification of Diseases (ICD) has been taken as the source of definitions for classifying the causes of maternal death. There have been nine revisions so far (with a tenth due in a few years) and each is slightly different from the previous revisions. Many conditions previously outside the maternity section are being re-classified into the maternity area as associated conditions or indirect obstetric causes and this widens the numerator of the ratio.

All the deaths within 1 year of an abortion or delivery count in the statistics of the Confidential Enquiry definitions of maternal mortality, thus differing from the definitions of the Fédération Internationale de Gynécologie et d'Obstétrique and the World Health Organisation, which only consider deaths within 42 days (6 weeks) of childbirth. This apparent large discrepancy in fact makes little difference in the proportions but does allow for a source of under-reporting if people forget to enter the pregnancy in the death certificate of a woman who dies some months after the event.

The denominator too has changed. Maternal deaths used to be expressed per thousand live births but in 1928 this was altered to total births by including stillbirths. In the examination of maternal deaths however, we now include deaths from abortion and ectopic pregnancy. Many consider that the denominator also should include all women with such conditions. Legal induced abortions may be fairly well categorised in England, Wales and Scotland but spontaneous abortions are an unknown quantity. There is no statutory obligation to report them, many do not reach hospital and some are not even known to the woman herself. Ectopic pregnancies are probably fairly well recognised and recorded for most would enter a NHS hospital and thus numbers might be obtained from the hospital in-patient enquiry (HIPE). Data are given per million estimated pregnancies. Because of these vagaries, the other denominators are probably best kept at total births on which data are reasonably precise.

Another simple factor is changing the way maternal mortality rates are expressed. With the smaller numbers of maternal deaths, rates per thousand mean little; the latest maternal mortality rate to be published in 1982 for England and Wales was 0.11 per thousand births. It is more convenient to shift the decimal point and so rates per 100 000 births are now commonly quoted (11/110 000). Since the minds of non-statistical humans often cluster on certain round numbers, like the million, it may well be that 110 per million will become the expressed maternal mortality rate as in Table 17.1 in the 1976–78 Report.

CONTENTS OF ENQUIRY

The flavour of each report varies slightly but an examination of the latest published will give an idea of what the working obstetrician can obtain from each. A copy of this report was sent to each consultant obstetrician in the country.

In the triennium covered (1976–1978) the maternal mortality rate for England and Wales was 11.9 per 100 000 total births. The report starts with data which should interest anybody associated with obstetrics; total numbers of births by socio-economic class and place of birth are included and maternities by age and parity are examined. Deaths by region are assessed and rates in the regions varied from 5.4 in the Wessex region to 18.0 per 100 000 in North East Thames during the 3 years. There were reduced numbers of deaths attributed to abortion and sepsis; the reduction in number of deaths from hypertensive disease was balanced by the rise in those from pulmonary embolism and haemorrhage. The last cause was examined in detail to include the usual maternal deaths from uterine haemorrhage, and other causes such as rupture of the uterus and ectopic pregnancy. Assessors recommended that each obstetric unit should have its own procedure for the treatment of catastrophic haemorrhage. Input from the Regional Assessors in Anaesthesia appears in this volume but not that of the Regional Pathologists for they were not in post during the triennium assessed here.

Deaths associated with pregnancy as opposed to those directly due to it have been divided into *indirect* and *fortuitous causes* following the 9th International Classification of Maternal Deaths. For each individual cause of death, a new statistical device has been used whereby the number of expected deaths (on the basis of age and parity from previous years) were compared with the number of actual deaths that occurred.

DEATHS BY CAUSE

The true maternal deaths are examined by cause. As always pulmonary embolism, hypertensive disease, haemorrhage and abortion are among the major causes of death in this report, and ectopic pregnancy has been included also. This is not due so much to an increase in the number of ectopic pregnancies that kill but a reduction in all the other causes. Anaesthesia is identified in this report as a specific cause of death following the recommendations of the 9th International Classification of Disease.

Hypertension

Fewer women died in association with eclampsia and the reduction in deaths from this cause was greater than that from pre-eclampsia. Cerebral haemorrhage was the commonest cause of death amongst the hypertensive women; 72% of the deaths directly caused by hypertensive disease was thought to have one or more avoidable factors.

Haemorrhage

A disturbing feature in the haemorrhage section was the increase in deaths from postpartum haemorrhage, many of them in the group of women having their first baby. Among the antepartum deaths, stress was placed upon the need for early blood transfusion in those with placental abruption. If a placenta praevia is diagnosed, the Caesarean section should be supervised by a consultant and not left to a junior doctor alone.

An increasingly important feature was that a disorder of blood coagulation was found in 17 out of 40 deaths associated with haemorrhage. In almost half these amniotic fluid embolism was suspected but only in a small number was the diagnosis confirmed histologically.

Emphasis has been placed upon the aggressive treatment of massive haemorrhage. If the bleeding cannot be controlled by manual compression of

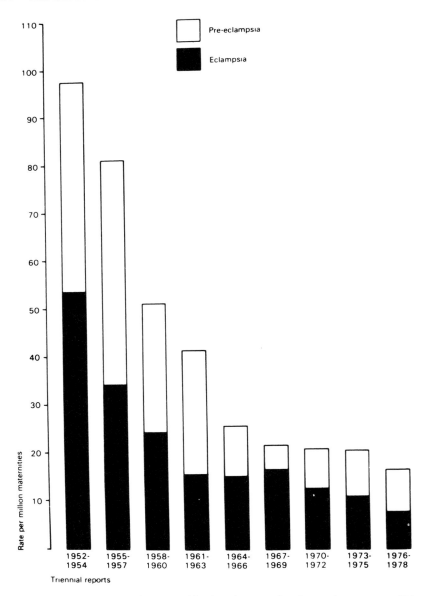

Fig. 12.2 Death Rates per million maternities from hypertensive diseases in pregnancy. Taken from the Reports of 1952–1978

the uterus and direct compression of the aorta then, after treatment of any coagulation disorder, either ligation or the internal iliac arteries or a hysterectomy must be done promptly. This requires an experienced obstetrician to be available. The value of a central venous pressure line in monitoring the patient's condition was stressed.

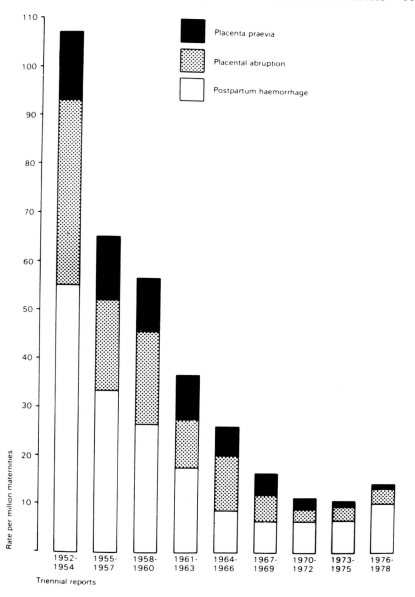

Fig. 12.3 Death rate per million maternities from haemorrhage. Note the lack of reduction in rates of postpartum haemorrhage compared with the continuing improvements in antepartum haemorrhage

Pulmonary embolism

The larger number of women who died in this section did so with no preliminary warning of thrombosis, particularly in the antenatal period. The increased risks of obesity and Caesarean section were shown and a small number of women died of pulmonary embolism after lactation had been suppressed by oestrogens after delivery. Attention was drawn to the failure to think of deep vein thrombosis as a diagnosis, the need to watch for this always and be prepared to act upon it speedily.

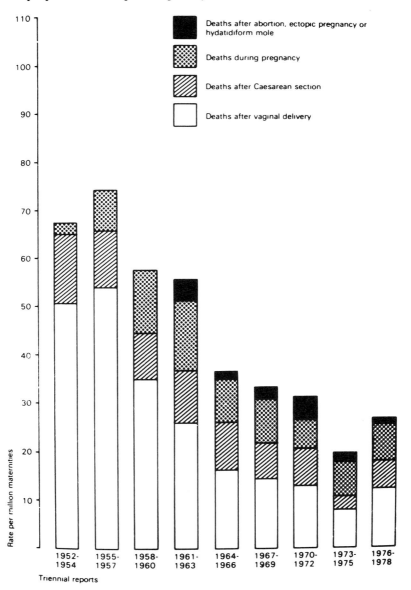

Fig. 12.4 Death rate per million maternities from pulmonary embolism. Note the steady rate in the antepartum period since 1964

Abortion

This section showed that deaths from all categories of abortion were much reduced on the previous triennium. Among deaths following a legal abortion, the majority were those in the mid-trimester of pregnancy. The report

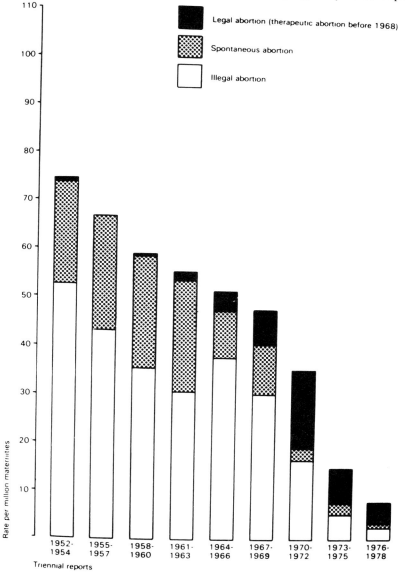

Fig. 12.5 Death rate per million maternities from abortion. Note the Abortion Act came into force in this country in 1969 and the following triennium had an increased death rate after legal abortions for the actual numbers went up enormously. From then on however, the rate has been decreasing

reiterated its concern about the continued use of Utus paste to perform abortions.

Caesarean section

Deaths connected with Caesarean section were examined; a mortality rate of 0.8 per thousand Caesarean sections performed in the National Health Service hospitals was derived. This is lower than the rate in the two previous triennia. The major individual causes were haemorrhage, pulmonary embolism and sepsis. The number of deaths associated with anaesthesia in Caesarean section showed no improvement from previous triennia and the problem of leaving a woman for Caesarean section to a junior anaesthetist was stressed.

In this section, the six postmortem Caesarean sections reported to the Confidential Enquiry were described; four of the infants were stillborn and two died within a week of delivery. This emphasises the futility of many postmortem Caesarean sections where, with much drama, a fetus is brought forth in an inappropriate place. Most women who die in pregnancy do so with an increasing hypoxia over the hours before death and so the fetus is considerably damaged before the Caesarean section starts. After birth paediatric facilities might not be at their best and the 100% perinatal mortality rate in even this small series should emphasise to the enthusiastic that postmortem Caesarean section very rarely results in good neonatal outcome.

Anaesthesia

In the section on anaesthesia, 38 out of 40 deaths were judged to have avoidable factors. Most of these were due to the lack of knowledge, inexperience or low standards of anaesthetic care in labour. Sixteen of the deaths were associated with difficulties with endotracheal intubation, eleven of whom died associated with Mendelson's syndrome. Four deaths were after epidural analgesia; an anaesthetist of some experience should not just be at the induction of anaesthesia but available for the whole of labour afterwards.

Rupture of the uterus

Attention was drawn to care in the use of oxytocic drugs, particularly among multiparae when there had been a previous Caesarean section. Clinicians were also warned that a continuing postpartum haemorrhage in the presence of a well contracted uterus should lead to a suspicion of a uterine tear leading to a senior doctor examining the cavity of the uterus and if he has any residual doubt, performing a laparotomy.

Ectopic pregnancy

Here it was stressed that since 1970 the mortality rate associated with this condition has not improved although the number of cases have been reduced greatly. A third of the women who died collapsed so suddenly there was no chance to give treatment. None of the deaths reported had an intra-uterine device in use but two of the women had previous tubal surgery. This high proportion, although not of statistical significance, should warn gynaecologists that when they perform plastic surgery on the Fallopian tubes they should indicate to the woman the increased risk of ectopic pregnancy following and discuss the early symptoms of this.

Infection

Mortality rates from this cause have continued to reduce after both childbirth and abortion. The risks of sepsis of the genital tract associated with anaerobic organisms are stressed. This condition can present in a variety of ways without the woman even being well enough to raise a pyrexia. There was an increase in the number of bowel perforations reported leading to peritoneal infection and death. The assessors also draw attention to uterine infections and septicaemia in association with cervical encirclage. Most obstetricians remove such a stitch as soon as the membranes rupture but sometimes it is kept in for clinically good reasons; the risks must be remembered.

ASSOCIATED CAUSES OF MATERNAL DEATHS

These are now divided into indirect and fortuitous. The former were deaths resulting from a previous existing disease which did not have a direct obstetrical cause but was aggravated by the physiological effects of pregnancy. An example would be mitral stenosis. Fortuitous deaths are those among well women who were pregnant at the time of death (or were within a year of it) but apparently the death was not related to or aggravated by the pregnancy, for example a road traffic accident. Differentiation depends upon the opinion of the clinical advisers; for example, of two women who died from septicaemia, one was considered to be an indirect death for she developed varicela at about the tenth week of pregnancy and threatened to abort. She was admitted to hospital but deteriorated and died soon. The death was considered to be due to viraemia and septicaemia with beta haemolytic streptocii being isolated in many sites. The source of this infection was not known so this was considered to be an indirect death because the pregnancy was unaffected. The other woman died from septicaemia due to haemolytic streptoccus in the puerperium. She however, had a graze on her elbow which was thought to be the source of the infection; this was therefore considered to be a fortuitous death. The differentiation between cases depends on how much information is available to the assessors and then on their clinical opinion. The Central Assessors will have to build up a core of case law to which they can refer back in order to get consistency in the future.

DOMICILIARY CONFINEMENTS

The death rate of women booked initially for a home confinement was reduced in this report in parallel with the diminution of births occurring in that locus. In the two previous reports there had been 44 and 10 such deaths reported whilst in the 1976–78 report there were only six. Of these only three were actually delivered at home and were due to an infection after an apparently normal delivery, to pulmonary embolism and to eclampsia. By the period of the review (1976–78) home deliveries made up only 2% of all births and so numbers are now so small that statistically valid correlations are hard to obtain.

AVOIDABLE FACTORS

A feature of the Reports of the Confidential Enquiry into Maternal Death has always been the attribution by the advisers of avoidable factors in groups of deaths These are cases where some aspect of the mother's care fell short of the accepted standards at that time and therefore contributed to the fatal outcome. It is not intended to mean that death could have been prevented or that the factor itself was a direct cause of the mother's death. This is obviously a subjective judgement and changes slightly as the advisers themselves change over the years. Further, the very publication of these reports has led to a rise in the level of what is considered to be normal care. In consequence, even though the standards of obstetrical care have risen in the 25 years under review, the percentage of deaths with avoidable factors has not dropped; it has stayed around 40% until 1966 and rose from thereon so that in the latest report it was 59%. This is as much a measure of the improved standards set by the observers as of lowered standards of the maternity services.

Attributing an avoidable factor implies some departure from generally accepted standards; it might therefore be used as a rough measure of care in that triennium, bearing in mind the way it is derived. A further subjective assessment is made when apportioning the responsibility of these factors among those concerned in childbirth (Table 12.1). In the antenatal period, the commonest single group responsible for an avoidable factor were the patients themselves (36.2%) whilst in labour it was the obstetrical staff (47.8%) and anaesthetists (32.3%). During the puerperium obstetricians again had the major proportion of 43.6%.

The apportionment of responsibility to administration is very low — only six out of 234 examined cases (2.6%). As the economic shortages in the Health Service become more evident, staff and service deficiencies may occur; the Regional Assessors should watch for these features and firmly allocate such avoidable factors to administration and not consider them to be the responsibility of the obstetrical and anaesthetic staff. Reference has already been made to under-supervised junior staff coping with emergency conditions; such problems may be associated with staff shortages, less well qualified locums and split appointments at several geographical sites.

Table 12.1 The apportionment of responsibility and the time in pregnancy of avoidable factors for maternal deaths. Taken from the 1976–1978 Enquiry series with permission from HMSO. Note that the numbers in this table are not mutually exclusive

Responsible person	Total	Antenatal period	Labour or operative procedure	Puerperium or post-operative period
Number(%)	Number(%)	Number(%)	Number(%)	Number(%)
Patient	54(23.1)	38(36.2)	7(7.8)	9(23.1)
General Practitioner	30(12.8)	21(20.0)	4(4.4)	5(12.8)
Consultant obstetric unit staff	95(40.6)	35(33.3)	43(47.8)	17(43.6)
Midwife	4(1.7)	2(1.9)	2(2.2)	0(0)
Anaesthetist	35(15.0)	3(2.9)	29(32.2)	3(7.7)
Other hospital staff	9(3.8)	4(3.8)	1(1.1)	4(10.3)
Other community staff	1(0.4)	0(0)	0(0)	1(2.6)
Administration	6(2.6)	2(1.9)	4(4.4)	0(0)
Total	234(100.0)	105(100.0)	90(99.9)	39(100.1)

The woman herself was attributed to be responsible for some avoidable factors, particularly if she would not come for or accept care. The doctors were not assessed on clinical judgement for this is so often a matter of individual judgement but when standards fell behind the norms of clinical management (set by the assessors) this has been attributed. Examples would be failure to treat fulminating pre-eclampsia, not calling an obstetrical flying squad or leaving junior staff to carry out more difficult obstetrics or anaesthesia when experienced help was available.

These criticisms should be borne in mind, particularly with the pressure to involve consultant obstetricians in more labour ward work in the next decade. When the quotations are used in isolation from the Confidential Enquiry, one would do well to return to the original definitions of the avoidable factors and then take the arguments from the beginning rather than just use the published figures superficially as they are published.

THE FUTURE

The pattern of the reports of the Confidential Enquiry are bound to show change. They have evolved over 25 years and altering obstetric management has changed rapidly inside this time. Numbers of maternal deaths are falling and fears of litigation are rising. The former allows problems of small figure variation to intrude and blur trends; the latter may cause staff to be reluctant to provide details of the clinical management. Bringing the definitions in line with international classifications will allow better comparisons with other countries. The Regional assessors in Pathology will be adding their comments more frequently and this will certainly change the pattern of the reports.

One is uncertain that the present system allows the Central Assessors to examine questions which are of great import in the future of obstetrics. For example, the increasing numbers of Caesarean sections in the United Kingdom is of concern to many inside and outside the profession. Perhaps a fuller assessment of the fatal risks to the mother would make obstetricians reflect before operating unthinkingly just to provide the neonatal paediatricians with a better small baby.

Another problem is the rate of death from post-partum haemorrhage which is now higher than it was in 1964. Careful examination of the deaths by the Central Assessors might lead to a fuller investigation of practice and any trends that may be appearing. Giving oxytocic drugs at the end of the second stage of labour to prevent bleeding in the third stage has become such a routine that details of timing, the drug used and the dosage may sometimes be relegated to junior midwifery staff. Further, there may be some movement against the use of oxytocics by the more vocative mothers who wish not to use pharmacology to help their childbirth. These influences need examination and the report on the Confidential Enquiry into Maternal Deaths could be a strong leader.

The apparent discrepancy with data generated from other countries could be diminished in future reports if a classification of Maternal Deaths was used with the cut-off point at 6 weeks (42 days) after childbirth. There are relatively few maternal deaths reported in the period 6–52 weeks and these might be reported in a separate section.

For many years the reports have been accepted as great examples of a national audit in which the profession looks at itself and is prepared to publish its results. If it is to go into the last decade of this century, the organisers should reflect the altered pattern of obstetrics which will be happening by then and mould the pattern of their future work to be of benefit to the woman having the babies and to obstetricians.

ACKNOWLEDGEMENTS

The author is grateful to the Comptroller of Her Majesty's Stationery Office for permission to re-publish Table 12.1 and Figures 12.2, 12.3, 12.4 and 12.5. He would also like to acknowledge his thanks to the Central and Regional Assessors over many years for, as a working obstetrician, he along with others has benefitted enormously from reading these reports every few years. The author is most grateful to Dr Elizabeth Cloake for her help with this chapter.

REFERENCES

Campbell J 1924 Maternal Mortality. Reports on Public Health and Medical Subjects 25. Her Majesty's Stationery Office, London

Chief Medical Officer 1953 On the State of Public Health. Her Majesty's Stationery Office, London

Department of Health and Social Security 1982 Report on Confidential Enquiries into Maternal Deaths in England and Wales 1976–78. Her Majesty's Stationery Office, London

PART TWO

Gynaecology

Jacques R. Ducharme

Puberty: physiology and physiopathology in girls

Puberty is the period which links childhood and adulthood. Under the influence of sex hormones, the adolescent is subjected to profound biological, morphological and psychological changes which all lead to full maturity and eventually fertility. These physiological events, controlled by the interaction of several complex neurohumoral secretory modifications, are depicted in Fig. 13.1; they appear to be part of a strict genetically determined programme most likely initiated during fetal life.

Several hormonal and humoral signals modulate the somatic adolescent growth spurt, the development of the gonads and that of sexual characteristics. In addition, heredity, nutritional, physical, psychological and environmental factors may all influence the age at which puberty will occur. Finally, love deprivation, sustained child abuse, prolonged stress including intensive competitive training and exercise, or more severe as in anorexia nervose, and chronic illnesses may all delay puberty. Physical as well as psychological stress may delay puberty of adolescents. In contrast, certain central nervous system (CNS) lesions in infancy and childhood may accelerate its onset.

The body of knowledge accumulated over the years concerning pubertal development has been summarised recently (Grumbach 1980, Ducharme 1981, Ducharme & Forest 1982, Reiter & Grumbach 1982). Although the extensive research carried out so far has permitted to characterise the humoral and hormonal secretory changes which occur throughout sexual development, the 'primum movens' or triggering mechanism which initiates puberty is still hypothetical.

It has now been clearly established that maturation of the hypothalamic neuroendocrine mechanisms which are responsible for the control of pituitary gonadotropin secretions plays a central role at puberty. The secretion of hypothalamic gonadotropin-releasing hormone (GnRH) increases and modulates gonadotropin secretion and secondarily that of gonadal sex steroids. In turn, the sex hormones will exert their biological effects at the periphery through the induction and regulation of specific receptors and the characteristic morphological changes of puberty will take place.

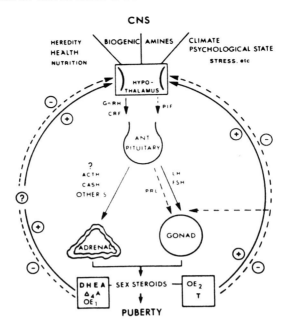

Fig. 13.1 Factors which regulate the onset and the course of pubertal development. (+, ———, positive feedback control; –, – – –, negative feedback control; ?, hypothetical; CRF, corticotropin-releasing factor; PIF, prolactin release-inhibiting factor; the other abbreviations are defined in the text (from Ducharme 1981, with permission)

HORMONAL CHANGES AT PUBERTY

Figure 13.2 is a schematic representation of regulatory and counter regulatory mechanisms intervening in the control of the hypothalamic-pituitary-gonadal axis (HPGA).

GnRH

The arcuate mucleus of the medial basal hypothalamus and its transducer neurosecretory neurons translate neural signals into a periodic oscillary chemical signal, gonadotropin-releasing hormone (GnRH) (Reiter & Grumbach 1982). This decapeptide is synthesised by the neurosecretory peptidergic neurons and released from the axon terminals at the median eminence to the anterior pituitary gland through the primary plexus of the hypothalamic-hypophyseal portal circulation. It appears that catecholaminergic and opioid neural pathways and sex steroids themselves modulate GnRH secretion. An increase in the amplitude and frequency of the GnRH pulse secretion likely takes place early in puberty and activates the pituitary-gonadal axis. Up to the present, however, such an increase has not been unequivocally demonstrated in the human. In contrast, the activation of

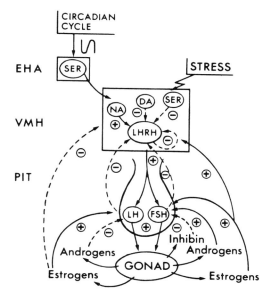

Fig. 13.2 Schematic representation of regulatory and counterregulatory mechanisms intervening in the control of the hypothalamic-pituitary-gonadal axis. DA, dopamine; EHA, extrahypothalamic areas; NA, noradrenalin; PIT, pituitary gland; SER, serotonin; VMH, ventral-medial hypothalamus (from Collu 1981, with permission)

pituitary gonadotropins through prior exposure to increasing amounts of GnRH is now well recognised. Indeed, no significant LH response to GnRH is observed in prepubertal children but during adolescence, the LH response to intravenous or subcutaneous administration of synthetic GnRH progressively increases up to adulthood. The difference in FSH response from childhood to adulthood is much less marked and, in adolescent girls, such an increase is not found (Job et al 1972, Grumbach et al 1974, Job 1977). Figure 13.3 illustrates the gonadotropin response obtained after intravenous GnRH administration during pubertal development in boys and girls respectively.

Gonadotropins

The first demonstrable biological change at puberty is likely the appearance of pulsatile LH release during sleep (Boyar et al 1972) and, albeit less marked, of FSH (Johanson 1974). As puberty progresses, LH secretory peaks increase in amplitude and extend during the wake period until adulthood when the difference between sleep and wake LH patterns disappears. These LH peaks seem to be in close correlation with the paradoxical phases of sleep (Weitzman et al 1975). This hypothalamic-pituitary activity seems independent of the negative feedback exerted by gonadal sex hormones since oestrogens are not essential for its occurrence as demonstrated in gonadal dysgenesis or Turner

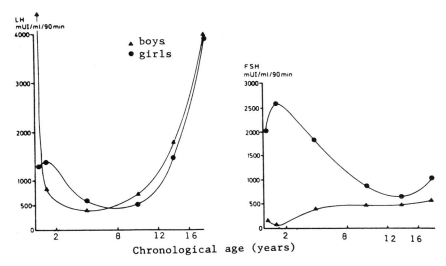

Fig.13.3 LH and FSH response to GnRH in the course of development (from Plauchu et al 1980, with permission)

syndrome (Boyar et al 1973, Grumbach et al 1974, Conte et al 1980). This finding is a remarkable example of the progressive maturation of the neuroendocrine control of the HPGA during puberty.

For the purpose of reference, Table 13.1 lists normal levels of gonadotropins and of gonadal steroids in girls at all stages of puberty. In general, circulating FSH levels increase approximately 1 year prior to those of LH. Plasma FSH rises by 10 to 11 years of age and although basal levels of gonadotropins increase gradually throughout puberty from stage 2, important fluctuations are observed in relationship to the menstrual cycle and more specifically with ovulation (Ducharme 1981, Ducharme & Forest 1982, Ducharme & Collu 1982). In order properly to assess gonadotropin secretion, ideally, plasma

Table 13.1 Plasma concentration of dehydroepiandrosterone (DHEA), androstenedione ($\triangle_4$A), FSH, LH, testosterone (T), oestrone (OE$_1$), and oestradiol (OE$_2$) in normal girls in relation to stages of puberty (P$_1$ to P$_5$) as measured by specific radioimmunoassays* (Adapted from Ducharme et al 1981, Fairman & Winter 1974)

	DHEA (ng/dl)	$\triangle_4$A (ng/dl)	FSH (ng/ml)	LH (ng/ml)	T (ng/dl)	OE$_1$ (ng/dl)	OE$_2$ (ng/dl)
P$_1$	133 ± 8	35 ± 22	82 ± 6	21 ± 1	11 ± 7	4 ± 4	2 ± 1
P$_2$	326 ± 151	72 ± 34	94 ± 9	21 ± 1	19 ± 5	5 ± 4	3 ± 3
P$_3$	427 ± 161	103 ± 43	142 ± 11	37 ± 3	28 ± 9	7 ± 4	13 ± 14
P$_4$	498 ± 90	176 ± 44	175 ± 12	76 ± 10	48 ± 12	12 ± 7	16 ± 14
P$_5$	741 ± 352	141 ± 83			38 ± 3	3 ± 1	8 ± 6

*Mean in nanograms (ng) per millilitre (ml) or decilitre (dl) ± s.d. For FSH and LH, the results are expressed as mean LER-907 standard concentration in ng/ml ± s.e.m. Steroid levels may be converted to nmol/l by multiplying T and DHA by 0.0347, DHT by 0.0344, $\triangle_4$A by 0.0349, OE$_1$ by 0.0370 and OE$_2$ by 0.0367. FSH can be converted from ng/ml to IU/l by multiplying by 0.05 and LH by 0.45 respectively.

gonadotropins should be measured at 20 min intervals for a minimum of three times to avoid fluctuations due to nyctohemeral variations. Twenty-four hour urinary gonadotropins are more reliable since they reflect total daily secretion and since values obtained from a 3 hour specimen correlate well with those from 24 hour urines, they are more practical and thus recommended (Kulin et al 1975).

Prolactin

Prolactin levels seem to increase by 14 to 15 years of age most likely due to the significant increase in plasma oestrogens which occurs (Frantz et al 1972, Ehara et al 1975). The physiological role, if any, of prolactin in the course of puberty is unknown. However, since prolactin is also secreted in a sleep-dependent manner, the concurrent sleep-related changes in LH, FSH and prolactin may suggest a common neuroendocrine modulatory mechanism for the three hormones.

Adrenal sex steroids

In prepuberty, the adrenal cortex is activated 'adrenarche' and a significant increase in plasma adrenal androgens takes place (Root 1973, Sizonenko 1978, Ducharme 1981, Ducharme & Forest 1982). In girls, dehydroepiandrosterone (DHEA) and its sulfate (DHEA-S) increase as early as 6 to 7 years of age followed within 1 to 2 years by a concomitant increase in $\triangle_4$androstenedione (A). This adrenal androgen production continues to rise throughout puberty and a second peak of these hormones occurs at approximately 12 to 13 years of age. Although these androgens are increased by ACTH and suppressed by dexamethasone confirming their adrenal origin (Forest et al 1973, Genazzani et al 1979), ACTH does not appear to be the sole regulatory factor of adrenarche. Parker & Odell (1979) have detected in the hypophysis a substance capable of stimulating androgen production by the adrenal reticularis (cortical androgen stimulating hormone or CASH) but its role in adrenarche remains to be determined.

Although these adrenal androgens are believed to induce the prepubertal growth spurt and the appearance of axillary and pubic hair in the adolescent, their role in the activation of the HPGA is less clear and speculative. The time sequence relationship between 'adrenarche' and the gonadal activation or 'gonadarche' together with the premature activation of the axis in certain conditions with high levels of circulating adrenal androgens such as congenital adrenal hyperplasia treated late (Boyar et al 1973b) would suggest that adrenal androgens may play a role at least permissive in this process (Ducharme et al 1976, Sizonenko 1978). If this hypothesis is correct, this action could be exerted either directly or by androgen metabolism to form other effective metabolites, androgenic or oestrogenic, which would exert a maturational effect on the hypothalamus and lead to the elevation of the threshold of sensitivity of the gonadostat to negative feedback exerted by gonadal steroids (see below). However, a number of observations in normal and agonadal patients (Conte et al 1980) and in precocious or delayed puberty (Sklar et al 1980) would cast doubt on this hypothesis. Indeed, these studies would rather suggest that the activation of HPGA or 'gonadarche' at puberty is totally independent of 'adrenarche'. In addition, puberty seems to occur at a relatively normal age in well treated addisonian patients (Urban et al 1980).

Gonadal sex steroids

The maturation of the ovary at adolescence has been well described by Ross et al (1981). Active follicle growth and atresia occur throughout infancy and childhood, controlled by three processes all of which contribute to the age-related progressive increase in ovarian weight: an increase (1) in the ovarian medullary stroma; (2) in the size of maturing follicles and (3) in the number of follicles attaining this larger size prior to atresia. As puberty nears, after 6–8 years, gonadotropins start to rise and the granulosa cells begin to secrete oestrogens in increasing quantities. Although follicular growth and oestrogen synthesis appear dependent on gonadotropin secretion, the trigger for the first ovulation remains unknown. The follicle ruptures and, after the ovum has been released, is rapidly transformed into corpus luteum secreting progesterone under LH stimulation.

In the follicular phase of the menstrual cycle, the synergic influence of LH and FSH increases oestrogen production which in turn induces endometrial development. In addition, as mentioned earlier, the oestrogens will eventually exert a positive feedback control on LH production. This phenomenon explains the rapid increase in oestradiol production in the week which precedes the LH peak, maximal oestradiol levels being reached 24 hours prior to this peak. An abrupt LH and oestradiol fall precedes immediately the rupture of the follicle and ovulation and, at the end of the cycle, a rapid and abrupt decrease in oestrogens and progesterone levels will allow shedding of the endometrium and menstruation.

Plasma oestrone will follow relatively closely plasma oestradiol; it is derived mainly from the metabolism of its prohormone $\Delta_4$androstenedione secreted both by the ovary and the adrenal. The small amounts of progesterone found during the proliferative phase of the cycle originates from the peripheral conversion of pregnenolone and its sulphate also secreted by the adrenal while 17α-hydroxyprogesterone is secreted in most part concomitantly to the pre-ovulatory LH and FSH peaks and parallels that of progesterone and oestradiol in the luteal part of the cycle.

Receptors

The target-organ response to trophic hormones will be dependent on the number of highly specific recognition sites — the receptors. For gonadotrophins, cell surface or membrane receptors will bind the hormone with high affinity and the hormone-receptor complex will induce a sequence of chemical steps: the activation of an adenylate cyclase system, the formation of the second messenger, cyclic adenosine 3', 5' monophosphate (CAMP) which, in turn, will influence in the cell milieu the phosphorylation of various proteins leading to steroidogenesis and the characteristic biological response of the hormones (Posner et al 1981).

As for steroid hormones, they enter the cytoplasm of the target cells by diffusion or facilitated transport, and bind to specific cytoplasmic receptors. The hormone-receptor complex is then activated and translocated into the nucleus, binds to the cell genome and stimulates RNA production; the transcription of specific mRNA is then exported into the cytoplasm where protein synthesis will take place. It is the change in the pattern of newly synthesised proteins that will alter cell function and condition the specific response of the cell to the hormone (Chan & Tindall 1981).

At the pre-antral stage, the granulosa cells of the ovary already have FSH, androgen and oestrogen receptors while receptors to both FSH and LH are found in the mature graffian follicle. The internal theca of both follicle stages and interstitial cells seem to have only LH receptors. *In vitro*, FSH seems to induce the appearance of LH receptors and the aromatisation of androgens to oestrogens which will stimulate the proliferation of granulosa cells and follicular growth. At the beginning of the menstrual cycle, FSH induces follicle growth and the appearance of LH receptors in the granulosa cells thus inducing the aromatisation of androgens to oestrogens. For appropriate follicular maturation to take place, steroid secretion *in situ* in addition to LH and FSH are essential, the latter modulating pituitary gonadotropin secretion (Channing & Kammerman 1974, Richards & Williams 1976).

INTEGRATED VIEW OF THE CONTROL

It is generally accepted that the hormonal changes characteristic of puberty result from an elevation of the threshold of sensitivity to circulating sex steroid of an hypothalamic centre which regulates gonadotropin secretion (Fig. 13.4).

During childhood, this centre or 'gonadostat' is extremely sensitive to the negative feedback exerted by small quantities of sex hormones, namely oestradiol and testosterone.

As puberty nears, this sensitivity decreases and some input from the central nervous system induces a progressive rise in GnRH secretion by hypothalamic cells leading to the synthesis and release of increasing amounts of gonadotropins and secondarily of sex steroids. While the latter hormones will induce the characteristic changes of puberty, a new equilibrium will gradually be reached and the negative feedback control exerted at a progressively lower level of hypothalamic sensitivity (Reiter & Kulin 1972). The existence of such a phenomenon is well illustrated by the fact that, in prepuberty, clomiphene citrate, an anti-oestrogen with mild oestrogenic activity, inhibits LH and FSH

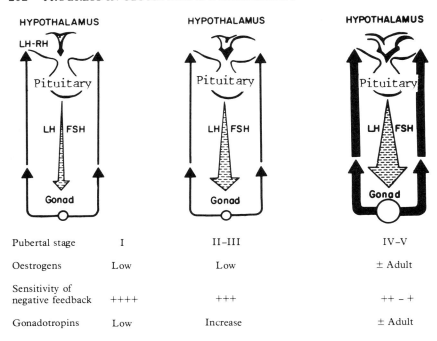

Pubertal stage	I	II–III	IV–V
Oestrogens	Low	Low	± Adult
Sensitivity of negative feedback	++++	+++	++ – +
Gonadotropins	Low	Increase	± Adult

Fig. 13.4 Modification of the threshold of sensitivity of the gonadostat to negative feedback exerted by oestrogen in the course of pubertal development in girls (from Reiter and Kulin 1981, with permission)

and, in boys, testosterone secretion in contrast to its stimulating effect during puberty and in the adult. This suggests that its action cannot be exerted until the threshold of sensitivity of the feedback mechanism has risen. However, as previously mentioned, the activation of the hypothalamic pituitary axis occurs in agonadal adolescents (Boyar et al 1973a, Grumbach et al 1974, Conte et al 1980) indicating that gonadal hormones are not essential for the maturation of the upper part of the axis to take place. Finally, it is only at some later stage of pubertal development that the positive feedback control exerted by oestrogens is observed (Kulin et al 1972, Kulin & Reiter 1976) presumably because the conditions essential to its actions are not present, mainly: the capacity of ovarian follicles to respond to FSH, the capacity of the central nervous system to induce synthesis and acute release of GnRH and a sufficient sensitivity of the hypophysis to GnRH to allow peak release of LH into the circulation. A positive feedback or increased LH response to circulating oestrogens, a function of circulating oestrogen levels, follows and becomes fully mature only after menarche has occurred (Winter & Faiman 1973a, Nakai et al 1978). The evolution of the gonadostatic control throughout humoral development from fetal to adult life is depicted in Fig. 13.5.

The nature of the biochemical event that is responsible for the changes in gonadostatic sensitivity and for the increase in frequency and amplitude of

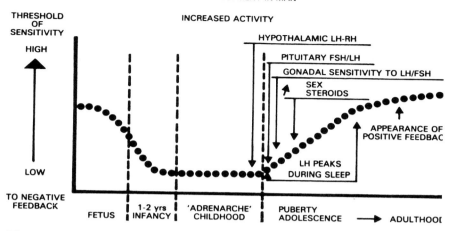

Fig. 13.5 Schematic representation of the various biological events that characterise the activity of the hypothalamic-pituitary-gonadal activity in the course of human development (from Ducharme, 1981, with permission)

GnRH discharges is still unknown. However, it appears that several brain neurotransmitters play a major role in such a phenomenon. Indeed, biogenic amines are known to exert a significant control on gonadotropin secretion (Collu 1981). Noradrenalin is able to stimulate gonadotropin synthesis and release, while dopamine, serotonin and melatonin appear to be inhibitory. Recent data, however, seem to indicate that melatonin is not involved in pubertal mechanisms (Lenko et al 1982, Ehrenkranz et al 1982) as had been previously postulated. Recently Adler et al (1983) have shown that both positive and negative feedback exerted by ovarian hormones on gonadotropin secretion may be mediated by modifications of hypothalamic catecholamine turnover. There is also accumulating evidence that endogenous opioid peptides may play a role in pubertal development. This is reviewed by Genazzani et al (1983). Extrahypothalamic areas of the central nervous system such as the amygdala and the hippocampus certainly also play a role in stimulating or inhibiting gonadotropin release through neurotransmitters (Gorski 1974).

In addition to the role exerted by various humoral factors possibly also including acetylcholine, and various peptides such as neurotensin and cholecystokinin, a number of other factors are at play in the regulation of the hypothalamic-pituitary-gonadal function. Indeed, in the course of sexual maturation, the pituitary response to hypothalamic neuro-hormones increases (Job et al 1972, Grumbach et al 1974, Job 1977, Plauchu et al 1980, Beck & Wutke 1980) while gonadal steroidogenesis also increases and some alteration in the peripheral metabolism of steroid hormones itself influenced by catechol-oestrogens takes place (Winter & Faiman 1973b, Faiman & Winter 1974, Ducharme et al 1976). In addition, the hormone receptors undergo a certain maturation and certainly determine in part the biological response of the target organs and tissues to trophic and/or steroid hormones. Finally, the maturation of the target organ itself conditions the response to trophic stimulation.

MORPHOLOGICAL CHANGES OF PUBERTY

Five stages of puberty have been described by Tanner and his colleague (P_1 to P_5). In girls, these reflect the progressive modifications of the breasts, the external genitalia and sexual hair which occur in the course of sexual development towards full maturity (Marshall & Tanner 1969, 1970, Tanner 1969). These progressive modifications are depicted in composite form in Table 13.2.

Secondary sex characteristics appear at a mean age of 10.5 years as an early budding of the breast which is usually the first clinical sign of puberty. These changes are commonly seen as early as 9 years or as late as 12 years and, within such ranges, these physiological variations in time are usually of no particular concern to the adolescent girl and her parents although the concomitant advance or delay in stature may bring the adolescent to medical attention. After a short-lived prepubertal slowing in growth, the typical adolescent growth spurt usually takes place between 11 and 14.5 years and coincides with sexual development. Breast budding in the form of a small sub-aerolar nodule is observed followed within approximately 6 months by the appearance of pubic hair and shortly after of axillary hair (Tanner stage 2). A gradual increase in breast size follows the development of the labia minora and labia majora and the vaginal mucosa become progressively reddened and secretory. A progressive

Table 13.2 Stages of sexual development at puberty in girls

Pubertal stages	
P_1	Prepubertal
P_2	Early development of subareolar breast bud Widening of aerolae, with or without small amounts of labial and axillary hair
P_3	Increase in size of palpable breast tissue and areolae Increased amount of dark pubic hair on mons veneris and of axillary hair, appearance of characteristic body odour
P_4	Further increase in breast size and areolae which protrude above breast level Adult amount of sexual hair but limited to pubis Acne Menarche may occur
P_5	Adult breast and areolar size Adult amount and distribution of pubic hair with extension to upper thigh Menarche

increase in axillary and pubic hair takes place and the characteristic body odour is found. The uterus increases in size up to Tanner stage 4 when the first menstruation occurs. By this time, the maximal growth rate has been reached (13 years of age) and acne is frequent.

Significant variations in this time sequence are common; when the sequence is reversed or when long intervals separate the appearance of one sex characteristic from the others, puberty is considered dissociated. Indeed, pubic hair and occasionally axillary hair may precede any evidence of breast or genital development. Such dissociation is of little significance and is usually accompanied by an increase in circulating levels of adrenal androgens, namely DHEA-S and A as in normal prepuberty (Sizonenko & Paunier 1975, Sizonenko et al 1975, Ducharme et al 1976, De Peretti & Forest 1978).

Initially, breast tissue may appear on one side only or one breast may remain larger for some time. This finding is usually transitory and is of no practical significance. However, when a significant size difference persists throughout puberty, it may become of cosmetic importance and eventually require plastic surgery. Within 3 or 4 years of its onset, pubertal sexual development will be completed and girls will reach their final height with complete fusion of the epiphyses within approximately 2 years after menarche. The age at which sex hormones, particularly oestrogens, start to exert their maturing effect on long bones will determine to a great extent the stature of the adult female.

ABNORMALITIES OF SEXUAL DEVELOPMENT

Ordinate pubertal development is dependent on the integrity of each of the complex components which regulate the hypothalamic-pituitary-ovarian axis.

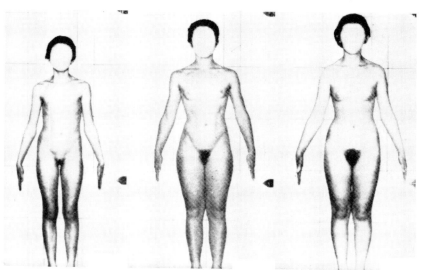

Fig. 13.6 12.75-year-old normal girls of different Tanner stage

Since the age of onset of puberty varies within a relatively wide range (Fig. 13.6), the term precocious puberty is reserved for girls who exhibit any secondary sex characteristic prior to 8 years of age. When no pubertal sign is apparent by 13–14 years, puberty is considered delayed. The first menstruation occurs at a mean age of 12.5 to 13 years, although menarche may appear as early as 10 or as late as 16.5 years in otherwise entirely normal girls.

These rather important physiological time variations are likely the result of variable differences in the kinetics of the mechanisms which trigger the onset and progression of puberty.

1. PRECOCIOUS PUBERTY

True or complete precocious puberty indicates an activation of the HPGA at an unusually young age. In contrast, pseudo-precocious puberty results from gonadotropic or sex steroid stimulation independent of this axis. Although complete sex precocity is always isosexual (in accordance with the sex phenotype), the occurrence of virilisation in girls points towards some abnormal sex steroid secretion by the adrenals or the gonads.

A classification of isosexual precocious pubertal development based on aetiological considerations is provided in Table 13.3.

Table 13.3 Aetiological classification of precocious puberty

1. Complete precocious puberty
   Idiopathic (sporadic or familial)
   Organic lesions of the hypothalamic-pituitary region
   (a) Congenital
   (b) Acquired
   — Tumours, hydrocephaly, injuries or infections
   Part of a specific syndrome
   — Neurofibromatosis of Von Recklinghausen
   — Polyostotic fibrous dysplasia of McCune Albright
   Others
   — Various anoxic, metabolic or endocrine disorders

2. Incomplete precocious puberty (dissociated puberty)
   Premature thelarche
   Premature adrenarche (pubarche)
   Premature menarche

3. Pseudo-precocious puberty
   Ovarian or testicular tumours
   Adrenal hyperplasia or tumours
   Gonadotrophin-producing tumours of non-endocrine sites (hepatoblastoma)
   Iatrogenic

Complete precocious puberty

Whatever the aetiology, the increase in circulating sex steroids will accelerate physical growth and bone maturation inducing budding and progressive enlargement of the breasts, increase in sexual hair and eventually menses. Acne will be frequently found. It must be emphasised that the intellectual or emotional development of these children will be that of their chronological age. Indeed, their physical development will lead one to consider these girls as older than they really are (Fig. 13.7) and impose of them requirements in skill and behaviour outside their reach which may seriously affect the child's emotional stability.

Precocious sexual development requires careful and thorough investigation although, contrary to the situation in boys where the incidence of space-occupying lesions of CNS is over 50%, no aetiology can be found and 75% to 95% of these cases are idiopathic. In addition, familial cases have been reported (Rosenfeld et al 1980). Nevertheless, complete hormonal and neuroradiological studies should be performed whenever the history or physical examination casts doubt on the aetiology. The pattern of pubertal development will follow essentially the same sequence as that of normal adolescent girls although

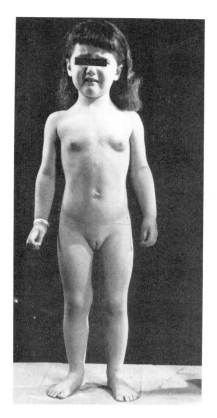

Fig. 13.7 2.75-year-old girl with early breast development (Tanner II), oestrogenisation of her vaginal mucosa and vaginal spotting. Her height (101 cm) was that of a 3.75-year-old and her bone age approximately 5 years

occasionally menses or sexual hair may be the first manifestation of puberty. Although the menstrual cycles are initially anovulatory as in older adolescents, ovulation and thus fertility will eventually occur at an early age. The ultimate result of such early onset of puberty will be short stature which will remain as the only stigma of its occurrence and menopause will occur at an appropriate age.

It is likely that some congenital or acquired hypothalamic or CNS dysfunction or lesion is responsible for the early onset of puberty, although no such lesion can usually be documented. EEG abnormalities, albeit minor, were described in some cases (Liu et al 1965) lending support to this view. It is possible that a more thorough neuroradiological investigation, if performed, may allow to establish an aetiological diagnosis in a higher percentage of cases.

If a CNS lesion is detected, a tumour most commonly localised in the posterior hypothalamus, the pineal gland, the median eminence, or tumours which exert pressure on the floor of the third ventricle are usually found. These tumours are generally hamartomas, teratomas or ependymomas; occasionally, optic gliomas, astrocytomas, chorioepitheliomas or neurofibromas as in phacomatoses, especially in the neurocutaneous syndrome of Von Recklinghausen, may also be aetiological. In the latter, characteristic multiple smooth edge small 'café au lait' spots are seen on all parts of the body and neurofibromata extending along the peripheral nerve pathways may be detected. In the McCune Albright syndrome, large irregular pigmented areas are found on the trunk and axilla and radiological evidence of typical bone lesions of polyostotic fibrous dysplasia will eventually be obtained. Occasionally isolated menses will precede any evidence of bone lesions and rarely autonomous oestrogen-secreting ovarian follicular cysts may develop and confuse the diagnosis (Fig. 13.8).

A history of head trauma, especially with severe brain concussion, loss of consciousness and seizures, of CNS infection, perinatal anoxia with or without prematurity, microcephaly or macrocephaly usually associated with hydrocephalus can also be uncovered. Other less common metabolic or endocrine dysfunctions such as hypothyroidism have been reported.

Incomplete or partial precocious puberty

Isolated breast development prior to 8 years of age (premature thelarche), of sexual hair (premature adrenarche or pubarche) is common and isolated menses (premature menarche) may occasionally be seen.

Premature thelarche occurs only in girls classically in the second year of life and is usually bilateral, without any evidence of oestrogenisation of the vaginal mucosa, of pubic or axillary hair and without concomitant increase in growth kinetics and bone maturation. After persisting several months, it regresses completely within 2 years in most cases and pubertal development will occur at the appropriate age. Nevertheless, initially these infants and children must be observed closely in order to be sure that complete sex precocity will not ensue.

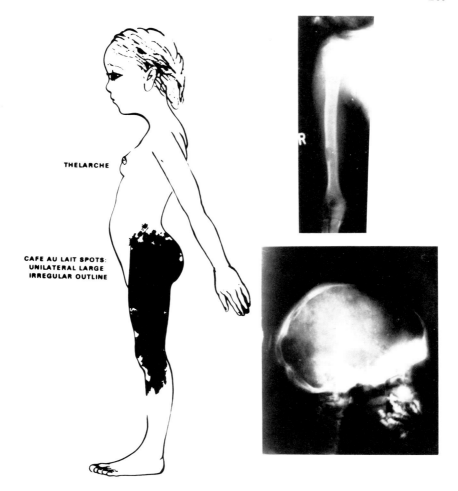

THELARCHE

CAFE AU LAIT SPOTS:
UNILATERAL LARGE
IRREGULAR OUTLINE

Fig. 13.8 Major clinical features of a child with the McCune-Albright Syndrome and precocious puberty (authorisation of doctors Deam & Winter 1981)

The cause of such isolated breast development is not clear. It has been attributed to a small increase of ovarian oestrogens in response to a transient elevation of circulating gonadotropins reported at this age (Bidlingmaier et al 1974).

The appearance as early as 5 years of age of pubic hair either isolated (premature pubarche) or concomitant with axillary hair (premature adrenarche) is also common. It may sometimes be associated with a slight increase in growth rate and bone maturation but does not progress towards complete sexual development until the appropriate age. Since adrenal androgens, namely DHA, DHA-S and A, correlate with the degree of sexual hair present (Korth-Schultz et al 1976), these hormones are thought to be aetiological. Periodic physical examination with measurement of androgen, gonadotropin and oestrogen levels will ensure that premature pubarche or adrenarche is not the expression of an androgen producing tumour or of the beginning of puberty.

Isolated vaginal spotting or premature menarche is occasionally seen but no satisfactory explanation is known for this occurrence. As mentioned above, it is most commonly found in the McCune Albright syndrome frequently before any typical bone lesion has appeared.

2. PSEUDO-PRECOCIOUS PUBERTY

An ovarian oestrogen producing tumour (granulosa cell tumour, thecal lipoid tumour or functional ovarian cyst) (Van der Werff ten Bosch 1975) is clinically indistinguishable from true early activation of the HPGA. A meticulous gynecological examination followed by plasma and/or urinary gonadotropin and oestrogen measurements will confirm the diagnosis. Since these tumours are usually palpable by abdominal and/or by rectal examination early after the onset of clinical signs, the diagnosis may be readily suspected in most cases. High oestrogen levels and suppressed gonadotropins will suggest the diagnosis. Fortunately, these tumours usually do not metastasize or do so slowly and late and a close initial follow-up will usually disclose the diagnosis and lead to early surgical removal and to complete cure.

Feminising adrenal tumours are extremely rare in childhood and adolescence and are of little practical significance in the differential diagnosis of sexual precocity in girls. Occasionally the accidental exposure to oestrogenic substances (namely contraceptive pills used by mother, relatives or siblings) may induce some pubertal manifestations and should be considered.

Treatment

Once a causal factor has been established, therapy aims at eliminating the factor. However in the more common idiopathic variety or other non tumoural cases, therapy aims essentially at arresting, inducing a regression or at least at slowing the rate of development of secondary sex characteristics and at preventing the accelerating effect of sex hormones on bone maturation. For this purpose 70–100 mg/m^2/day of oral cyproterone acetate (Rager et al 1973, Werder et al 1974), 30 mg daily of medroxy-progesterone acetate (MPA) orally (personal data, unpublished) or 100–200 mg of depo-MPA intramuscularly every 2–4 weeks (David et al 1972) have been used. Although the efficacy of these compounds on suppressing the development of secondary sex characteristics is well documented, their efficacy in delaying the progression of bone maturation and early fusion of the epiphyses in order to increase the adult height of these children remains controversial. Recently, the use of LHRH agonists in this condition has been used and seems promising (Comite et al

1981, Mansfield et al 1982). Guidelines in the assessment of cases of precocious pubertal development are provided in Table 13.4.

Table 13.4 Guidelines in the assessment of precocious puberty (PP)

A. General
    — Medical personal and family history
    — Complete physical examination
    — Ophthalmological and anthropometric examination
    — Bone maturation
    — Skull X-ray including spot films of sella turcica
    — EEG
    — Serum FSH, LH, T, OE$_2$
    — 24 h urine FSH, LH, 17-ketosteroids
    — Vaginal cytology for maturation index

B. Specific

    The initial assessment:
    1. Is negative: follow-up at 3–6 months
        — Progression and adolescent FSH and LH response to 100 μg GnRH i.v.: idiopathic PP
        — No progression: premature adrenarche (pubarche) or thelarche

    2. Suggests an intracranial tumour:
        — Axial tomodensitometry
        — Pneumo- and/or angioencephalography if necessary
        — Neurosurgery

    3. Suggests a gonadal tumour:
        — Serum and/or urinary HCG (trophoblastic tumour: ←)

    4. Suggests an intra-abdominal tumour:
        — Echography
        — Tomodensitometry (CAT SCAN)
        — Serum HCG and α-foetoproteins

3. DELAYED PUBERTY

Puberty is considered delayed when breast tissue and/or sexual hair by approximately 13–14 years have not appeared.

An aetiological classification of delayed puberty is given in Table 13.5.

Constitutional

In these patients, the pubertal activation of the HPGA is delayed together with their physiological development as evidenced by height, genital development and bone maturation. Since a similar history among siblings or the parents is frequently obtained, a strong genetic influence seems to be at play. Levels of plasma and urinary gonadotropins and of adrenal and gonadal sex steroids will be appropriate for their developmental age (bone maturation). Although some overlapping in LH response to GnRH between prepuberty and early puberty may be found (Job et al 1976), their response will usually be characteristic of

Table 13.5 Aetiological classification of delayed puberty

1. Constitutional

2. Chronic malnutrition of systemic disease
   — Endocrine
   — Non-endocrine

3. Gonadal insufficiency
   (a) Primary (hypergonadotrophic):
        — Turner's syndrome
        — Pure gonadal dysgenesis
        — Resistant ovary syndrome
        — End-organ insensitivity to androgens
        — Autoimmune ovarian failure
        — Others
   (b) Secondary (hypogonadotrophic):
        — Panhypopituitarism
          (i) Congenital (idiopathic)
          (ii) Acquired (CNS tumours)
        — Congenital isolated gonadotrophin deficiency
        — As part of CNS dysfunction:
          (i) Prader-Willi Syndrome
          (ii) Laurence-Moon-Biedl syndrome
          (iii) Holoprosencephaly
          (iv) Others

prepuberty. Since this delay does not constitute a disease per se and is time-limited, the teenager must be reassured as to its outcome and no hormonal therapy is usually required.

Secondary to chronic disease

Chronic endocrine (hypothyroidism) or non-endocrine diseases (cardiac, gastrointestinal, pulmonary, renal, etc) may result in delayed sexual development; the correction when possible of the underlying cause will usually resume growth and development and result eventually in triggering of the HPGA.

True gonadal insufficiencies

Hypogonadism can be divided in two major groups:

1. primary hypogonadism, which will lead to an early increase in circulating gonadotropins, and
2. secondary hypogonadism which results from lack of endogenous gonadotropic stimulation.

1. Primary (hypergonadotropic) hypogonadism

Gonadal insufficiency with inhability of the ovary to secrete adequate amounts of oestrogens will result in sexual infantilism and early triggering of the hypothalamic-pituitary-axis with hypergonadotropism due to inadequate negative feedback control (Conte et al 1980).

Prepubertal gonadectomy or gonadal failure secondary to radiation or chemotherapy usually for neoplastic diseases may also be causal.

Turner's syndrome (gonadal dysgenesis) In these patients a negative or low positive chromatin pattern is found together with a 45 XO chromosomal anomaly, an XX/XO mosaicism or some other numerical (XO/XXX; XO/XX/XXX) or structural anomalies of the X chromosome (such as 46-isochromosome X_p-, X_q-). It is the most common cause of primary hypergonadotropic hypogonadism in phenotypic females with an incidence of 1:2000–3000 live births (Rimoin & Schimke 1971, Therman et al 1980). In general, aplasia or hypoplasia of the ovaries (gonadal streaks) is present and short stature is the rule. Variable degrees of other stigmata such as a characteristic facies with low-set and malformed ears, low hair-line, high arched palate, cubitus valgus, short and/or webbed neck, shielded chest with microthelia and wide spaced nipples and numerous pigmented naevi are characteristic (Fig. 13.9). Coarctation of the aorta and congenital renal anomalies, found in more than 50% of cases, usually as a horseshoe kidney, are frequent. A certain number of these children may show some moderate to mild mental retardation. In such patients, usually XO/XX mosaics, a certain degree of ovarian development will induce puberty, menses and exceptionally fertility although early menopause will result (Styne & Kaplan 1979).

XO/XY chromatin negative gonadal dysgenesis females have a similar phenotype but a variable degree of masculinisation depending on the amount of functional testicular tissue present. In Noonan's syndrome, contrary to the male equivalent, no ovarian dysfunction is present.

Pure gonadal dysgenesis. These patients have a normal female phenotype but absent or rudimentary gonads (Sohval 1965) confirmed at laparoscopy and occasionally congenital deafness. Serum and urinary gonadotropins are high. The karyotype is 46XX in approximately half of the cases while in the others a 46XY karyotype is found. The 46XX variety is transmitted by an autosomal recessive gene (Simpson 1972) and several members of a sibship may be affected. Sporadic or occasional familial cases of the so-called rudimentary ovary syndrome are likely a variant of this disorder. The 46XY variant can also occur in sibships and appears transmitted by an X-linked recessive or as an autosomal dominant gene expressed in females only (Espiner et al 1970); since it carries a 25% risk of gonadal malignant degeneration (Schellhas 1974), gonadectomy must be performed.

Resistant ovary syndrome In this syndrome, primary compiete ovarian follicular maturation is lacking due presumably to some defect in gonadotropin receptors (Starup & Pedersen 1978) and amenorrhoea in otherwise normally appearing 46XX adolescent or adult females is the presenting complaint.

Androgen insensitivity syndrome An X-linked recessive gene is responsible for this previously called testicular feminisation which results from a severe quantitative deficiency of target cells androgen receptors or from qualitative

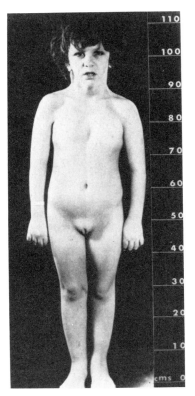

Fig. 13.9 Nine-year-old girl with XO Turner's syndrome. Height age: 6 years; bone age: 7 years 9 months. Note the characteristic and triangular facies, low-set ears, shielded funnel chest, and low and wide-spread nipples. This child also had a horseshoe kidney and coarctation of the aorta

defects of these same receptors or of chromatin where specific binding of the androgen-receptor necessary to initiate the androgenic response takes place (Pinsky 1981). Plasma testosterone and oestrodiol levels are somewhat higher than in normal males of comparable age because the same insensitivity to circulating androgens is found in the hypothalamus and in the absence of efficient T negative feedback control, elevated LH release and excessive Leydig cell stimulation will ensue. Since the peripheral action of oestrogen is not impaired, normal breast development will take place. Normal female external genitalia are found and usually absent or sparse axillary and pubic hair. Labial, inguinal or intra-abdominal testes are found together with rudimentary Wollfian ducts but Müllerian derivatives are absent or rudimentary. The vagina is usually short and no uterus is present. Unless other members of the family are known to be affected, inguinal or labial masses and/or amenorrhoea will bring the patient to the physician. If the receptorial defect is incomplete, a variable degree of masculinisation will occur. A typical case of complete insensitivity to androgens is shown in Fig. 13.10.

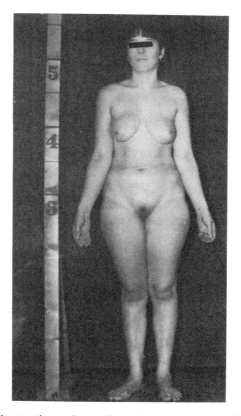

Fig. 13.10 A case of the complete end-organ insensitivity to androgens. Note the well-developed breasts, fine and sparse pubic hair. The testes were in the inguinal canals

Autoimmune ovarian failure. As part of a multiple endocrine autoimmune disease, autoimmune ovarian failure may also occur (Ruehsen et al 1972) in addition to Addison's disease, hypoparathyroidism and lymphocytic thyroiditis.

Others. An anomaly of the genital tract, particularly uterine, vaginal and/or hymeneal atresia, may be suspected when a normal girl of pubertal age with appropriate sex characteristics and normal gonadotropin levels is seen. Finally, a variety of problems of sexual differentiation may be responsible for sexual infantilism such as true hermaphroditism, mixed gonadal dysgenesis, enzymatic deficiencies (17α-hydroxylase, 5α-reductase, 17-ketoreductase, etc) but are outside the scope of this paper.

2. Secondary (hypogonadotropic) hypogonadism

Gonadotropic insufficiency, isolated or part of several trophic hormone deficiencies, will delay sexual development: idiopathic or secondary to a tumour of the pituitary or hypothalamus. In isolated gonadotropin deficiency, the girl will be of normal or of tall stature since the effect of sex hormones on bone maturation and epiphyseal fusion is lacking or delayed. Adrenal androgens will induce a moderate quantity of axillary and pubic hair. A space-occupying lesion in the hypothalamic-pituitary region, mainly cranio-pharyngiomas and chromophobe adenomas can be detected by conventional means. Otherwise, the use of GnRH or chlomiphene stimulation may be of value to differentiate primary hypogonadism from simple constitutional delay of puberty. It must be recognised that a long-standing deficit of endogenous GnRH stimulation may hamper gonadotropin response unless GnRH is administered for several days.

A number of syndromes or systemic diseases with gonadotropin deficiency have been described including the Laurence-Moon-Biedl syndrome, an autosomal recessive disease characterised by retinitis pigmentosa, polydactily, severe obesity, mental retardation, hypogonadotropic (or hypergonadotropic) hypogonadism and occasionally diabetes insipidus and diabetes mellitus; *the Prader-Willi Syndrome* with a hypothalamic defect, partially responsible for bulimia leading to severe obesity, and hypogonadism. In these patients, infantile hypotonia, a characteristic round facies, small broad hands and feet and mental retardation are found. Finally, anorexia nervosa, severe stress such as that related to competitive sports or a number of chronic diseases may all affect the HPGA and delay the onset or progression of puberty or bring about a regression of sexual characteristics.

Investigation

Guidelines for the assessment of delayed puberty are given in Table 13.6.

All patients with significantly delayed or arrested puberty require an investigation of their HPGA, the extent of which will be determined according to the case history and clinical findings. If there is evidence of impairment of some other pituitary-end-organ function, the biological evaluation will be made accordingly. The diagnostic approach will include basal plasma and urinary hormone determinations, radiological and cytogenetic studies. In addition, GnRH testing will be found useful in the assessment of LH and FSH pituitary reserve (Conte et al 1980) and a 4-hour stimulation with GnRH can usually differentiate hypogonadotrophic hypogonadism from constitutionally delayed puberty, the former exhausting its gonadotropin reserve with time (de Lange et al 1978). However, since oestrogens and androgens are known to potentiate the effect of GnRH on gonadotropin release (Greeley et al 1976, Mahesh & Mazian 1979), the results must thus be interpreted in relationship to levels of circulating sex steroids. In adolescent patients with anorexia nervosa, the response to GnRH will revert to that of prepubertal children (Marshall & Kelch 1979).

Clomiphene citrate administered to children prior to puberty suppresses LH, FSH and testosterone secretion; from mid-puberty however this

Table 13.6 Guidelines in the diagnosis of delayed puberty

Medical, personal and family history

Complete physical and anthropometric examination

Ophthalmological examination and evaluation of hearing and of smell

Bone maturation

Skull X-ray including spot films of the sella turcica

Serum FSH, LH, T, OE_2

Chromatin pattern and karotype

LH and FSH response to 100 μg GnRH i.v.

LH and FSH response to chomiphene citrate: 100 mg/day $\times$ 5

Pituitary function tests

Others

Follow-up at 6 months: constitutional delay or hypogonadotrophic hypogonadism if all tests negative

antioestrogen with low oestrogenic activity will stimulate LH release presumably by positive feedback action (Kulin et al 1972, Grumbach et al 1974).

Treatment

Therapeutic considerations of delayed puberty are given in Table 13.7. Constitutional delay of puberty requires no therapy. However, in primary

Table 13.7 Treatment of delayed puberty

1. Constitutional

    Reassurance — no specific Rx

2. Primary hypogonadism

    Initially ethinyl OE_2 0.02-0.05 mg/day p.o. or equivalent followed by 3 wks/mo. + medroxyprogesterone acetate 5 mg/day $\times$ 5 days (cycle days 21–25)

3. Secondary hypogonadism

    1. Ethinyl OE_2 as above
    2. Clomiphene citrate 50–100 mg/day $\times$ 5 days
    3. HCG 2000–4000 IU 3 $\times$ /week i.m.

hypogonadism, patients are given oestrogen and progestational agents are added once vaginal bleeding has been induced in order that regular cyclic menses are established. When full sexual maturation has been reached, combined oestrogen-progestin as found in most contraceptive pills is adequate.

In secondary hypogonadism, treatment should consist ideally of the replacement of the hypothalamic factor by synthetic GnRH or an agonist and, in the case of a pituitary deficiency, replacement with FSH (or human menopausal gonadotropin: hMG) and or LH (or human chorionic gonadotropin: hCG) in order to preserve fertility. However, although GnRH agonists are promising, treatment with these agents is at the moment still in the experimental phase and meanwhile, oestrogen replacement or the use of hCG and hMG is used.

Acknowledgments

The author's research is supported by the Medical Research Council of Canada and La Fondation Justine-Lacoste-Beaubien. The secretarial assistance of Ms S. Tassé and Ms G. Jacob is gratefully acknowledged.

REFERENCES

Adler B A, Johnson M D, Lynch C O, Crowley W R 1983 Evidence that norepinephrine and epinephrine systems mediate the stimulatory effects of ovarian hormones on luteinizing hormone and luteinizing hormone-releasing hormones. Endocrinology 113: 1431

Beck W, Wuttke W 1980 Diurnal variations of plasma luteinizing hormone, follicle-stimulating hormone and prolactin in boys and girls from birth to puberty. Journal of Clinical Endocrinology & Metabolism 50: 635

Bidlingmaier E, Versmold H, Knorr D 1974 Plasma oestrogens in newborns and infants. In: Forest M G, Bertrand J (eds) Colloques Sexual Endocrinology of the Perinatal Period, 32, p. 35. INSERM, Paris

Boyar R, Finkelstein J W, Roffwarg H et al 1972 Synchronization of augmented luteinizing hormone secretion during sleep. New England Journal of Medicine 287: 582

Boyar R, Finkelstein J W, David R et al 1973a Twenty-four luteinizing hormone and follicle-stimulating hormone secretory patterns in gonadal dysgenesis. Journal of Clinical Endocrinology and Metabolism 37: 521

Boyar R, Finkelstein J W, David R et al 1973b Twenty-four secretory patterns of luteinizing hormone and follicle-stimulating hormone in sexual precocity. New England Journal of Medicine 289: 282

Chan L C B, Tindall D J 1981 Steroid hormone action. In: Collu R, Ducharme J R, Guyda H (eds) Pediatric Endocrinology, Comprehensive Endocrinology Series, p. 63. Raven Press, New York

Channing C, Kammerman S 1974 Binding of gonadotropins to ovarian cell. Biology of Reproduction 10: 179

Collu R 1981 Neuroendocrine control of pituitary hormone secretion. In: Collu R, Ducharme J R, Guyda H (eds) Pediatric Endocrinology, Comprehensive Endocrinology Series, 1, p. 28. Raven Press, New York

Comite F, Cutler G B, Rivier J, Vale W W, Loriaux D L, Crowley W F 1981 Short-term treatment of idiopathic precocious puberty with a long-acting analogue of luteinizing hormone-releasing hormone. New England Journal of Medicine 305: 1546

Conte F A, Grumbach M M, Kaplan S L, Reiter E O 1980 Correlation of luteinizing hormone-releasing factor-induced luteinizing hormone and follicle-stimulating hormone

release from infancy to 19 years with the changing pattern of gonadotropin secretion in
agonadal patients: Relation to the restraint of puberty. Journal of Clinical Endocrinology
and Metabolism 50: 163

David M, Bovier Lapierre M, Sempé M 1972 Le traitement des pubertés précoces par
l'acétate de médroxyprogestérone. Pédiatrie 27: 623

Dean H J, Winter J S A 1981 Abnormalities of pubertal development. In: Collu R, Ducharme
J R, Guyda H (eds) Pediatric Endocrinology, Comprehensive Endocrinology Series, p. 327.
Raven Press, New York

De Lange W E, Snoep M C, Doorenbos H 1978 The effect of LHRH infusion on serum LH,
FSH and testosterone in boys with advanced puberty, delayed puberty and
hypogonadotrophic hypogonadism. Acta Endocrinologica 89: 209

De Peretti E, Forest M G 1978 Pattern of plasma dehydroepiandrosterone sulfate levels in
humans from birth to adulthood: evidence for testicular production. Journal of Clinical
Endocrinology and Metabolism 47: 570

Ducharme J R 1981 Normal puberty: clinical manifestations and their endocrine control. In:
Collu R, Ducharme J R, Guyda H (eds) Pediatric Endocrinology, Comprehensive
Endocrinology Series, p. 293. Raven Press, New York

Ducharme J R, Collu R 1982 Pubertal development; normal, precocious and delayed. Clinics
of Endocrinology and Metabolism 11: 57

Ducharme J R, Forest M G 1982 Développement pubertaine normal. In: Bertrand J,
Rappaport R, Sizonenko P C (eds) Endocrinologie Pédiatrique, Physiologie-
Physiopathologie Clinique, p. 315. Editions Payot, Lausanne

Ducharme J R, Forest M G, De Peretti E, Sempé M, Collu R, Bertrand J 1976 Plasma
adrenal and gonadal sex steroids in human pubertal development. Journal of Clinical
Endocrinology and Metabolism 42: 468

Ehara Y, Yen S S C, Siler T M 1975 serum prolactin levels during puberty. American
Journal of Obstetrics and Gynecology 121: 995

Ehrenkranz J R L, Tamarkin L, Comite F & al 1982 Daily ryth of plasma melatonin in
normal and precocious puberty. Journal of Clinical Endocrinology and Metabolism 55: 307

Espiner E A, Veale A M, Sands V E, Fitzgerald P H 1970 Familial syndrome of streak
gonads and normal male karyotype. New England Journal of Medicine 283: 6

Faiman C, Winter J S D 1974 Gonadotropin and sex hormone patterns in puberty: clinical
data. In: Grumbach M M, Grave G D, Mayer F E (eds) Control of the Onset of Puberty,
p. 32. John Wiley, New York

Forest M G, Saez J M, Bertrand J 1973 Present concept in the initiation of puberty-neonatal
and prepubertal hormonal influences. In: Schattwaer F K (ed) Some Aspects of
Hypothalamic Regulation of Endocrine Functions, p. 339. Springer Verlag, Stuttgart

Frantz A G, Kleinberg D L, Noel G L 1972 Studies on prolactin in man. Recent Progress on
Hormone Research 28: 527

Genazzani A R, Pintor C, Fanchinette F, Inaudi P, Maci D, Corda R 1979 Changes
throughout puberty in adrenal secretion after ACTH. Journal of Steroid Biochemistry 11:
571

Genazzani A R, Facchinette F, Petroglia F, Pintor C, Puggioni R, Bagnoli F, Corda R 1983
Circulating opioid and prepubertal development (Abstract). Neuroendocrinology Letters 5:
326

Gorski R A 1974 Extrahypothalamic influences on gonadotropin regulation. In: Grumbach M
M, Grave G D, Mayer E E (eds) Control of the Onset of Puberty, p. 182. John Wiley,
New York

Greeley G H, Allen M B, Mahesh V B 1976 Potentiation of LH release by oestradiol at the
level of the pituitary. Neuroendocrinology 18: 233

Grumbach M M 1980 The neuroendocrinology of puberty. In: Krieger D T, Hughes J C
(eds) Neuroendocrinology, p. 249. Sinauer Assoc., Sunderland

Grumbach M M, Roth J C, Kaplan S L, Kelch L P 1974 Hypothalamic-pituitary regulation
of puberty in man: Evidence and concepts derived from clinical research. In: Grumbach M
M, Grave G D, Mayer F E (eds) Control of the Onset of Puberty, p. 115. John Wiley,
New York

Job J C 1977 The neuroendocrine system and puberty. In: Martini L, Besser G M (eds)
Clinical Neuroendocrinology, p. 487. Academic Press, New York

Job J C, Garnier P W, Chaussain J L, Milhaud G 1972 Elevation of serum gonadotropins

(LH and FSH) after releasing hormone (LH-RH) injection in normal children and in patients with disorders of puberty. Journal of Clinical Endocrinology and Metabolism 35: 473

Job J C, Chaussain J L, Garnier P W, Toublanc J-E 1976 Effect of synthetic luteinizing hormone-releasing hormone on the release of gonadotropins in hypophysogonadal disorders of children and adolescents. Constitutional delay of puberty in males. Journal of Pediatrics 88: 494

Johanson A 1974 Fluctuations of gonadotropin levels in children. Journal of Clinical Endocrinology and Metabolism 39: 154

Korth-Schultz S, Levine L S, New M I 1976 Evidence for the adrenal source of androgens in precocious adrenarche. Acta Endocrinologica 82: 342

Kulin H E, Bell P M, Santen R J, Ferber A J 1975 Integration of pulsatile gonadotropin secretion by timed urinary measurements: an accurate and sensitive 3 hour test. Journal of Clinical Endocrinology and Metabolism 40: 783

Kulin H E, Grumbach M M, Kaplan S L 1972 Gonadal-hypothalamic interaction in prepubertal and pubertal man: Effect of clomiphene citrate on urinary follicle-stimulating hormone and plasma testosterone. Pediatric Research 6: 162

Kulin H E, Reiter E O 1976 Gonadotropin and testosterone measurements after estrogen administration to adult men, prepubertal and pubertal boys, and men with hypogonadotropism: Evidence for maturation of positive feedback in the male. Pediatric Research 10: 46

Lenko H L, Lang U, Aubert M L, Paunier L, Sizonenko P C 1982 Hormonal changes in puberty. VII. Lack of variation of daytime plasma melatonin. Journal of Clinical Endocrinology and Metabolism 54: 1056

Liu N, Grumbach M M, de Napoli R A, Morishima A 1965 Prevalence of EEG abnormalities in idiopathic precocious puberty and premature pubarche: bearing on pathogenesis and neuroendocrine regulation of puberty. Journal of Clinical Endocrinology and Metabolism 25: 1296

Mahesh V B, Mazian S J 1979 Role of sex steroids in the initiation of puberty. Journal of Steroid Biochemistry 11: 587

Mansfield M J, Loughlin J S, Crawford J D, Bode H H, Crowley W F 1982 Effects of an LHRH agonist D-Trp^6-Pro^9-NET-LHRH (LHRH) on growth and skeletal maturation in central precocity. Pediatric Research 16: 141A

Marshall J C, Kelch R P 1979 Low dose pulsatile gonadotropin-releasing hormone in anorexia nervosa: a model for human pubertal development. Journal of Clinical Endocrinology and Metabolism 49: 712

Marshall W A, Tanner J M 1969 Variations in the pattern of pubertal changes in girls. Archives Diseases in Childhood 44: 291

Marshall W A, Tanner J M 1970 Variations in the pattern of pubertal changes in boys. Archives Diseases in Childhood 45: 13

Nakai Y, Plant T M, Hess D L, Keogh E J, Knobil E 1978 On the sites of the negative and positive feedback actions of estradiol in the control of gonadotropin secretion in the rhesus monkey. Endocrinology 102: 1008

Parker L, Odell W 1979 Evidence for existence of cortical androgen-stimulating hormone. American Journal of Physiology 236: E616

Pinsky L 1981 Sexual differentiation. In: Collu R, Ducharme J R, Guyda H (eds) Pediatric Endocrinology, Comprehensive Endocrinology Series, p. 231. Raven Press, New York

Plauchu H, Claustrat B, Betend B, David M, François R 1980 Le test à l'hormone hypothalamique synthétique LHRH chez l'enfant normal de la naissance à l'âge adulte. Pediatrie 35: 119¹

Posner B I, Khan M N, Bergeron J J M 1981 Mechanism of polypeptide action: current concepts. In:Collu R, Ducharme J R, Guyda H (eds) Pediatric Endocrinology, Comprehensive Endocrinology Series, p. 29. Raven Press, New York

Rager K, Huenges R, Gupta D, Bierich J R 1973 The treatment of precocious puberty with cyproterone acetate. Acta Endocrinologica 74: 399

Reiter E O, Grumbach M M 1982 Neuroendocrine control mechanisms and the onset of puberty. In: Edelman I S, Berne R M (eds) Annual Review of Physiology, p. 595. Annual Reviews, Palo Alto

Reiter E O, Kulin H E 1972 Sexual maturation in the female. Pediatric Clinics of North America 19: 581

Reiter E O, Kulin H E, Hamwood S M 1974 The absence of positive feedback between estrogen and luteinizing hormone in sexually immature girls. Pediatric Research 8: 740

Richards J S, Williams J J 1976 Luteal cell receptor content for prolactin (PRL) and luteinizing hormone (LH): regulation by LH and PRL. Endocrinology 99: 1571

Rimoin D L, Schimke R N 1971 Genetic disorders of the endocrine glands, p. 285. Mosby C V, St Louis

Root A W 1973 Endocrinology of puberty. I. Normal sexual maturation. Journal of Pediatrics 83: 1

Rosenfeld R G, Reitz R E, King A B, Hintz R L 1980 Familial precocious puberty associated with isolated elevation of luteinizing hormone. New England Journal of Medicine 303: 859

Ross G T, Vande Wiele R, Frantz A G 1981 The ovaries and the breasts. In: Williams R H (ed) Textbook of Endocrinology, 6th edn, p. 358. W. B. Saunders, Philadelphia

Ruehsen M, Blizzard R M, Garcia-Bunnuel R, Jones G S 1972 Autoimmunity and ovarian failure. American Journal of Obstetrics and Gynecology 112: 693

Schellhas H F 1974 Malignant potential of the dysgenetic gonad. Obstetrics and Gynecology 44: 298

Simpson J L 1972 Genetic aspects of gynecology disorders occurring in 46 XX individuals. Clinical Obstetrics and Gynecology 15: 157

Sizonenko P C 1978 Endocrinology in preadolescents and adolescents. I. Hormonal changes during normal puberty. American Journal of Diseases of Children 132: 704

Sizonenko P, Paunier L 1975 Hormonal changes in puberty: III. Correlation of plasma dehydroepiandrosterone, testosterone, FSH and LH with stages of puberty and bone age in normal boys and girls and in patients with Addison's disease of hypogonadism or with premature or late adrenarche. Journal of Clinical Endocrinology and Metabolism 41: 894

Sizonenko P C, Paunier L, Carmignac D 1975 Hormonal changes during puberty. IV. Longitudinal study of adrenal androgen secretions. Hormone Research 7: 288

Sklar C A, Kaplan S L, Grumbach M M 1980 Evidence for dissociation between adrenarche and gonadarche: studies in patients with idiopathic precocious puberty, gonadal dysgenesis, isolated gonadotropin deficiency, and constitutionally delayed growth and adolescence. Journal of Clinical Endocrinology and Metabolism 51: 548

Sohval A R 1965 The syndrome of pure gonadal dysgenesis. American Journal of Medicine 38: 615

Starup J, Pedersen H 1978 Hormonal and ultrastructural observations in a case of resistant ovary syndrome. Acta Endocrinologica 89: 744

Styne D M, Kaplan S L 1979 Normal and abnormal puberty in the female. Pediatric Clinics of North American 26: 123

Tanner J M 1969 Growth and endocrinology of the adolescent. In: Gardner L I (ed) Endocrine and Genetic Diseases of Childhood, p. 19. W. B. Saunders, Philadelphia

Therman E, Denniston C, Sarto G E, Ulber M 1980 X-chromosome constitution and the human female phenotype. Human Genetics 54: 133

Urban M D, Lee P A, Gutai J P, Migeon C J 1980 Androgens in pubertal males with Addison's disease. Journal of Clinical Endocrinology and Metabolism 51: 925

Van der Werff ten Bosch J J 1975 Isosexual precocity. In: Gardner L I (ed) Endocrine and Genetic Diseases of Childhood, p. 619. W. B. Saunders, Philadelphia

Weitzman E D, Boyar R M, Kapen S, Hellman L 1975 The relationship of sleep and sleep stages to neuroendocrine secretion and biological rhythms in man. Recent Progress in Hormone Research 31: 399

Werder A, Murset G, Zachman M, Brook C G D, Prader A 1974 Treatment of precocious puberty with cyproterone acetate. Pediatric Research 8: 248

Winter J S D, Faiman C 1973a The development of cyclic pituitary gonadal function in adolescent females. Journal of Clinical Endocrinology and Metabolism 37: 714

Winter J S D, Faiman C 1973b Pituitary-gonadal relations in female children and adolescents. Pediatric Research 7: 948

Intersex

INTRODUCTION

The doctor of today should have a broad understanding of sex differentiation and its failures. Careful study of pathological states can elucidate normal physiology and contribute to the reduction of psychological distress, the most serious clinical aspect.

A prosaic but useful definition of sex is that it is a species dimorphism represented at different planes by chromosomes, gonads, sex ducts, external genitalia, bodily habitus, secondary sex characteristics and behaviour or psychological attitude. The terms 'chromosomal' or 'gonadal' sex are self-explanatory. 'Phenotypic' sex refers to the apparent sex of the individual as judged by external characteristics. The term 'intersex' is applied to cases in which there is some contradiction between the manifestations or they are so poorly developed as to leave doubt as to the appropriate sex designation.

A few fundamental points facilitate understanding of anomalies of human sex differentiation:

1. Sex is not, as society regards it, a simple grouping of individuals into two entirely distinct classes. Biologically, it is a *spectrum* ranging from the very masculine to the very feminine. While most individuals are easily classed as male or female, there are in the intermediate zone some who biologically are neither male nor female. In other words, sex is not a binary phenomenon but a set of characteristics with a bimodal distribution. The doctor must assign such cases to one or other sex, but this is an administrative simplification of biological reality.

2. The chromosomal complement of a zygote will normally determine the sex of the gonads. If for any reason the gonad has differentiated contrary to the chromosomal sex, then all subsequent sex development can be expected to accord with the gonadal sex.

3. If a Y chromosome is present, no matter the number of X chromosomes, its influence will tend to dominate and some masculine development result.

4. In the human, the female state corresponds closely to the neuter. In other words if there is no second or 'differentiating' sex chromosome (XO) and/or no gonadal development, the individual's phenotype will be female. It follows that masculine development requires some positive influence.

This meams that given a normal and compatible chromosome and gonadal sex constitution only two basic types of physical intersex occur — incomplete masculinisation of chromosomal and gonadal males and partial masculinisation of females.

There are cases with no demonstrable anatomical or physiological abnormality, but psychologically there is contradiction to the physical sex. Such cases rarely present in gynaecological practice.

Cases may be grouped according to the level at which the abnormality appears to operate:

1. *Chromosomal*
2. *Gonadal*
3. *Partial masculinisation of chromosomal and gonadal females*
4. *Incomplete masculinisation of chromosomal and gonadal males*
5. *Cerebral*

With complex cases it is wise to detail the sexual state — chromosomal, gonadal, etc — as far as possible.

The method of chromosomal analysis and the apparent mechanisms whereby the sex chromosomes induce gonadal differentiation which ultimately lead to development of sex ducts and secondary characteristics have been established for some time and are detailed in biological texts (see Scott 1984). Currently the precise sex-determining mechanism involving the Y chromosome is a matter of debate.

H-Y ANTIGEN

Sometimes discrepancies were noted between Y chromosomal status and testicular development. In experiments on inbred mice, male-derived grafts were rejected by females but not female-derived by males or male-to-male grafts. It was concluded that this was due to a weak transplantation antigen carried by male mice but not females. This was called the H-Y (or serologically determined male, SDM) antigen, thought to be possibly the product of the testis-determining gene on the Y chromosome (Wachtel et al 1975). It was discovered to be present in other animals, including humans.

Ohno (1978) has shown that the H-Y antigen is present on the plasma membrane of the cell. By removing the H-Y antigen from the cell surface and by applying excess of H-Y antibody it was demonstrated in tissue culture that a gonadal cell of a type which prior to this procedure would organise seminiferous tubules around it would on the contrary organise follicular-like structure. However, XX human males have been found to express the H-Y antigen and also a Turner's syndrome patient with ovarian function (Haseltine et al 1984).

Over the years after its discovery much evidence came forward to support the idea that the H-Y antigen was the essential factor for testicular development and was controlled by a gene on the Y chromosome. Where chromosomes and gonadal sex were discordant the H-Y status was usually in keeping with the gonadal findings and this gave much support for the idea that it was the product of the key sex-determining gene. The methodology of detecting H-Y was complex and poorly reproducible, involving an assay with an end-point of mouse sperm cytotoxicity. More recently monoclonal antibody to H-Y has become available and has improved detection but not removed all the problems. Discordant observations have accumulated that cast doubt on the validity of the simple explanation that the H-Y gene and its product cause testicular development. Findings in wood lemmings and in humans with XO and deletion of the short arm of the X chromosome and with isochromosomes of the long arm of the X, all of whom were H-Y positive, have necessitated revision of the idea that the H-Y was carried on the Y chromosome (Wachtel et al 1980).

It came to be appreciated that graft rejection and serological sperm cytotoxicity methods used for determining H-Y status may not measure the same factor (Polani & Adinolfi 1983). It seemed at first that there might be two factors: (1) H-Y, the male-specific *transplantation* antigen involved in graft rejection, and (2) the target of the serological assay — SDM antigen (Silvers et al 1982). However, further animal studies have revealed even more complex H-Y anomalies (Simpson et al 1982), suggesting that more than two factors may be involved, and it has even come to be questioned whether there *are* sex-differentiating antigens.

Polani & Adolfini (1983) have suggested that the H-Y antigen is controlled by a structural gene on an autosome which produces a precursor molecule (H-Yp). Currently work is proceeding to try to determine the precise role of the H-Y antigen and the way it may interact with other factors (Nakamura et al 1984).

CHROMOSOMAL INTERSEX

Turner's syndrome

Turner's syndrome is a term which has been used with reference to a range of conditions. Shortness of stature, usually less than 5 feet, is the outstanding physical characteristic. Streak gonads are the rule with amenorrhoea and poorly developed secondary sex characteristics. Webbing of the neck and a peculiarly straight, low hair line are common. Lymphoedema of the extremities present at birth may first arouse suspicion of the condition.

Jones et al (1966) proposed that the term be applied to the female showing infantilism due to streak gonads and retardation of growth; additional somatic features might or might not be present. Patients with sexual development between normal female and normal male but who are short in stature and show other somatic features often associated with Turner's syndrome they suggested be referred to by the term 'Turner's phenotype'.

Most patients with classical Turner's syndrome have either a 45,X complement in all cells or deficient chromosome material involving the short arm of an X. This may be due to deletions of the short arm (46,XXp-) or its absence with a long-arm isochromosome (46,XXqi). Alternatively, there may be mosaicism with such a cell-line contributing. Where the abnormal cell-line affects non-gonadal tissue, it may cause Turner's stigmata without gonadal dysgenesis.

The analysis by Ferguson-Smith (1965) of the relationship between phenotype and karyotype in Turner's syndrome variants showed that where the sex chromosome complement deviated from XO, the classical Turner's clinical picture deviated towards normal maleness or normal femaleness to left or right of the XO median.

Ford (1969) reviewed the evidence in relation to chromosome mosaicism in cases of Turner's syndrome. In a collected series of 163 cases, 28 were mosaics of various sorts. An XO cell-line was nearly always present, but very rarely a normal one.

The absent sex chromosome in 45,X cases of Turner's syndrome need not necessarily have been an X, as is indicated by the report of 45,X Turner's syndrome in one of uniovular twins, the other being a male with 46,XY karyotype (Lejeune 1964). Monozygosity was determined by complete concordance for blood group and other genetic markers.

The evidence suggests that genes are present on both long and short arms which are necessary for the development of a functioning ovary. However, short stature and the other somatic abnormalities frequently found in cases of 45,X Turner's syndrome are *not* found in individuals with a 46,XXpi or 46,XXq-complement. From this it can be deduced that the genes responsible for normal development of these physical features are situated in the short arm of the X chromosome and that the short arm of two X chromosomes must be present in the female for normal development to take place (Jacobs 1969).

Polani (1981) argues that Turner's syndrome cases with a full range of associated deformities (neck webbing, increased carrying angle, short neck, etc) should be differentiated from those that have as the only association of the gonadal agenesis a degree of dwarfism. In that category only about 50% have an XO chromosome complement, but many have structural or mosaic chromosomal abnormalities, and normal sex chromosomes are almost never present.

In view of the relatively gross somatic anomalies displayed in postnatal Turner's syndrome it would not be surprising if some examples had features incompatible with survival. Many embryos with an X sex chromosome complement destined to be cases of Turner's syndrome perish before reaching viability (Smith et al 1969). Reported incidences of 45,X vary from about 2% in induced abortions to 20% in spontaneous abortions. These figures support the view that most chromosomally abnormal embryos abort. Hecht & Macfarlane (1969) concluded that between 96 and 98% of X conceptuses are *not* born alive. Polani (1970) suggested that the incidence of 45,X in spontaneous abortions is 200 times higher than in a population of extra-uterine survivors.

The streak gonads postnatally usually contain only fibrous tissue, but occasionally such patients menstruate and give birth to a normal child. These occurrences emphasise the fact learnt from the study of XO abortuses that germinal follicles are present at the early fetal stage but tend to undergo resorption before birth in most XO cases. King et al (1978) recorded what they claimed was the sixth reported non-mosaic XO individual to achieve a pregnancy. There was a high fetal wastage (22 of 46) and a high incidence of chromosome abnormality in the surviving infants (8 of 26 live-borns had an abnormality, three showing trisomy 21). They recommended pre-natal and amniotic chromosome studies in such patients. The matter is further reviewed by Dewhurst (1978) and Simpson (1981), who conclude that because of biased reporting the actual risk of chromosomal abnormality is not in reality as high as the above figures suggest.

The dwarfism of Turner's syndrome has been something of a mystery. The fusion of epiphyses which arrests growth normally occurs as a consequence of gonadal hormone production at puberty. It might therefore be expected that if individuals without gonads showed any variation in height it would be towards excessive growth. Growth hormone is not deficient.

Simpson & Lebeau (1981) reported that cell culture division time of fibroblasts from 45,XO individuals is slow. They suggest this may account for the short stature, the retarded intra-uterine growth and the high abortion rate. However, there must be some other factor(s) operating as, if this were the only explanation, it would be expected that Turner's syndrome patients would ultimately attain full height.

Klinefelter's syndrome (seminiferous tubule dysgenesis)

Klinefelter's syndrome in phenotypic males is characterised by azoospermia, gynaecomastia and atrophic testes. Histologically the testes show hyalinisation and degeneration of the seminiferous tubules with apparent overgrowth of Leydig cells. They are chromatin positive and the usual chromosome pattern is 47,XXY. In some cases no chromosome abnormality can be detected. In these the testicular abnormality is less pronounced and some tubules usually show some spermatogenesis. These cases are sometimes referred to as 'chromatin-negative Klinefelter's syndrome'.

The chromatin-positive cases are eunuchoid, the sole-to-pubic length being considerably greater than in normal males. They have small testes and prostates, diminished body and facial hair, raised gonadotrophin levels and tendency to lowered intelligence. Mosaicism is common, but at least a proportion of cells contain X and Y chromosomes *plus at least one additional X chromosome.*

The frequency is of the order of two cases per 1000 phenotypic male births. Higher incidences are found in populations of mentally defective males. Clinically, males with seminiferous tubular dysgenesis frequently present at infertility clinics. About 10% azoospermic or severely oligospermic males have seminiferous tubular degeneration or about 1–2% of all males attending subfertility clinics. This is not to say that every chromatin-positive male is infertile. In XY/XXY cases, if some XY cells are involved in the composition of the testes, sperm production may occur.

The diagnosis can readily be confirmed by checking the buccal smear. Once diagnosed, there is little to be done except possibly plastic surgery to the breasts where these are embarrassingly large. These individuals have led normal, active sex lives as males and have had no suspicion that they were 'intersexes'. Consequently the psychological aspect has to be handled with great delicacy. *Nothing is usually to be gained by explaining the diagnosis to the patient in precise terms.* Sufficient to say that there is some 'incomplete glandular development' and hint that the infertility problem may not easily be solved. It is neither necessary nor appropriate to state that sterility is absolute; if there is a small, undetected XY cell-line it may not be.

Phenotypic females with extra X chromosomes

Cases have been described of females with three X chromosomes (Court-Brown et al 1964). There are no remarkable features and fertility is possible. They may be suspected by finding more than one chromatin body in some cells.

This complement is found less frequently in normal populations compared with mentally defective populations. There may be a differential mortality between XX and XXX females at a certain stage of life.

Abnormal Y chromosome complements

In the 'XYY (or 'YY') syndrome' there is a 47,XYY constitution or XXYY. They tend to be taller than normal males and are found more frequently in institutions for mentally defective males. This is common to other extra sex chromosome conditions including Klinefelter's syndrome.

Long-term follow-up results have been published (Lancet 1982). Klinefelter's syndrome cases have shown no unexpected physical features, and mental retardation was absent, though there was a marginally reduced IQ. Homosexual tendencies were not evident. The picture with XYY seems similar. The future for these children is apparently far from gloomy. Knowledge of the anomaly may help teachers to be alert to institute any special help which may be needed to cover any difficulties.

Some cases have been recorded in which there was abnormality of the external genitalia. The most constant feature with structural abnormalities of the Y is infertility. Patients with small fragments of Y may have normal testicular development. It was concluded that the masculinisation genes responsible lay near the centromere, probably on the short arm (Jacobs 1969).

XX/XY chimerism

The words 'mosaic' and 'chimera' both describe subjects with cells of different chromosomal constitutions. In a chimera the cells derive from two acts of syngamy (union of gametes), while in a mosaic they arise from a single act of gamete fusion and the error develops at mitotic divisions subsequent to fertilisation. Chimeras may be from two entirely distinct zygotes (e.g. binovular twins) or from two separate acts of syngamy involving a single ovum (e.g. dispermic conceptions with participation of ovum nucleus and nucleus of the second polar body, or daughters of the ovum nucleus by mitotic division, and fusion of one daughter of the zygote nucleus with the nucleus of the second polar body, see Ford 1969, for review. It is only in relation to XX/XY mixtures that such situations can readily be identified, but they may exist when both cell strains are XY or XX. It may be impossible to say whether a mixed population of cells is due to mosaicism or chimerism but most are mosaic. However, if the complement is 46,XX/46,XY it is probably chimerism as it requires a most unlikely sequence of mitotic errors to produce only two cell-lines, 46,XX/46,XY. XX/XY chimerism can be produced artificially, e.g. with intra-uterine transfusion for rhesus isoimmunisation. A minority of XX/XY cases are hermaphrodites and are considered under 'Gonadal intersex'. In an XX/XY phenotypic female with primary amenorrhoea one gonad was a streak, while the other was the seat of a disgerminoma.

Mixed gonadal dysgenesis

'Mixed gonadal dysgenesis' describes cases in which the gonad on one side is a testis and on the other a 'streak' ('asymmetrical gonadal dysgenesis'). There may be unilateral Mullerian development and partial masculinisation of the external genitalia. The chromosome constitution is often 45,X/46,XY mosaic.

GONADAL INTERSEX

Ovotesticular states

The presence of both ovarian and testicular tissue is a form of sexual neutrality labelled 'hermaphroditism'. The term has been much misused and now it is best to specify details. ('Pseudohermaphroditism', a term widely used in the older literature, has no specific meaning). The arrangement of the ovarian and testicular tissues can vary widely, as may other aspects of genital development. Most cases are chromatin-positive and 46,XX. The *expected* chromosome complement — XX/XY — is the exception rather than the rule.

It is particularly common amongst the Bantu tribe (van Niekerk 1974). Three-quarters of 302 cases had been reared as males; the external genitalia were ambiguous and 50% menstruated, but spermatogenesis was exceptional. Five patients had developed disgerminomas. Pregnancy has occasionally been reported (Williamson et al 1981).

It was assumed that for testicular differentiation a Y chromosome was essential. As in many ovotesticular cases the chromosome complement was XX with no evidence of a strain of Y-containing cells, the correctness of this assumption came to be questioned. Sufficient cases had been recorded with only XX cells found, so that a hidden XX/XY mosaicism was unlikely to be the explanation in all. Interchange of material may take place between the X and the Y chromosome when they are associated at prophase in the first meiotic division in the primary spermatocyte. The fertilisation by a sperm carrying an X chromosome to which male-determining alleles from the Y are transferred will give a zygote whose sex chromosome constitution can be designated XX^Y. Random X inactivation during early embryogenesis according to Lyon's hypothesis could lead to testicular differentiation in cells with the X chromosome carrying Y material active and any with the ordinary X active to ovarian differentiation. Alternative explanations are the occurrence of a mutation in the sex genes or of an autosomal mutation which dominates the influence of the sex chromosomes.

Pure gonadal dysgenesis

In distinction to Turner's syndrome there is a group of individuals with gonadal dysgenesis who, apart from the expected sexual infantilism, have no other physical stigmata. These are classed as having 'pure gonadal dysgenesis'. The chromosomal constitution may be 46,XY (Swyer's syndrome) or 46,XX. If it is remembered that when no gonads develop a female phenotype is to be expected *regardless* of the chromosome complement, it will be understood why such cases may be XX or XY. Polani (1972) suggested that some cases may be examples of what he describes as sex inversion, which corresponds to the category of 'contrary gonadal development' discussed later. Galactosaemia can lead to a streak gonad as in gonadal dysgenesis or cause premature ovarian failure (Kaufman et al 1979, 1981).

Absence of the H-Y antigen (see page 223) is usual in X-Y pure gonadal dysgenesis cases (Ghosh et al 1978, Wachtel 1979) but is not invariable. H-Y positive cases probably result from mutation of the gene(s) concerned with H-Y receptors, the mutation rendering them unresponsive to the testicle-developing action of H-Y (Simpson et al 1981). Some XY cases have a non-fluorescent Y chromosome and absence of the H-Y antigen (Curtis et al 1980).

Contrary gonadal development (sex inversion)

Some phenotypic males with testes have a 46,XX constitution representing sex reversal, deviation or inversion (Polani 1972) between chromosome and gonadal level. Mice display sex reversal (Sxr) and the chromosomal sex is discordant with the gonadal and phenotypic sex. Polani (1972) reviewed around 30 human 46,XX phenotypic males. A possible explanation is that there has been an XXY zygote from which a Y chromosome has been lost. Alternatively the paternally-derived X may carry some translocated Y material which is not part of the fluorescent terminal portion. Support for the idea of deletion and translocation has come from studies with the Xg blood-group factor. Other explanations are a mutant abnormal masculinising autosome or a translocation from a Y to an autosome. It is possible that a strong, temporary androgenic influence at the time of gonadal differentiation may operate.

The opposite type of contrary gonadal development, i.e. an XY subject with ovaries, female sex ducts and phenotype has apparently not been detected in humans. It is, however, possible that the cases of XY pure gonadal dysgenesis referred to above are in biological terms the opposite of XX males but they lack active ovaries (Polani 1981).

PARTIAL MASCULINISATION OF CHROMOSOMAL AND GONADAL FEMALES

Congenital adrenal hyperlasia

'Adrenogenital syndrome'; steroid synthesis defects

'Adrenogenital syndrome' refers to cases in which alterations in the genital organs and their function are apparently due to pathology in the adrenal gland. This includes (a) a variety of neoplasms, (b) an ill-defined group of cases with hirsutism and menstrual disorders, and (c) 'congenital adrenal hyperplasia' due to inborn errors of adrenal steroid metabolism. The cases of intersex with an adrenal basis are almost all in the last category.

It is one form of intersex in which the aetiology is clearly defined and for which specific therapy is available in most cases. Diagnosis is very important, for if treated appropriately, they may fulfil their full sexual role, including childbearing. The cause is a metabolic enzyme deficiency inherited as a recessive gene.

'Congenital adrenal hyperplasia' covers a range of abnormalities of steroid synthesis. The common form, 21-hydroxylase deficiency, results in a build-up of androgens with virilisation of female children. Other very rare types may have the opposite effect, e.g. 3β-hydroxysteroid-dehydrogenase deficiency causes failure in production of androgen with lack of masculinisation of a male fetus. It is incompatible with survival, so such clinical presentations do not occur after the perinatal phase, but *the important point is to realise that quite different effects can be produced depending on the enzyme involved.* There is a complete spectrum of rare intersexual forms from masculinised females to unmasculinised males, but it is only the former group that present as problems of clinical management. The enzymatic defect is not necessarily confined to the adrenal gland, but will involve the ovaries or testes if the relevant metabolic step occurs there (Hall et al 1980).

They include in order of their position on the biosynthetic pathway from cholesterol: (1) *Cholesterol to pregnenolone block* (probably 20,22 desmolase deficiency, adrenal filled with lipoid; female phenotype; die early). (2) *3β-hydroxysteroid-dehydrogenase deficiency* (female child may be virilised due to dehydroepiandrosterone build up; males may be incompletely so due to deficiency of androstenedione). (3) *17α-hydroxylase deficiency* (block at progesterone level also affects gonads; females lack sex characteristics while males are incompletely masculinised; hypertension and hypokalaemia). (4) *21-hydroxylase deficiency* (the common type; 17α-hydroxyprogesterone build up; may be salt losing or non salt losing). (5) *11β-hydroxylase deficiency* (11-desoxycortisol build up; virilisation and hypertension). (6) *18-hydroxylase and 18-dehydrogenase deficiency* (corticosterone raised; aldosterone deficient; electrolyte affects).

Clinical aspects of 21-hydroxylase deficiency

Presentation may be at birth but rarely with hirsutism around puberty; 17α-hydroxyprogesterone is the key metabolite but this may not be elevated at birth though it becomes so within a few days. A convenient 'blood-spot' radioimmunoassay has been developed (Riordan et al 1984) which may be used for screening between days 5 and 10; urinary pregnanetriol is elevated; pregnanetriol is measured in the 17-ketogenic steroid (KGS) assay; thus in the 'late onset' cases the KGS will be high (of the order seen in Cushing's syndrome) in sharp contrast to the normal values seen in most other cases of hirsutism. ACTH stimulation may be employed in difficult cases to facilitate identification of the specific enzyme defect. If a newborn infant with an intersex problem becomes systemically ill, the blood chemistry should be checked. The blood urea and serum potassium rise; later the standard bicarbonate falls and finally the serum sodium. These changes may be very rapid and ECG monitoring may be wise.

Treatment consists of giving cortisol (hydrocortisone) to suppress the excessive ACTH production, about 0.15 mg/kg of body weight per day. The dose required approximates to 150% of physiological requirements (Hall et al 1980). It is titrated against the steroid levels and growth charts. The daily dose should be divided, approximately 6 hourly, with a larger dose at night to cover the ACTH suppression till the morning. Complete suppression of 17α-hydroxyprogesterone levels is not possible without excessive cortisol dosage (Antony 1984). In the salt-losing type a salt-retaining hormone (fludrocortisone 50 to 100 μg/day) is also required with intravenous saline at first.

If not diagnosed and treated, nowadays most likely in the male, the consequences are accelerated skeletal maturation and early epiphyseal fusion with resultant dwarfism; precocious puberty and excessive libido with aggressive behaviour occur in some cases, and eventually inhibition of gonadotrophin production with sterility. Cortisol therapy will control these undesirable effects.

For a woman who has borne a child with 21-hydroxylase deficiency, prenatal diagnosis in a subsequent pregnancy may have relevance; treatment might possibly be started while the child is still *in utero* and would hopefully minimise masculinisation. This was first attempted measuring the ratio of ketosteroids to hydroxycorticosteroids. Measurement of 17αOH progesterone has been reported as helpful (Hughes & Laurence 1979). An alternative approach is to take advantage of the fact that the gene involved displays linkage with definable markers (Pollack et al 1979). The gene or genes controlling the expression of 21-hydroxylase have been located on the short arm of chromosome 6 which carries HLA antigens, and associations were shown with HLA antigens, particularly the B group (Levine et al 1978). Fleischnick et al (1983) report on extended MHC haplotypes showing shared genotypes in unrelated patients.

Exogenous hormone-induced masculinisation of females

Masculinisation can occur from exogenous steroids administered to the mother in pregnancy. This has been reported with testosterone derivatives and nortestosterone-derived progestogenic steroids. Many patients with a tendency to abortion were given such preparations, and a number of virilised females were born. The virilising effects are not progressive after delivery, unlike those due to inborn errors of metabolism. The only treatment is plastic surgery.

Androgenic maternal tumours

Very rarely maternal tumours producing androgen occur in association with pregnancy and these may have the same effect as exogenous androgens.

INCOMPLETE MASCULINISATION OF CHROMOSOMAL AND GONADAL MALES

This may be due to four basic types of defect. In the commonest there is normal production of testosterone and Müllerian inhibiting factor (MIF), but failure of peripheral action of the androgens; the second involves failure of androgen production; the third failure of conversion of testosterone to its active form peripherally and the fourth is failure of MIF production.

Testicular feminisation — or androgen insensitivity — syndrome

In the 'testicular feminisation syndrome' 46,XY individuals have a female phenotype (Morris 1953). Testicles are present and amenorrhoea is the rule as there is merely a short, blind, vagina. In the light of studies on the pathogenesis the term 'androgen insensitivity syndrome' came to be used but it is not applicable to all forms.

Unless older relatives have had the condition or surgical exploration of the abdomen or genital tract has been necessitated for some coincidental reason, few cases are encountered before puberty, as those affected are usually regarded as entirely normal girls till then. Breast development occurs at puberty and may even be excessive. Pubic and axillary hair is usually absent or scant. The external genitals are female. The clitoris is not hypertrophied. The blind vagina is about 5–6 cm in length but is usually adequate for coitus. The uterus is absent or represented only by a fibrous band. Testes may lie in the inguinal region or the abdomen. Histologically, they are similar to undescended testes in otherwise normal males. The tubules are lined by primitive germ cells with some Sertoli cells. Leydig cells are present in large numbers and these are similar to adult Leydig cells both on light and electron microscopy. The chromosome complement is 46,XY. Psychologically these patients are usually extremely bright and alert, with a strongly feminine disposition and are usually happily integrated in life. They can achieve complete intercourse with orgasm in the female role. Their confident, positive demeanour contrasts markedly with that of Turner's syndrome patients.

There is an X-linked recessive inheritance. Carrier females may have diminished axillary and pubic hair and a history of late menarche.

The diagnosis once suspected can usually be confirmed by checking that the individual is chromatin-negative. The concentration of testosterone in the peripheral plasma is within or above the range for normal males. Gonadectomy is frequently performed because of the high incidence of neoplasia. Apart from this the main problem of management is usually to avoid the patient discovering that she is, or has been, the possessor of testicles.

Wilkins (1965) postulated that the underlying abnormality was the inability of the end organs to respond to androgens. Tissue incubation studies demonstrated that androstenedione and dehydroepiandrosterone can be produced by the testes and they can be converted to testosterone. That Müllerian inhibition takes place indicates that MIF production is normal. Nearly all the later evidence points to target organ non-responsiveness.

The free testosterone enters cells and can then be converted by 5α-reductase to dihydrotestosterone. These two hormones bind with receptors and then diffuse into the nuclei and interact with acceptor sites to produce a response in the cell. The testosterone-receptor complex regulates gonadotrophin secretion, spermatogenesis and Wolffian-duct differentiation, while the dihydro-testosterone-receptor complex controls external virilisation at puberty. Circulating testosterone and androstenedione are interconvertible and they can undergo peripheral conversion to oestradiol and oestrone respectively. In turn the oestrone and oestradiol can undergo some interchange while the testes produce a small amount of oestradiol.

The androgen resistance appears often to be related to diminished high-affinity receptors for dihydrotestosterone (Keenan et al 1974), as in mice with the analogous disorder (Tfm mice). There may be partial receptor deficiency at 37°C but normal binding at 26°C; at 42°C the binding diminishes — 'receptor instability'.

When enzyme deficits are suspected before puberty, a test dose of chorionic gonadotrophin may be given; the failure to produce testosterone should be matched with an elevation of hormone level at the site of synthesis at which the relevant enzyme operates.

The feminising influence is not fully explained. The receptor deficiency probably extends to cerebral centres and feedback is impaired. There is some oestrogen feedback which can be shown to reduce LH levels (Naftolin et al 1983). Most reports indicate there is an increase in the testicular production of oestrogen, while the peripheral conversion from androgens may also be on an increased scale (Walsh et al 1974).

Incomplete forms of androgen insensitivity syndrome

In some of these the degree of androgen insensitivity is incomplete, while in others the feminising component is absent. Two distinct types are referred to as types 1 and 2 (Wilson et al 1974, Walsh et al 1974).

Type 1

The whole group represents a mild partial form of the testicular feminisation syndrome. They have been given a variety of syndrome labels (Reifenstein, Rosewater, Gilbert-Dreyfus, Lubs, etc). Different members of the same affected family can show each of the syndromes, so the terms have ceased to have value.

The spectrum ranges from gynaecomastia and azoospermia to hypospadias and presence of a pseudo-vagina in more severe cases. Chest and facial hair is usually minimal, as is temporal hair-line regression. The testes are small, often cryptorchid, and the voice does not 'break'. Germ cell maturation is arrested and the vas deferens may be absent or hypoplastic. There may be other Wolffian duct differentiation defects: gynaecomastia at puberty and partial male secondary sex character development. Complete Müllerian duct inhibition is the rule, indicating normal MIF production. There is androgen-receptor deficit in genital skin. Feminisation at puberty is not usually striking.

Some apparently normal males may be infertile because of androgen receptor abnormality (Aiman et al 1979). Diagnosis should be suspected when azoospermia is associated with elevated levels of plasma LH and testosterone. There may be clitoral enlargement. Further virilising effects will occur at puberty and therefore there is a case for carrying out early gonadectomy.

Type 2 (5α-reductase deficiency)

5α-reductase deficiency is well known due to reports on families in the Dominican Republic (Imperato-McGinley et al 1979). The defect operates peripherally at intracellular level due to lack of conversion of testosterone into dihydrotestosterone. Facial and body hair is reduced and there is lack of temporal baldness. No prostatic tissue is palpable. It is inherited as an autosomal recessive condition. There are normally virilised Wolffian structures which terminate in the vagina. There is sometimes a change in gender-role at puberty when a degree of masculine development of the external genitalia occurs — erroneously regarded as 'sex change'.

Plasma testosterone is normal and LH moderately elevated, but dihydrotestosterone is low in adults. Elevated testosterone/dihydro-testosterone ratios can be induced with a chorionic gonadotrophin stimulation test before puberty. Deficient 5α-reductase activity can be demonstrated in genital skin.

Receptor-positive androgen insensitivity

There is a small group of cases with androgen insensitivity but neither 5α-reductase nor androgen receptors are deficient. The defect appears to be beyond receptor level, in the hurly-burly of nuclear chemical activity. It may well be a heterogeneous group chemically, and certainly the clinical range is as great as that for classical receptor-deficiency testicular feminisation (Griffin & Wilson 1980, Wilson et al 1981).

Defective androgen production syndrome

Various enzymatic defects result in failure of testosterone production and consequent lack of masculinisation. These include 20,22-desmolase, 3β-hydroxysteroid dehydrogenase, 17-hydroxylase, 17,20-desmolase and 17-ketosteroid reductase (otherwise known as 17β-hydroxysteroid dehydrogenase) (Wilson et al 1974). The clinical manifestations may range from partial to complete failure of masculinisation depending on the quantitative abnormality in testosterone production and the biological effects of the precursor steroids which accumulate because of the metabolic block. Certain of these enzymatic defects are common between the testis and adrenal and have already been referred to under 'congenital adrenal hyperplasia'.

Defective Müllerian regression syndrome

There have been occasional reports of apparently normal 46,XY individuals who have shown persistent Müllerian duct structures — sometimes in the form 'hernia uteri inguinali' (Brook et al 1973, Wilson et al 1974). The condition is probably due to MIF deficiency and is inherited as a recessive trait, autosomal or X-linked.

CEREBRAL INTERSEX

Homosexuality, transvestism and transsexuality are forms of intersex which involve atypical sexual drive and behaviour which rarely come within the province of gynaecologists as there are no biochemical or physical abnormalities. However, transsexuals may be referred with a view to surgery to convert physical sexual features.

INTERSEX STATES AND GONADAL MALIGNANCY

Intersexual individuals have an increased propensity to gonadal neoplasms, some malignant. This is mainly related to cases in which at least some cells bear a Y chromosome and there are intra-abdominal gonads. The malignancy risk is greatest when the gonads are dysgenetic (see Scott 1984). Consideration must be given to appropriately timed gonadectomy in cases at high risk.

MANAGEMENT

It is usually the *psychological* aspect of the situation which is of prime importance. Full investigation is appropriate before any intelligent advice or guidance can be given. Good advice, however, may be entirely in contradiction to the biological findings. It must be couched in terms which will not increase psychological disturbance. No rules can be laid down for correct management beyond the need for a sympathetic and compassionate understanding of the individual patient's social and psychological problems.

If it becomes necessary to explore the abdomen and biopsy the gonads, it is desirable to have facilities available for the immediate production and interpretation of frozen sections. If gonadal tissue contrary to the phenotypic sex is present removal is usually appropriate; the surgeon should have come to a clear decision as to his line of action for each possible eventuality.

Rarely the question of re-registration of sex arises. This is sometimes accepted by the Registrar General if he is persuaded that the original sex registration has been an error. The criteria for assignation of sex is the body phenotype — not the chromosomal or gonadal status.

REFERENCES

Aiman J, Griffin J E, Gazak J M, Wilson J D, MacDonald P C 1979 Androgen insensitivity as a cause of infertility in otherwise normal men. New England Journal of Medicine 300: 223–227

Antony G 1984 Management of Congenital Adrenal Hyperplasia. Lancet i: 1073

Brook C G D, Wagner H, Zachmann M, Prader A, Armendares S, Frenk S, Aleman P, Najjar S S, Slim M S, Genton N, Bozie C 1973 Familial occurrence of persistent Mullerian structures in otherwise normal males. British Medical Journal I: 771–773

Court-Brown W M, Harnden D G, Jacobs P A, Maclean N, Mantle D J 1964 Medical Research Council Special Report Series No. 305. HMSO, London

Curtis W R S, White B J, Lucky A W, Roche-Bender N, Knab D R, Johnsonbaugh R E 1980 Gonadal dysgenesis with mosaicism and a nonfluorescent Y chromosome: Report of two cases with correlation of clinical, pathologic, and cytogenetic findings. American Journal of Obstetrics and Gynecology 136: 639–645

Dewhurst Sir J 1978 Fertility in 47,XXX and 45,X patients. Journal of Medical Genetics 15: 132–135

Ferguson-Smith M A 1965 Karyotype-phenotype correlations in gonadal dysgenesis and their bearing on the pathogenesis of malformations. Journal of Medical Genetics 2: 142–155

Fleischnick E, Raum D, Alosco S M, Gerald P S, Yunis E J, Awdeh Z L, Granados J, Crigler J F Jr, Giles C M, Alper C A 1983 Extended MHC haplotypes in 21-hydroxylase-deficiency: shared genotypes in unrelated patients. Lancet i: 152–156

Ford C E 1969 Mosaics and chimeras. British Medical Bulletin 25: 104–109

Ghosh S N, Shah P N, Gharpure H M 1978 Absence of H-Y antigen in XY females with dysgenetic gonads. Nature 276: 180

Griffin J E, Wilson D 1980 The syndromes of androgen resistance. New England Journal of Medicine 302: 198–209

Hall R, Anderson J, Smart G A, Besser M 1980 Fundamentals of Clinical Endocrinology, 3rd edn. Pitman Medical, London

Haseltine F P, Breg W R, Genel M 1984 Oocyte production in a Turner syndrome patient with serologically detectable male antigen. Journal of Reproductive Immunology 6: 19–24

Hecht F, Macfarlane J P 1969 Mosaicism in Turner's syndrome reflects the lethality of XO. Lancet ii: 1197–1198

Hughes I A, Laurence K M 1979 Antenatal diagnosis of congenital adrenal hyperplasia. Lancet ii: 7–9

Imperato-McGinley J, Peterson R E, Gautier T, Sturla E 1979 Androgens and the evolution of male-gender identity among male pseudo-hermaphrodites with 5α-reductase deficiency. New England Journal of Medicine 300: 1233–1237

Jacobs P A 1969 Structural abnormalities of the sex chromosomes. British Medical Bulletin 25: 94–98

Jones H W, Turner H H, Ferguson-Smith M A 1966 Turner's syndrome and phenotype. Lancet i: 1155

Kaufman F, Kogut M D, Donnell G N, Koch R, Goebelsmann U 1979 Ovarian failure in galactosaemia. Lancet ii: 737–738

Kaufman F R, Kogut M D, Donnell G N, Goebelsmann U, March C, Koch R 1981 Hypergonadotropic hypogonadism in female patients with galactosemia. New England Journal of Medicine 304: 994–998

Keenan B S, Meyer W J III, Hadjian A J, Jones H W, Migeon C J 1974 Syndrome of androgen insensitivity in man: absence of 5α-dihydrotestosterone binding protein in skin fibroblasts. Journal of Clinical Endocrinology and Metabolism 38: 1143–1146

King C R, Magenis E, Bennett S 1978 Pregnancy and the Turner syndrome. Obstetrics and Gynecology 52: 617–624

Lancet 1982 Leading article, Long-term outlook for children with sex chromosome abnormalities. Lancet ii: 27

Lejeune J 1964 The 21 trisomy-current stage of chromosomal research. Progress in Medical Genetics 3: 144–177

Levine L S, Zachmann M, New M I, Prader A, Pollack M S, O'Neill G J, Yang S Y, Oberfield S E, Dupont B 1978 Genetic mapping of the 21-hydroxylase-deficiency gene within the HLA linkage group. New England Journal of Medicine 299: 911–915

Morris J M 1953 The syndrome of testicular feminisation in male pseudo-hermaphrodites. American Journal of Obstetrics and Gynecology 65: 1192–1211

Naftolin F, Pujol-Amat P, Corker C S, Shane J M, Polani P E, Kohlinsku S, Yen S S C, Bobrow M 1983 Gonadotrophins and gonadal steroids in androgen insensitivity (testicular feminization) syndrome: effects of castration and sex steroid administration. American Journal of Obstetrics and Gynecology 147: 491–496

Nakamura D, Wachtel S S, Gilmour D 1984 Gonad-specific uptake of H-Y antigen in the chicken. Journal of Reproductive Immunology 6: 11–17

Ohno S 1978 The role of H-Y antigen in primary sex determination. Journal of the American Medical Association 239: 217–220

Polani P E 1970 The incidence of chromosomal malformations. Proceedings of the Royal Society of Medicine 63: 50–52

Polani P E 1972 Errors of sex determination and sex chromosome anomalies. In: Ounsted C, Taylor D C (eds) Gender Differences: Their Ontogeny and Significance, pp 13–39. Churchill Livingstone, Edinburgh

Polani P E 1981 In: Austin C R, Edwards R G (eds) Mechanisms of Sex Differentiation in Animals and Man, pp 465–590. Academic Press, London

Polani P E, Adinolfi M 1983 The H-Y antigen and its functions: a review and a hypothesis. Journal of Immunogenetics 10: 85–102

Pollack M S, Maurer D, Levine L S, New M I, Pang S, Duchon M, Owens R P, Merkatz I R, Nitowsky H M, Sachs G, Dupont B 1979 Prenatal diagnosis of congenital adrenal hyperplasia (21-hydroxylase deficiency) by HLA typing. Lancet i: 1107–1108

Riordan F A I, Wood P J, Wakelin K, Betts P, Clayton B E 1984 Bloodspot

17α-hydroxyprogesterone radioimmunoassay for diagnosis of congenital adrenal hyperplasia and home monitoring of corticosteroid replacement therapy. Lancet i: 708–711

Scott J S 1984 Intersex and sex chromosome abnormalities. In: Macdonald R (ed) Scientific Basis of Obstetrics and Gynaecology, 3rd edn, p. 201. Churchill Livingstone, Edinburgh

Silvers W K, Gasser D L, Eicher E M 1982 H-Y antigen, serologically detectable male antigen and sex determination. Cell 28: 439–440

Simpson J L 1981 Pregnancies in women with chromosomal abnormalities. In: Schulman J D, Simpson J L (eds) Genetic Diseases in Pregnancy, pp 439–471. Academic Press, New York

Simpson E, Chandler P, Pole D 1981 A model of T-cell unresponsiveness using the male-specific antigen H-Y. Cellular Immunology, 62: 251–257

Simpson E, McLaren A, Chandler P 1982 Evidence for two male antigens in mice. Immunogenetics 15: 609–614

Simpson J L, Lebeau M 1981 Gonadal and statural determinants on the X chromosome and their relationship to in vitro studies showing prolonged cell cycles in 45,X; 46,X,del(X)(p11); 46,X,del(X)(q13); and 46,X,del(X)(q22) fibroblasts. American Journal of Obstetrics and Gynecology 141: 930–940

Smith M, Macnab J, Ferguson-Smith M A 1969 Cell culture technics for cytogenic investigation of human abortus material; analysis of 45 cases and report of 3 specimens with gross chromosomal aberrations. Obstetrics and Gynecology 33: 313–323

van Niekerk W A 1974 True Hermaphroditism; Clinical, Morphologic and Cytogenic aspects. Harper & Row, London

Wachtel S S 1979 The Genetics of Intersexuality: clinical and theoretic perspectives. Obstetrics and Gynecology 54: 671–684

Wachtel S S, Ono S, Koo G C et al 1975 Possible role for H-Y antigen in the primary determination of sex. Nature 257: 235–236

Wachtel S S, Koo G C, Breg W R, Genel M 1980 H-Y antigen in X,i(Xq) gonadal dysgenesis. Evidence of X linked genes in testicular differentiation. Human Genetics 56: 183–187

Walsh P C, Madden J D, Harrod M J, Goldstein J L, MacDonald P C, Wilson J D 1974 Familial incomplete male pseudohermaphroditism, type 2: decreased dihydrotestosterone formation in pseudovaginal perineoscrotal hypospadias. New England Journal of Medicine 291: 944–949

Wilkins L 1965 The Diagnosis and Treatment of Endocrine Disorders in Childhood and Adolescence, 3rd edn. Charles C Thomas, Springfield, Illinois

Williamson H O, Phansey S A, Mathur R S 1981 True hermaphroditism with term vaginal delivery and a review. American Journal of Obstetrics and Gynecology 141: 262–265

Wilson J D, Harrod M J, Goldstein J L, Hemsell D L, MacDonald P C 1974 Familial incomplete male pseudohermaphroditism, type 1; evidence for androgen resistance and variable clinical manifestations in a family with the Reifenstein syndrome. New England Journal of Medicine 200: 1097–1103

Wilson J D, George F W, Griffin J E 1981 The hormonal control of sexual development. Science 211: 1278–1284

Psychosexual counselling

One of the major reasons for which patients often consult doctors is related to psychosexual problems. Whilst the medical profession acknowledges that problems exist in this field and that these problems may adversely affect their patients, very few doctors are adequately trained to assist in influencing their symptoms, their behaviour and their interpersonal relations. Some medical practitioners do recognise that a woman is suffering from a psychosexual problem but because of their lack of training and lack of confidence in their ability to help they choose to ignore the symptoms, or dismiss them with some attempt at humour or even sarcasm. The acute embarrassment of discussing personal sexual problems is such that if a doctor does not display immediate sympathy, empathy and understanding, the patient will feel hurt, rejected or will withdraw from further consultation. The insecure and poorly trained doctor often prescribes antidepressants, tranquilisers or sedatives, rather than attempting to counsel a woman regarding a sexual problem.

Sexual counselling can be regarded as a method whereby problems which a patient may possess are identified, clarified and explored in such a manner that they reflect, like a mirror, the patient's own psyche. Only after such an exploration can the areas which require redirection, re-education or retraining, be determined.

Before deciding that a sexual problem exists and counselling is needed, it is important to realise how sexual attitudes and behaviour are acquired. In the same way that individuals have differing beliefs regarding religion, politics or social behaviour so do people have varied attitudes and expectations regarding moral and sexual behaviour. These attitudes and expectations are learned in a variety of ways, not least of which is the influence of parents, family, religion, school, peers and the media.

Sexual attitudes may be influenced by society and by its laws as well as by the actions and behaviour of friends and acquaintances. This complex mass of information with its mix of myths, beliefs, truths and distortions all combine to influence an individual's perception and development of attitudes to sexuality. Education regarding basic anatomy and physiology is often lacking, but even when this is supplied in one form or another, there is seldom a formalised

239

attempt to incorporate this information into the broader concept of interpersonal growth and development.

Because of these educational neglects, men and women often reach maturity, marry, procreate or develop other relationships without achieving enjoyment or satisfaction from their sexual activities. They may feel guilty about their thoughts and activities, or they may feel frustrated in not achieving certain levels of response. Their particular attitudes to sexuality may cause bitter and acrimonious disruption of their interpersonal relationships. When this occurs, patients often begin a search for help. An aware medical practitioner may be in an ideal position to help by identifying that a sexual problem exists and then either directing the patient to a trained counsellor or performing that task himself.

The types of problems which may present to a medical practitioner can be conveniently divided into four general groups but it is important to realise that there is often considerable overlap between one group and another.

Loss of libido

Libido is the feeling or desire for sexual activity and is an affective response to environmental stimuli. Like the feeling of joy or sadness, happiness or anxiety, libido is influenced by a number of factors, some of which will be discussed further. A good, close and loving interpersonal relationship leads to a feeling of contentment and enjoyment in each other's company. When this positive interpersonal relationship is reinforced by words, physical stimuli and sexual foreplay, then libido and sexual activity is increased. Libido may also be enhanced by thoughts, fantasies and visual stimuli such as erotic literature, films or observing sexual activity. However, there are a number of factors which produce a negative effect on libido and these must be fully explored when taking a counselling history.

(a) *Failure to communicate.* Communication is a process involving two or more people whereby verbal or non-verbal messages are passed and feedback is obtained regarding ideas, feelings and physical actions. When one person only is involved in such a process while the other remains passive, providing either no or negative feedback, then a sense of frustration and anger becomes a dominant feature. This situation often occurs between married couples who have neglected each other's needs. Typical is a young couple with young children. The husband may work by day in an occupation which is neither interesting nor rewarding. His wife stays at home looking after the children, washing, cleaning, cooking, shopping and feeling lonely. She looks forward to the nightly return of her husband but he is tired, bored and frustrated with his work situation. He has little to say and neglects to enquire how his wife is feeling or how she spent her day. Their evenings together develop into a routine of getting the children bathed, fed and into bed, preparing the evening meal, clearing away, watching television and then finally retiring for the night. There is little opportunity for conversation, communication or touching. When bed eventually brings them into close physical contact, sexual activity is brief and joyless. Very soon one or both become bored with their partner's sexual needs and responses. This leads to apathy, or to frustration, resulting in a gradual drift into a non-sexual partnership or alternatively to arguments and acrimony.

(b) *Boredom and failure of emotional arousal.* This is often closely allied to lack of communication, particularly in those instances when arousal and foreplay are neglected. The method of intercourse is usually very predictable and brief. Often the male ejaculates prematurely leaving his partner frustrated and bitter. Rather than continue such sexual activity she will avoid intercourse by going to bed late (or early) or, when he attempts to have intercourse, she lies passive and non-responsive. If she pleads some mythical pelvic discomfort or pain she is said to suffer from vaginismus; if she attempts to resist intercourse or says she gains no pleasure from the act, she is said to suffer from frigidity. A male with similar problems of lack of libido may have erectile impotence or on occasions suffer from premature or retarded ejaculation. It is therefore important to take a careful history of interpersonal communication and domestic activity before attempting to treat the cause.

(c) *Lack of sexual knowledge and experience.* This may affect libido in several ways. When neither partner in a sexual union has any great understanding of the psychological forces nor of the physiological mechanisms which are necessary to achieve a satisfactory sexual response then there develops a feeling of disenchantment with the sexual relationship. Most often, the male achieves an early or premature ejaculation, leaving his partner feeling totally dissatisfied. This dissatisfaction eventually leads to a rejection of sexual activity and the anorgasmic female is labelled as being frigid.

(d) *Aversion to a sexual partner.* Couples often marry prematurely in response to psychological, physical or financial needs and then regret their decision. As the years pass one of them may see their partner in a less favourable light or their partner actually changes in physical appearance or personality. When this occurs it may produce such aversion and dislike that sexual activity is impossible. A woman who becomes grossly obese after several children may find that her partner can no longer display affection or sexual arousal in her presence. A man who becomes an alcoholic may so offend his wife that she cannot tolerate his physical presence. There are many other forms and causes of aversion which reduce considerably the ability to react to sexual advances and these must be explored in a careful history.

(e) *Children.* The fear of pregnancy may cause some women to refrain from intercourse, thus setting in chain a sequence of sexual denials and frustrations which can cause disruption to an otherwise satisfactory relationship. However, more common is the desire to avoid children seeing or hearing any sexual activity. This fear of displaying close sexual contact in the presence of children may so inhibit couples that repression of sexual urges results. Intercourse is often rushed and unsatisfactory. Premature ejaculation is common and loss of libido, orgasmic failure and frustration leads to avoidance of further sexual activity.

(f) *Differences and difficulties in social, religious and cultural beliefs.* These may adversely affect the interpersonal relationships of a couple. Often the gap between the couple is so great that within a few years the previously close, loving couple will begin to criticise each other for imagined shortcomings and failures. A 'war' breaks out in an attempt to gain a superior moral position — so the physical and sexual relationship disintegrates.

(g) *Sexual aberrations.* Another major cause in a breakdown in sexual relationships and resultant loss of libido is that related to sexual aberrations. Whilst there is no doubt that each person should be encouraged to regard their own sexuality and their style of sexual behaviour as part of their individuality, it is important to understand that some people have been taught to believe that certain sexual behaviours are abnormal or perverted. To ask a reluctant partner to indulge in an abhorrent sexual act may produce such disgust and distaste as to destroy a relationship. Under these circumstances, loss of libido is rapid and may be total for the relationship.

Orgasmic failure

The second major group of sexual problems which may present to a medical practitioner are those of orgasmic failure. Masters and Johnson have produced elegant studies which describe the four phases of the orgasmic response cycle, the physiological mechanisms being similar for men and for women. These physiological mechanisms correspond to the phases of sexual arousal induced by psychological and physical stimulation during normal sexual intercourse. Arousal is achieved following psychological and physical stimulation which may include sexual thoughts, fantasies, words, visual stimuli, music, alcohol or drugs. The period of time necessary to achieve a normal sexual response cycle including an orgasm can be shortened or prolonged depending on the influence of the psychological stimulation. Indeed, psychological influence can be so strong that both men and women have achieved a normal orgasm without any physical stimulation. The converse of this psychological stimulation is the inhibition which may occur due to various actions and thoughts, which lead to suppression of erotic fantasies. Under these circumstances, physical stimulation over a number of hours may produce nothing but a sore clitoris and a frustrated female.

There are a number of reasons why women may be anorgasmic and the list below is far from exhaustive.

(a) *Lack of knowledge and experience.* A number of men and women have little or no knowedge of the sensate areas on the genitals which when stimulated will enhance orgasmic response. Each person has their own responsive erotic areas which must be explored and learned by both the male and the female. No two women respond in identical ways so that it is important that each female 'teach' her partner which areas on her body respond best to various forms of stimulation. This requires that the male be aware of his need to learn, that he learns best from his partner and that positive directive feedback be provided during each phase of sexual arousal. The female should be encouraged to guide and instruct her partner regarding those erotic areas which enhance her arousal.

The knowledge that the clitoris and labia are the most sensitive and responsive areas is probably understood by most, but the quality of stimulation is an individual matter. Unfortunately a large number of women believe their role is to be a passive partner to their 'experienced' mate whilst in turn the male is often ashamed to admit he is a novice in sexual activity. If this couple are not educated early in their relationship, it may result in anorgasmia and a frustrating interpersonal experience and finally to marked reduction in libido by one or both partners.

(b) *Attitudes and beliefs*. These are developed during the formative years and may profoundly influence the ability to achieve an orgasm. Children taught rigid, moral, religious and social codes as they grow, who are taught to fear and avoid sexual contact and activity often develop orgasmic dysfunction. Guilt, anxiety and fear of performance failure may all play a part in inhibiting the ability to reach a normal orgasmic response.

(c) *Hostility* to one's partner and poor interpersonal relations can so inhibit the normal response cycle that orgasm is prevented. The ability to communicate both verbally, physically and sexually is a most important pre-requisite to a good sexual relationship.

(d) *Boredom and monotony* are common causes of orgasmic failure. A routine and monotonous approach may cause one partner to feel bored to the point of distraction and under these conditions orgasm may never occur.

Impotence or ejaculatory failure

Other problems are impotence, retarded ejaculation and premature ejaculation. Men may have premature ejaculation because of excitement, anxiety or through habit. Once premature ejaculation occurs the thought of further premature ejaculation leads to anxiety and fear of further loss of ejaculatory control. This in turn induces a vicious cycle of repeated failure, feelings of frustration, anxiety and eventually avoidance of sexual activity.

Retarded or delayed ejaculation may also occur because of anxiety, low arousal levels or to inhibitory stimuli. These men with worries, fears and anxieties or with an insufficient level of sexual arousal may fail to achieve a satisfactory erection and therefore will not be able to initiate the normal ejaculatory response mechanisms.

Sexual aberrations

Problems relating to homosexuality, transvestism, sado-masochism, and other aberrant sexual activities may present to a medical practitioner but these will not be discussed in this chapter.

Presentation of problems

Women who wish to discuss a sexual problem will seldom present their symptoms or their worries to their doctor in such a manner that they are readily identified. There are several modes of presentation but in almost all instances the patient will 'test' the doctor to determine whether he is likely to respond in an appropriate manner to their embarrassing problem.

A common set of symptoms includes headaches, insomnia, nervousness, palpitations, feelings of depression or anxiety. The children, their finances, arguments with their partner or physical abuse are often given as causes for disharmony. Other presenting symptoms may be vaginal discharge, pelvic pain, dyspareunia or dysmenorrhoea. If a careful history is not elicited patients may be given tranquilisers, anti-depressants or sedatives; or, alternatively, be referred for unnecessary investigations and operations of a gynaecological nature.

The medical practitioner must be aware that a large number of such symptoms have a psychosexual cause and be prepared to ask sufficient appropriate questions to allow his patient to express her real concerns.

Taking a history

It is important to give time to the patient. Because of the sensitive and embarrassing nature of the problem, a number of women may take some time to present the whole story. If they are rushed or cut short they fail to give a true picture and then a wrong diagnosis may result. Once it is realised that a psychosexual problem exists it is imperative that the sexual partner be involved in the exploration. Try to set a time when both can attend and the doctor can listen in an uninterrupted manner to their story.

1. First find out from each partner what the problem appears to be. Check with each one that they perceive the problem in the same way.

2. Determine what the couple would like to achieve. This is important, for the gap between the actual and the desired achievement is what the doctor/therapist must help the couple to achieve. Explore the problem in full — when it first began, under what circumstances, what makes it worse, what makes it better.

3. Determine from each partner their background. What was their family upbringing, their schooling, their religion, the influence of peers and personal relationships and how these affected their attitudes and knowledge.

4. Obtain a daily profile on each partner. From the time each wakes till each goes to sleep try to determine what they do individually. It is surprising how little time couples spend together, unable to share thoughts and activities nor learn about each other's needs. Only by obtaining a complete daily and weekly profile can a clear picture of a mismatch in activities be identified.

5. Determine difficulties in their interpersonal relationship and their ability to communicate and share their personal feelings.

6. Enquire about their sexual techniques and knowledge. Endeavour to determine the types of past sexual experiences — whether these were pleasurable or distressing — whether they spend sufficient time in the arousal phase — do they attempt to 'pleasure' their partner — can they abandon themselves to the enjoyment of sexual activity with their partner?

Having obtained a history there should now have emerged a clear picture of the problem, how it is affecting each one of the couple and how it occurred. At this stage explanation and education may be all that is required to improve or change the underlying situation. However, a large number of couples will require further counselling and a progressive re-education in techniques.

Improving interpersonal relations

For those couples who have a problem in interpersonal relations it is important to explain the importance of communication.

Communication is the process whereby a person sends a message to another who not only receives the message but provides feedback to the sender.

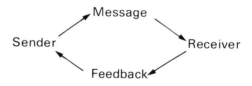

Communication Model

In describing the communication model it is important to emphasise the significant role of the receiver and the feedback which is provided. Positive feedback enhances further messages whilst negative or passive responses by the receiver can inhibit communication.

Discussion of communication usually begins with a description of verbal communication but is quickly extended to physical and sexual communication. At all times the importance of the receiver and the type of feedback is emphasised. To reinforce the importance of good communication it is sometimes helpful to use a videotape of the couple during a counselling session. After the initial distraction and awareness of the videocamera a series of well-directed questions can often initiate a dialogue involving the couple. When these segments are played back to the couple they may see themselves as others do, and rapidly become aware of deficiencies in their style of communication. I have found the use of the videocamera to be of the greatest value when dealing with a couple, one of whom cannot perceive he/she is obstructing good interpersonal relations.

Improving sexual techniques

When it is realised that the problem is one of technique it is often best to use a series of behaviour modification exercises which are aimed at improving physical arousal or to control sexual responses.

1. Sensate focus can be used as a pleasuring exercise and to learn about each other's body. Using the communication model to provide feedback at all times, the couple take it in turns to explore their partner's body, by stroking touching or kissing, finding out just what sensate activity will produce the greatest pleasure.

2. Genital focus is an extension of sensate focus activity but here the emphasis is placed on the genital organs with the clitoris, labia, perineum and peri-anal region in the female and the penis, scrotum and peri-anal region of the male being explored.

3. Squeeze technique may be employed to assist with problems of premature ejaculation.

4. Masturbation and the use of vibrators may be employed to enhance arousal and orgasmic responses.

Counselling sessions

Dual counselling sessions should, ideally, last between 45 and 75 minutes with most time devoted to exposing the problem and clarifying it in such a manner that the causes can be clearly seen by each of the couple. If no progress is made during two sessions then further counselling should be terminated. If progress is being achieved then an attempt must be made to complete all further counselling within five sessions. To prolong counselling sessions beyond this number without justification is to produce a generally negative reaction and provoke a resistance to change.

Success rate for counselling

The success of any regime of therapy is usually measured by some finite point such as elimination of a disease or a specific symptom, by improved mobility or some such clinical mark which can be clearly identified. Sexual counselling however is much more difficult to evaluate in such terms. The ability to achieve the desired end point can be taken as the standard of success but the maintenance of this level of achievement depends on the continuing interest and motivation of the couple.

In our counselling programme we have found almost universal improvement in every couple who are both motivated and eager to improve. However, the success rate for therapy declines sharply when one or both of the couple reject the notion that he/she is partly responsible or if one of the couple has no commitment or motivation. In spite of demonstrating that the 'client/couple' can improve, a number eventually slip back into their negative attitude and so their relationship founders again.

Short-term success in counselling is usually reasonably good for the motivated couple, but long-term improvement depends on the amount of change and the effort which has been put into achieving the change.

Generally about 50% of couples will demonstrate good improvement in the short-term but of these, about half will eventually regress. The best results which can be expected is permanent improvement in about 30% of couples.

Summary

Sexual problems are common and are often caused by lack of proper education and by poor interpersonal relations. Counselling should be directed at exploration, improving communication and re-education. It is important to give the couple permission to indulge and abandon themselves to pleasure without guilt. When poor technique is present there are a series of behaviour modification exercises which, when correctly and judiciously used, will improve and correct a great number of problems. Gynaecologists should be aware of the magnitude of sexual problems in the community and be prepared to counsel and treat people with these problems.

Suggested reading list of books and articles related to sexual counselling

Textbooks

Argyle M 1975 Bodily Communication. Methuen & Co Ltd, London
Kaplan H S 1976 The Illustrated Manual of Sex Therapy. Souvenir Press Ltd, London
Kaplan H S 1976 The New Sex Therapy. Balliere Tindall, London
Kolodny R C, Masters W H & Johnson V E 1979 Textbook of Sexual Medicine. Little, Brown & Co, Boston
Masters W H & Johnson V E 1970 Human Sexual Inadequacy. Little Brown & Co, Boston

Articles

Betts T 1982 Psychosexual Problems in the Female In: Studd J (ed) Progress in Obstetrics and Gynaecology. Vol. 2, pp 252–263. Churchill Livingstone, Edinburgh
Hallstrom T 1977 Sexuality in the Climacteric. Clinics in Obstetrics and Gynaecology, 4: 227–239
Kagan N 1971 Influencing Human Interaction. Instructional Media Centre East Lansing, Michigan
Pion R, Annon J 1975 Office Management of Sexual Problems: Brief Therapy Approaches. Journal Reproductive Medicine, 15: 127–144
Wren B G, Robertson R 1976 A Technique of Sexual Counselling. Medical Journal of Australia, 2: 641–643
Wren B G 1978 Sexual Counselling — A Dual Counselling Approach. Australian and New Zealand Journal of Obstetrics and Gynaecology, 18: 250–252

Recurrent abortion

Approximately 15% of clinically recognised pregnancies abort spontaneously (Warburton & Fraser 1959) so that about 2% of women would be expected to have two spontaneous abortions in any two successive pregnancies purely by chance. Huisjes (1984) cogently argues that the term habitual abortion implies a systematic maternal or paternal cause, but this is not always the case. Most recurrent abortions are fortuitous. Warburton & Fraser (1959) estimated the risk of further abortion as 20% after one abortion, 23% after two abortions and 26% for women with three previous abortions. The former definition of recurrent abortion as being three consecutive abortions has been superceded by two consecutive abortions with most clinicians. The vigour with which the gynaecologist will attempt to elucidate the cause after two consecutive abortions will inevitably depend on the pressure exerted on him by the anxious couple. These investigations will need to consider the following possible factors.

CHROMOSOMAL ABNORMALITIES

Fetal chromosomal abnormalities

About 55% of first trimester spontaneous abortions are due to a chromosomal abnormality (Lauritsen 1976). Autosomal trisomy accounts for about half of the abnormalities, while polyploidy and monosomy X each account for a further 20%. Boué & Boué (1973), in a study of 43 women from whom two consecutive abortions were karyotyped, showed that when the first abortion was chromosomally normal the second abortion also tended to be normal. When the karyotype of the first abortion was abnormal, the second abortion tended likewise to be abnormal. However, there was no correlation between the two karyotypes. Unfortunately they did not examine the karyotype of the couples concerned.

Parental chromosomal abnormalities

The reported incidence of chromosomal abnormalities amongst couples with repeated spontaneous abortions varies according to the population studied.

Ward et al (1980), reporting on 100 couples, found no balanced translocations, but as no term pregnancies were reported amongst these couples the authors concede that they may have selected against translocation carriers, since these would be expected to have at least one successful pregnancy. Most studies have reported an increased incidence of parental chromosomal abnormalities. Sant-Cassia & Cooke (1981) in a study of 182 couples with a history of two or more spontaneous abortions consecutively referred for karyotyping, detected 17 abnormal karyotypes, a frequency of 4.67% of individuals studied. The pregnancy outcome in those with normal and those with abnormal karyotypes was compared in 105 of the couples. The distribution of confirmed pregnancies, confirmed spontaneous abortions, live births, stillbirths, ectopic gestation and medically induced abortions was not significantly different in the two groups. Despite this apparent lack of difference in outcome it would be reasonable to suspect a genetic basis for recurrent abortion. For instance, women have more chromosomal abnormalities than men amongst these couples, and in particular, abnormalities involving chromosome 7 seem to occur more frequently (Sant-Cassia & Cooke 1981). The clinician looks forward to the development of further techniques in genetic investigation, which would differentiate between those couples with a bad pregnancy pattern and those in whom a more favourable outcome could be expected.

Because of the increased incidence of chromosomal abnormalities in couples with repeated spontaneous abortions, parental chromosomal analysis is an important investigation. If a parental balanced translocation carrier is detected, amniocentesis ought to be offered in the next pregnancy to exclude an unbalanced fetal translocation. In theory the chance of a translocation carrier producing a chromosomally unbalanced gamete is 1:2, with the chance of a balanced translocation gamete being 1:4 and a gamete with a normal complement 1:4. Stevenson & Davison (1976) reported an actual incidence of 1:15 for live births with an unbalanced translocation when the father was a carrier, but they found the incidence to be as high as 1:10 when the mother was the carrier. A possible explanation for this dissimilar incidence is the strong selection against the abnormal gamete in the male before conception.

There is no reason to suppose that normal variants such as pericentric inversions, long Y chromosomes, or satellites on acrocentric chromosomes are a cause of recurrent abortion.

UTERINE ABNORMALITIES

Abnormal Müllerian development

Although abnormal Müllerian tube development has been implicated in recurrent abortion and pre-term labour, it must be emphasised that the exact causal relationship is not clear. There are numerous reports associating congenital uterine abnormalities with a poor pregnancy outcome, but there are many women who have unrecognised abnormalities and have uneventful pregnancies. Jones & Jones (1953) reported that 25% of women with a double uterus will have serious reproductive problems, such as pre-term labour and repeated abortions. Most of the reports have been on small numbers. Heinonen et al (1982) investigated the reproductive performance of a large series of 182 women with uterine anomalies. The reproductive performance was best in the complete septate group, when the fetal survival rate was 86%. Women with a unicornuate uterus had the worst fetal survival rate at 40%, while patients with complete bicornuate uteri fared little better with 50% survival. Following metroplasty for septate and bicornuate uteri, not only was the fetal survival rate increased from 10% before the operation to 88% after the operation, but the spontaneous abortion rate was reduced from 84% to 12%. This fetal survival rate following metroplasty was similar to that reported by Strassman (1966).

Because of the frequent association with renal tract anomalies and occasionally a pelvic kidney, an intravenous urogram is essential, especially if any corrective surgery is being considered. It is noteworthy that in the Heinonen et al (1982) study, an intravenous urogram was carried out in only 29% of patients. Of the women investigated 23% had abnormal urograms. Hysteroscopy and a hysterogram are important diagnostic aids. Numerous different classifications of abnormal Müllerian tube developments have been drawn up, but the best description is a diagram and a simple explanation. Other causes of recurrent abortion must be excluded and a reasonable aetiological association established before embarking on an operative correction. Two main techniques of doing a metroplasty have been described. The operation described by Strassman (1966) involves a transverse incision between the round ligaments, the uterine cavities are opened and the partition between them split down the middle and a single cavity formed. The septum is incised not excised. The transverse incision is converted into an anterior-posterior suture line to prevent the raw edge of the septum from growing together and forming adhesions. A rudimentary horn should be removed to prevent haematometra of pregnancy in it (Strassman 1966). Jones & Jones (1953) described a different technique — the muscular septum is resected with a sagittal wedge excision resulting in a single suture line sagittaly over the upper segment. This incision avoids injury to the cornual ends. As metroplasty involves an incision in the upper segment of the uterus, such a scar carries the risk of uterine rupture in a subsequent pregnancy, similar to upper segment Caesarean section scars. An elective section is mandatory in the subsequent pregnancy.

Endometrial steroid receptors

Sant-Cassia et al (1984) reported that women who had unexplained primary subfertility had significantly less cytoplasmic oestradiol and progesterone receptors in the secretory phase generally and in the mid-secretory phase in particular, when compared to normal fertile women. It may be that a lack of progesterone and oestradiol receptors at a time when implantation would be expected to occur may prevent implantation or continuation of the pregnancy beyond a few days. This lack of receptors may be a cause of a number of subclinical abortions.

Uterine blood supply

Burchell et al (1978) injected radio-opaque dye into the uterine arteries of 119 uteri removed at hysterectomy. They then correlated the vascular configuration with the patients previous reproductive history. Patients whose uterus had two ascending uterine arteries on one side had significantly more abortions and smaller newborn babies than those with one artery. Amongst patients with a single ascending branch of the uterine artery 15% had spontaneous abortions. When the ascending branch was divided into anterior and posterior uterine arteries the incidence of women experiencing spontaneous abortion increased to over 45% when the bifid artery occurred on one side only, and to 60% when the uterine artery was double on both sides. The authors postulate that if vascular configuration is a factor in placentation, an abnormal uterine arterial pattern would fail to provide an adequate foundation for the developing placenta in early pregnancy and an inadequate blood flow in late pregnancy.

Intra-uterine adhesions

Intra-uterine synechiae have been implicated in recurrent abortion. The abortions may occur because of a reduced uterine cavity or a lack of sufficient endometrium. The condition, known throughout the world as Asherman's syndrome, was in fact first described by Heinrich Fritsch in 1894. The incidence of intra-uterine adhesions is increasing and is particularly prevalent in Israel, Greece and South America (Schenker & Margalioth 1982). These workers reported significantly that in 91% of cases pregnancy was a predisposing factor. This highlights the importance of avoiding vigorous curettage in the post-abortion or post-partum period. Bergquist et al (1981) in a study of 25 patients with intra-uterine adhesions reported that the majority presented with repeated pregnancy loss. The patients were treated either by curettage or lysis of the adhesions via a hysteroscope, and the insertion of an intra-uterine contraceptive device for up to 2 months or an intra-uterine Foley catheter for about 7 days. Post-operatively they were given antibiotics and cyclic oestrogens and progesterones. The spontaneous abortion rate improved from 78% to 20% following treatment and the successful pregnancy rate increased from 32% to 52%. They interestingly reported that successful pregnancy following therapy was as likely to occur following mild forms of the disease and after severe adhesions, and they could not establish any correlation between the severity of intra-uterine adhesions and scanty periods. However, they urged the adoption of a uniform classification based on findings at hysteroscopy so that the severity of the adhesions could be compared with pregnancy outcome.

Cervical incompetence

The diagnosis of cervical incompetence is difficult to establish objectively. It is usually based on a history of a previous dilatation and curettage, or a termination of pregnancy followed by mid-trimester spontaneous abortion or early pre-term delivery. Classically the mid-trimester abortion or pre-term delivery is rapid, painless and without any bleeding, but this is not inevitable. The condition can follow cervical amputation, cone biopsy and laceration occurring at the time of delivery. Congenital cervical incompetence has been described and Jennings (1972) in describing four pairs of sisters with this condition suggested a familial tendency. While Cousins et al (1980) in a controlled study of reproductive outcome in women exposed to diethyl-stilboestrol (DES) found an increased incidence of pre-term delivery and subsequent perinatal loss. In some of the patients the pre-term delivery was associated with cervical incompetence. Unfortunately because of the small numbers involved, the authors could not establish whether uterine anomalies, known to be associated with DES therapy, were the cause of the pre-term labour. It is possible that the increased incidence of cervical incompetence in such patients is due to an alteration in the components of the cervical tissue itself, rather than to gross anomalies in the upper genital tract.

The passage of a Hegar 8 dilator without difficulty in the non-pregnant patient, a pre-menstrual hysterogram, ultra-sound examination of the cervix in early pregnancy (Brook et al 1981) and the measurement of cervical resistance (Anthony et al 1982) have all been described as aids to diagnosis. Floyd (1961) concluded that cervical dilatation of 1–3 cm in the second trimester *per se* does not signify cervical incompetence and imminent abortion or delivery.

There are two basic techniques of cervical cerclage. The Shirodkar (1955) encerclage involves a transverse incision on the anterior fornix. The bladder base is reflected upwards. A similar incision is made posteriorly and an unabsorbable tape, such as Mersilk, is used to encircle the cervix. Both incisions are closed and therefore the knot is buried. This implies that an anaesthetic would be required to remove the suture. This method of cerclage is usually performed prior to pregnancy, and very often the suture is left *in situ* at term and the child is delivered by Caesarean section. The McDonald (1957) suture involves a simple cerclage without any dissection of the bladder, the knot is tied anteriorly and is not buried. This method of cerclage is usually performed early in the second trimester.

Harger (1980) reviewed just over 250 cervical cerclage procedures. The fetal survival rate after elective McDonald or Shirodkar suture was 78% and 87% respectively. The difference was not statistically significant. Because the McDonald technique is much simpler, and equally effective, the Shirodkar method is now less used. To date no randomised control trial on the effectiveness of cervical cerclage in cervical incompetence has been reported.

Interestingly Weekes et al (1977) reported that cervical cerclage did not prolong the duration of pregnancy in uncomplicated twin pregnancies. Because of the uncertainty about the efficacy of the procedure, the Medical Research Council and the Royal College of Obstetricians and Gynaecologists are currently organising a prospective controlled trial in the United Kingdom.

IMMUNOLOGY

One hypothesis to explain why the fetus, despite possessing antigens foreign to the mother, survives pregnancy without rejection has postulated the production of a plasma blocking factor. The suggestion is that this factor prevents sensitised maternal lymphocytes from reacting with and destroying fetal cells. Rocklin et al (1976) reported that women who experience recurrent abortion lacked IgG blocking factor which is present in normal multiparous women. McIntyre & Faulk (1979) suggested that the blocking activity is localised within the trophoblast membrane. One suggestion for this lack of blocking factor in women suffering repeated abortion is the presence of histocompatibility between the women and their partners, and therefore the stimulus for its production is insufficient. Little is known about the aetiology of blocking factors in normal pregnancy or how important they are in preventing rejection of the fetus.

It has been proposed that habitual abortion could result from inadequate immunological recognition of the implanting blastocyst. The hypothesis is that if a couple have similar antigens, the mother could not recognise embryonic tissue as foreign; a degree of parental histoincompatibility is important for successful reproduction (Taylor & Faulk 1981). These workers reported on four women with a history of repeated unexplained spontaneous abortion who appeared to share with their husband more HLA antigens of the A, B, C and DR loci than would be expected by chance. These women were transfused throughout pregnancy with leucocyte enriched plasma from at least 16 different erythrocyte compatible donors. All four pregnancies proceeded to term. The proposition that antigenic differences between mother and fetus could lead to reproductive advantages (Billington 1964) was attractive and interesting. However, as McLaren (1975) has pointed out in an excellent study on inbred animals and after careful analysis of the published data, the experimental foundations on which this hypothesis are based were insecure and unlikely to be correct. It is possible, however, that although the hypothesis is incorrect, the infusion of pooled histoincompatible leucocytes could still be beneficial for other reasons which are not clear at present. The number of patients treated by Taylor & Faulk (1981) and Beer et al (1981) is small and a study with good controls has yet to be reported. Scott (1983, personal communication) studied HLA antigen sharing in 12 couples with a history of three or more consecutive abortions and 77 fertile couples as controls. The degree of HLA antigen sharing did not define a population with increased pregnancy wastage or predict subsequent pregnancy outcome. At present a relationship, if any, between unexplained recurrent fetal loss and parental antigen sharing has still to be elucidated.

Systemic lupus erythematosus

Patients with systemic lupus erythematosus may present with recurrent abortion before the disease becomes overt (Grigor et al 1977). The mechanism for the spontaneous abortions in these patients may well be immunological (Bresniham et al 1977).

HORMONE ABNORMALITIES

Thyroid

Although inadequate thyroid function has been proposed as a cause of recurrent abortion, there has been no convincing evidence. Winikoff & Malinek (1975) in a detailed study, reported that normal women reached a typical pregnancy thyroid profile at 7–8 weeks gestation, while patients with a history of recurrent abortion did not reach this profile until 14–15 weeks and patients who miscarried never reached it at all. All these patients were free from overt thyroid disease and probably had normal thyroid function in the non-pregnant stage. These workers treated four women with a history of previous abortions with thyroxine throughout six pregnancies. The thyroid profile had previously shown a lag in response, but this returned to normal and the pregnancies were carried to term. As in all other reports, the numbers studied are small. If hypothyroidism is present it should be treated, but there is no good evidence to suggest treatment of euthyroid patients with thyroxine.

Diabetes

Most textbooks suggest a glucose tolerance test as part of the investigations for recurrent abortion; however, in practice this is invariably normal. There is no reported series that implicates an abnormal glucose tolerance test as a cause of recurrent abortion.

Progesterone

A great deal has been written about progesterone deficiency in recurrent abortion. Most of the earlier studies highlighted the low progesterone and pregnanediol levels in pregnancies undergoing spontaneous abortion. However, the low levels were recorded only after the onset of vaginal bleeding. These low levels of progesterone were probably the result of the spontaneous abortion, rather than the cause. The studies reporting on the use of progesterone or progestational agents once a pregnancy was established, failed to demonstrate their effectiveness as compared to placebo.

Corpus luteum deficiency

In recent years the concept of the inadequate corpus luteum has been proposed. This has been defined as a deficiency in the amount and or duration of progesterone steroidogenesis. The diagnosis is made by dating the endometrium 2 or more days out of phase with the subsequent period in at least two cycles. This defect manifests itself either by primary subfertility or repeated first trimester abortions. The incidence amongst habitual aborters has been reported as to be as high as 35% (Jones 1976). The author concedes that her population may have been unrepresentative, as she has a special interest in this problem. Horta et al (1977) reported that women with a history of three previous consecutive spontaneous abortions had significantly lower levels of plasma progesterone during the luteal phase and early pregnancy as compared with normal fertile women. Despite their lower levels of plasma progesterone, patients with habitual abortion did get pregnant. Those who went on to abort spontaneously had low levels of plasma progesterone before vaginal bleeding or abortion occurred. These workers suggested that although ovulation occurred, the progesterone steroidogenesis was deficient at the time of implantation. There may be many causes for this syndrome and clinically it is often impossible to determine a single aetiology. It has been suggested that patients with this condition who suffer recurrent abortion should be treated with progesterone before the missed menstrual period and during the first weeks of pregnancy. However, though this is an interesting concept, there have been no controlled studies demonstrating that progesterone therapy prior to the missed menstrual period will prevent an abortion due to an inadequate luteal phase. It is interesting that Johansson (1971) reported that the administration of synthetic gestagens from the third day after ovulation depressed the plasma levels of progesterone. This depression did not appear to be a true luteolytic effect, as injections of human chorionic gonadotrophin caused an increase in the level of plasma progesterone.

INFECTIONS

Listeria monocytogenes

There is some evidence that this gram-positive bacillus may be a cause of recurrent abortion. If either the vaginal swabs or the semen culture are positive, the couple ought to be treated with Ampicillin (Leading Article 1980).

Mycoplasm

This organism is frequently found in the vagina and cervix in the absence of disease. Although some reports have suggested that this organism may be a cause of primary subfertility and repeated abortion, the series of patients studied have been small. The role of this organism and of chlamydia trachomatis in recurrent abortion is unclear.

Toxoplasmosis

Toxoplasma gondii may in the acute stage of the disease lead to spontaneous abortion. The significance of toxoplasmosis in recurrent abortion has yet to be established (Stray-Pederson & Lorentzen-Styr 1977).

THE MALE

Veterinarians have long been aware of the role of the male in recurrent abortion. This male factor amongst couples with repeated spontaneous abortion is not clear. Polyspermia is an ill defined condition, there are no standard criteria for diagnosis, indeed, some workers doubt that it is a pathological entity. Rehan et al (1975) found an incidence for this condition amongst 1.2% of fertile couples. Glazerman et al (1982) defining polyzoospermia as a sperm count of 250 × 10^6/ml found an incidence of 4.2% amongst infertile couples. They reported an abortion rate of 25% amongst 30 couples where the man had polyspermia. They had no explanation for the reported increased incidence of spontaneous abortion and subfertility. It did not appear to be related to the ability of the sperm to penetrate the cervical mucus.

CONCLUSION

While medical investigation of the couple with repeated spontaneous abortion often fails to reveal a cause, it is important to have a basic plan for investigation. A careful clinical history including details of when the previous abortions occurred is essential. The special investigations which are suggested in most textbooks include blood counts, urine analysis, blood urea, glucose tolerance tests, thyroid function tests and seriological tests for syphilis. These tests rarely reveal anything abnormal. The two most important primary investigations are chromosomal analysis of the couple and a hysterogram. It is justified to assume an optimistic prognosis as even after three spontaneous abortions there is approximately a 75% chance that the following pregnancy will succeed. This encouraging news should be put to the couple concerned and borne in mind by the clinician when assessing any suggested beneficial treatment for this problem.

Stray-Pederson & Stray Pederson (1984) showed that psychological support alone may lead to a marked improvement in the outcome of pregnancy. Among couples with repeated spontaneous abortions with no abnormal findings, women receiving specific antenatal counselling and psychological support had a pregnancy success rate of 86% as compared to a success rate of 33% observed in women of similar couples who received no specific antenatal care.

Acknowledgments

I am indebted to Mr A J Tyack, Consultant Obstetrician and Gynaecologist at the City Hospital, Nottingham for his help in the preparation of this chapter.

REFERENCES

Anthony G S, Calder A A, MacNaughton M C 1982 Cervical resistance in patients with previous spontaneous mid trimester abortion. British Journal of Obstetrics and Gynaecology 89: 1046–1049

Beer A E, Quebbeman J F, Ayers J W T, Haines R F 1981 Major histoincompatibility complex antigens, maternal and paternal immune responses and chronic habitual abortions in humans. American Journal of Obstetrics and Gynecology 141: 987–999

Bergquist C A, Rock J A, Jones H W Jr 1981 Pregnancy outcome following treatment of intra-uterine adhesions. International Journal of Fertility 26: 107–111

Billington W D 1964 Influence of immunological dissimilarity of mother and fetus on size of placenta in mice. Nature 202: 317–318

Boué J, Boué A 1973 Chromosomal analysis of two consecutive abortions in each of 43 women. Humangenetik 19: 275–280

Bresniham B, Grigor R R, Oliver M, Lewkonia R M, Hughes G R V 1977 Immunological mechanism for spontaneous abortion in systemic lupus erythematosus. Lancet ii: 1205–1207

Brook I, Feingold M, Schwartz A, Zakut H 1981 Ultrasonography in the diagnosis of cervical incompetence in pregnancy: a new diagnostic approach. British Journal of Obstetrics and Gynaecology 88: 640–643

Burchell R C, Creed F, Rasoulpour M, Whitcomb M 1978 Vascular anatomy of the human uterus and pregnancy wastage. British Journal of Obstetrics and Gynaecology 85: 698–706

Cousins L, Karp W, Lacey C, Lucas W E 1980 Reproductive outcome of women exposed to diethylstilboestrol in utero. Obstetrics and Gynecology 56: 70–76

Floyd W S 1961 Cervical dilatation in the mid trimester of pregnancy. Obstetrics and Gynecology 18: 380–381

Fritsch H 1894 Ein fall von volligem Schwund der Gebarmutterhohle nach auskratzung. Zentralblatt fur Gynakologie 18: 1337–1342

Glazerman M, Beinstein D, Zakut C, Misgav N, Inslen V 1982 Polyzoospermia: a definite pathological entity. Fertility and Sterility 38: 605–608

Grigor R R, Shervington P C, Hughes G R V, Hawkins D F 1977 Outcome of pregnancy in systemic lupus erythematosus. Proceedings of the Royal Society of Medicine 70: 99–100

Harger J H 1980 Comparison of success and morbidity in cervical cerclage procedures. Obstetrics and Gynecology 56: 543–548

Heinonen P E, Saarikoski S, Pystynen P 1982 Reproductive performance of women with uterine anomalies: an evaluation of 182 cases. Acta Obstetrica and Gynaecologica Scandinavica 61: 157–162

Horta J L H, Fernández J G, De León B S, Cortés-Gallegos V 1977 Direct evidence of luteal insufficiency in women with habitual abortion. Obstetrics and Gynecology 49: 705–708

Huisjes 1984 Spontaneous abortion, pp 13–14 Clinical Reviews in Obstetrics and Gynaecology. Churchill Livingstone, Edinburgh

Jennings C L Jr 1972 Temporary submucosal cerclage for cervical incompetence: report of forty eight cases. American Journal of Obstetrics and Gynecology 113: 1097–1102

Johansson E D B 1971 Depression of the progesterone levels in women treated with synthetic gestagens after ovulation. Acta Endocrinologica 68: 779–792

Jones G S 1976 The luteal phase defect. Fertility and Sterility 27: 351–356

Jones H W Jr, Jones G E S 1953 Double uterus as an etiological factor in repeated abortion: indications for surgical repair. American Journal of Obstetrics and Gynecology 65: 325–339

Lauritsen J G 1976 Aetiology of spontaneous abortion. Acta Obstetrica et Gynecologica Scandinavica Suppl. 52: 1–29

Leading Article 1980 Perinatal listeriosis. Lancet i: 911

McDonald I 1957 Suture of the cervix for inevitable miscarriage. Journal of Obstetrics and Gynaecology of the British Empire 64: 346–350

McIntyre J A, Faulk W P 1979 Maternal blocking factors in human pregnancy are found in plasma not serum. Lancet ii: 821–823

McLaren A 1975 Immunology of trophoblast. Edwards R G, Howe C W S, Johnson H (eds) Clinical and Experimental Immunoproduction. Cambridge University Press, Cambridge

Rehan N E, Sobrero A J, Fertig J W 1975 The semen of fertile men: statistical analysis of 1300 men. Fertility and Sterility 26: 492–502

Rocklin R E, Kitzmiller J H, Carpenter C B, Garovoy M R, David J R 1976 Maternal-fetal relation; absence of an immunological blocking factor from serum of women with chronic abortions. New England Journal of Medicine 295: 1209–1213

Sant-Cassia L J, Cooke P 1981 Chromosomal analysis of couples with repeated spontaneous abortions. British Journal of Obstetrics and Gynaecology 88: 52–58

Sant-Cassia L J, Symonds E M, Johnson J, Selby C, Baker P, Maynard P V 1984 Endometrial oestradiol and progesterone receptors in normal and subfertile women. Proceedings of the Nuffield Obstetrical and Gynaecological Society. Journal of Obstetrics and Gynaecology 4: 204

Schenker J G, Margalioth E J 1982 Intra-uterine adhesions: an updated appraisal. Fertility and Sterility 37: 593–610

Strassmann E O 1966 Fertility and unification of double uterus. Fertility and Sterility 17: 165–176

Stray-Pederson B, Stray Pederson S 1984 Etiologic factors and subsequent reproductive performance in 195 couples with a prior history of habitual abortion. American Journal of Obstetrics and Gynecology 148: 140–146

Stray-Pederson B, Lorentzen-Styr A 1977 Uterine toxoplasma infections and repeated abortions. American Journal of Obstetrics and Gynecology 128: 716–721

Shirodkar V N 1955 A new method of operative treatment for habitual abortion in second trimester of pregnancy. Antiseptic 52: 229–235

Stevenson A C, Davison B C C (eds) 1976 Disorders due to Chromosomal Anomalies, p. 129. William Heinemann Medical Books, London

Taylor C, Faulk W P 1981 Prevention of recurrent abortion with leucocyte transfusions. Lancet ii: 68–69

Warburton D, Fraser F C 1959 Genetic aspects of abortion. Clinical Obstetrics and Gynaecology 2: 22–35

Ward B E, Henry G P, Robinson A 1980 Cytogenetic studies in 100 couples with recurrent spontaneous abortions. American Journal of Human Genetics 32: 549–554

Weekes A R L, Menzies D N, de Boer C H 1977 The relative efficacy of bed rest, cervical suture and no treatment in the management of twin pregnancy. British Journal of Obstetrics and Gynaecology 84: 161–164

Winikoff D, Malinek M 1975 The predictive value of thyroid 'test profile' in habitual abortion. British Journal of Obstetrics and Gynaecology 82: 760–766

Hormonal methods of contraception and their adverse effects

Considerable attention is focused from time to time on serious disorders associated with taking contraceptive pills. The latest episode followed publications relating to neoplasia (Pike et al 1983, Vessey et al 1983). Two points, however, need always be borne in mind:

1. Serious adverse effects are rare events. This raises particular difficulties in statistical analysis of reports which almost inevitably lead to controversies over their interpretation.

2. All reports of serious adverse effects have dealt overwhelmingly with studies of women taking combinations of oestrogen and progestogen. There seems more safety in other methods of hormonal contraception, for example, those using the progestogen component on its own. This could be an illusion, however, arising from the scarcity of studies on progestogen-only methods.

VARIETIES OF HORMONAL CONTRACEPTIVE METHOD

The combined oestrogen-progestogen pill

This is the model that emerged from the earliest considerations by Pincus and others of how hormone-like substances could be used for highly effective contraception, relying principally for its effectiveness on the regular inhibition of ovulation.

Progestogen-only pills

These pick up the actions of the combined pill other than ovulatory inhibition. A small dose of progestogen throughout the cycle, so that endogenous oestrogen is never 'unopposed', will disrupt endometrial development, prevent the cervical mucus 'window' of sperm acceptance at mid-cycle and possibly also interfere with the hormonally dependent mechanisms of tubal transport. Some individuals will experience ovulatory inhibition in some cycles and some may have progesterone production reduced should ovulation occur. All these effects combine to reduce fecundability.

Depot injections of progestogens

The principle of this mode of administration is that, shared with other kinds of drugs, of providing a reservoir of material in the body from which the active agent is distributed systemically at a slow release rate. One preparation, depot medroxyprogesterone acetate (DMPA), is provided in a microcrystalline aqueous suspension. The other, norethisterone oenanthate (NETO), is dissolved in castor oil. Both are given by deep intramuscular injection.

In long-term use they have not been associated with any serious adverse effects. Experience in this country has, however, been relatively limited.

Post-coital pills

Two tablets of relatively high dose combined pills (Ovran/Eugynon 50) are taken at once followed by two tablets 12 hours later (Yuzpe & Lancee 1977). These are taken when unprotected intercourse occurs near the time of ovulation and are effective if taken up to 72 hours later.

Another hormonal method is to use a very high dose of oestrogen only, for example ethinyloestradiol 5 mg a day for 5 days (Haspels & Andriesse 1973). Both of these, especially the oestrogen only method, cause nausea and vomiting. Neither are associated with serious morbidity. There has been one case of acute non-fatal pulmonary oedema reported using the high dose oestrogen method. A relatively high dose of progestogen, using 600 μg of levonorgestrel, is currently under clinical trial. The first method, using combined pills, is the only one approved for a product licence by the Committee on Safety of Medicines (CSM).

Hormone-releasing intrauterine devices

There has been little use of these in this country. The progesterone-releasing T-device, the Progestasert, has been used in some centres but there appeared to be an unusually high risk of ectopic pregnancy among method failures (Snowden 1977). There is no other hormone-related morbidity reported and it is likely that similar devices releasing levonorgestrel will be introduced in Britain. Much of the research and development work has been done in Finland and Sweden (Nilsson et al 1981).

Vaginal rings

Rings to be placed in the upper vagina for several weeks at a time are likely to be introduced for general use soon. They are made of porous silastic and release progestogens such as levonorgestrel (LNG) into the upper vagina from which absorption takes place through lymphatic channels to act on the cervix, uterus, tubes and ovaries (Burton et al 1979). This mode of administration avoids the first passage through the liver. The dose required is therefore very much lower

Table 17.1 Use of hormonal substances in contraception

Combined pill:	oestrogen and progestogen
Progestogen-only pill:	progestogen
Depot progestogen injection:	progestogen
Post-coital pills:	oestrogen and progestogen
	oestrogen only
	progestogen only
Intrauterine devices:	progestogen
Vaginal rings:	progestogen
Implants:	oestrogen
Male contraception:	progestogen and androgen
Nasal/conjunctival instillation:	LH/RH analogue

than with systemic administration (e.g. 20 μg of LNG per day) and the risk of side-effects is reduced.

Subcutaneous implants

Oestradiol implants have been used to suppress ovulation and therefore act contraceptively. A progestogen by mouth must always be given simultaneously to offset a hyperplastic effect on the endometrium by unopposed oestrogen. Experimentally, work is being carried out on combined implants.

Male contraception

A combination of hormonal substances can be given to the male, analogously with the female combined pill. One component, for example medroxy-progesterone, will act on the hypothalamus to inhibit the output of pituitary gonadotrophins and an androgen such as methyltestosterone can be be added to replace endogenous testosterone, as not only the seminiferous tubules but also the Leydig cells will remain unstimulated. These methods are at present still under trial.

Other experimental methods

Hormones have been given into the conjunctival sac and also, by insufflation, on to the olfactory epithelium. From both these sites effective concentrations can reach the hypothalamus and pituitary, affecting gonadotrophin production. It is possible that a method using a LH/RH analogue may be found effective for the inhibition of ovulation (Bergquist et al 1979). Here again, major systemic absorption is avoided and therefore the risk of unwanted side-effects is reduced.

BENEFICIAL EFFECTS OF THE COMBINED PILL

Prescribers have a natural concern for the risks of adverse effects, which if serious are of paramount importance and every effort is needed to minimise these risks. In discussing them, it must also be remembered that there are many beneficial effects of hormonal contraceptives, particularly the combined oestrogen-progestogen pill.

Apart from highly effective fertility control by an easy method of administration and the benefits flowing from this, most women are rendered free from the discomforts of the natural menstrual cycle — mittelschmerz, dysmenorrhoea, pre-menstrual tension, heavy and perhaps unpredictable bleeding. The withdrawal bleeding is predictable and can even be avoided when it would be inconvenient by manipulation of the pill-taking regime, for example running two or more packets together consecutively. There is also a reduction in benign breast lesions (Vessey et al 1971) and protection against ovarian cysts, ovarian cancer and endometrial cancer (for a review see Vessey 1984). There is protection against acute salpingitis (Weström et al 1976, Burkman 1981) and endometriosis. There is a reduced risk of rheumatoid arthritis in pill users (RCGP Oral Contraception Study 1978) and some reduction in thyroid disorders (Frank & Kay 1978).

Table 17.2 Combined pill: beneficial effects

High effectiveness against conception	
Cycle stabilisation	
Reduced risk of:	ovarian cancer
	endometrial cancer
	ovarian cysts
	endometriosis
	benign breast lesions
	iron deficiency
	salpingitis
	rheumatoid arthritis
	thyroid disorders

ADVERSE EFFECTS OF HORMONAL CONTRACEPTIVES

Study methods

Evidence of adverse effects may be gathered from epidemiological studies, from simple case reports, or from laboratory findings of disturbed biomedical variables. Often a search is initiated from theoretical considerations or more often theory may suggest that a certain adverse effect should occur without it being found in practice to do so. The usual pattern has been a cluster of case reports which, after appropriate hypotheses have been generated, are followed by structured epidemiological studies. The results of studies may be supported by evidence from national routinely gathered statistics. Serious adverse effects from hormonal contraceptives have been so uncommon that large groups of users and controls have had to be recruited; statistical analysis has been difficult and to some extent the conclusions have been controversial.

In the early days of the combined pill in Britain, an association between use of the pill and deep vein thrombosis was noticed (Inman & Vessey 1968). As the incidence of risk and the risk factors were worked out, it became clear that large prospective, longitudinal or 'cohort' studies would be required to study the adverse effects of the pill. Accordingly in the mid-1960s two large studies were initiated in this country as follows:

1. Family Planning Association Oxford — Family Planning Association Study — Oxford Study

Findings were collated from women attending FPA clinics first in High Wycombe, then a number of other centres and recorded in a central unit at Oxford University Social Medicine Department, directed by Professor Martin Vessey (Vessey et al 1976). 17 032 women were recruited as established users of different contraceptive methods, 56% of whom were on the contraceptive pill. The sample consisted of white, married, women aged between 25 and 39 at entry who had used their initial method for at least 5 months.

2. Royal College of General Practitioners Oral Contraceptive Study

23 000 pill users and an equal number of never-user controls were recruited from the lists of 1400 general practitioners from all over the British Isles (Kay 1974). Details of age, parity, social class and smoking habit were recorded at entry. A central unit in Manchester directed by Dr Clifford Kay, collates and records this and continuing incidental morbidity data.

Somewhat later, cohort studies were initiated in the United States, for example, the Walnut Creek Contraceptive Drug Study (1974) recruiting from users of the Keyser-Permanente Health Care System in California and oral contraceptive data were included in the Boston Collaborative Drug Surveillance Programme (1973).

In more recent times, the Centres for Disease Control (CDC) in the U.S.A. have set up a large cohort study on Cancer and Steroid Hormones (CASH Study). This group has made significant observations on the relationship between the combined pill and neoplastic conditions (CDC 1983a, 1983b).

Large cohort studies such as these make an outstanding contribution to the study of adverse effects provided that the organisation and recording methods are efficient and that the sampling technique provides valid information with minimal bias, the extent of which if present at all should be capable of reasonably accurate estimation. For example, in the RCGP Study pill users attend their doctor at regular intervals, but controls do not. Therefore there will be an increased reporting of all symptoms among pill users. Kay estimates this bias to be 19% and is very cautious about the significance of excess reporting below this figure. The great advantage of cohort studies is that they indicate the risk of an effect as an absolute predicted incidence.

Retrospective or case-control studies are organised on the basis of a group of subjects suffering an adverse effect or event being compared, as to their use of the pill, with a comparable group not suffering in this way. Cohort bias is much more difficult to eliminate and statistical analysis requires more complicated techniques. Results are expressed in the form of 'relative risks' and not in absolute incidences. They are smaller and therfore less costly than control studies. They can also produce useful evidence much more rapidly and are thus helpful in determining whether a series of case reports of an effect is likely to be due to chance or to a true association with the medication. Much scorn has been applied in the literature to the findings of such surveys, particularly in the United States (Goldzieher & Dozier 1975, Macrae 1980), but the importance of the findings depends to a large extent on the use to which the reader puts them. Retrospective studies need confirmation and relative risk ratios need to be numerically high to be convincing.

Table 17.3 Combined pill: serious risks

Venous thrombosis and embolism
Coronary artery thrombosis
Cerebral artery thrombosis
Other arterial thromboses (e.g. retinal, mesenteric)
Subarachnoid haemorrhage
Hypertension
Gall bladder disease
Psychological depression
Increased risk of neoplasia in:

                                    liver
                                    cervix
                                    breast (? unconfirmed)

Circulatory

The combined oestrogen-progestogen pill increases cardiac output by reducing peripheral resistance (Lehtovirta 1974a, 1974b), increases certain blood coagulation factors (Poller et al 1971, Sagar et al 1976), leads to a hypertensive reaction in a small proportion of cases (Woods 1967, Kay 1974), and in an even smaller group is associated with increased risks of arterial lesions including myocardial infarction and cerebrovascular events (Vessey & Doll 1976).

The haemodynamic effect is of little importance in the physiologically healthy user but requires caution before prescribing combined pills for those with cardiac disorders. The coagulation effect adds the need for caution in cardiac disease with valvular deformity or replacement, or with dysrhythmias.

One of the earliest adverse effects discussed was the increased risk of deep vein thrombosis (Royal College of General Practitioners 1967, Vessey & Doll 1969) more often in calf muscles, but also seen in unusual sites such as the arms. A proportion of women with undiagnosed DVT developed pulmonary embolism and this became a tragic cause of sudden death in women prior to 1969. In December of that year it was publicly announced by the Chairman of the CSM (then Committee on Safety of Drugs) that certain pill combinations were more likely to lead to venous thromboembolism, these being pills with more than 50 μg of oestrogen in the daily dose (Inman et al 1970). Prescribers were advised not to prescribe combined pills in which this amount was exceeded. There was a precipitate fall in the incidence of DVTs and pulmonary embolism in pill takers and these conditions have become rare in young women (Vessey & Inman 1973). Later Meade demonstrated that reducing the oestrogen level to 30 μg daily reduced the risk even further (Meade et al 1980).

The status of superficial venous thrombosis as a pill risk was less certain. Some studies (RCGP, Kay 1974) demonstrated this; others could not observe an effect (for review see Vessey 1980).

The mechanism of the DVT risk remains controversial. Changes in the venous wall of leg veins have been noted (Irey et al 1970). Numerous studies also demonstrated changes in blood coagulation variables (Poller et al 1971) and a state of mild hypercoagulability of the blood has been described (Meade 1982). It is suggested that such an effect only arises from the synthetic oestrogens used in the pill and not from the 'natural' oestrogens used in the perimenopausal hormone replacement therapy. However in HRT the effective dose is markedly lower than is needed for contraception.

One consequence of the coagulability effect is the need for caution with major surgical operations. Frequently women are advised to stop combined pills for 4 weeks before and 2 weeks after a major elective procedure under general anaesthesia. When this is not possible, low dose heparin, dextran infusion and inflatable stockings may be used. It is vital to warn patients to use an alternative method pre-operatively as this is not a time for early pregnancy to be considered with equanimity.

'Pill hypertension' is shown in cohort studies to be uncommon but nevertheless always observable. The RCGP study showed a first year incidence of 1% increasing to 2.5% over 5 years of use (Kay 1974). The frequency is clearly related to the amount of progestogen in the type of combined pill taken, for a fixed dose of oestrogen. For this reason progestogen dose should be minimised and blood pressure taken at intervals during monitoring. The rise is normally slow, benign in the early stages and reversible. Rarely, death has occurred from malignant hypertension (Beral & Kay 1977). Before blood pressure monitoring became a wide-spread practice, there were case reports of patients severely affected by the complications of hypertension. It is possible that the blood pressure effect is linked to an increase in angiotensinogen in the blood, but as with many observed biochemical changes only a small proportion of subjects affected show any evidence of a disease process.

The venous thrombotic effect alerted observers to the possibility of arterial lesions and these also were noted from similarly early times (Bickerstaff & Holmes 1967, Doll 1970). However, reduction of oestrogen *per se* did not reduce the risk of stroke and myocardial infarction, a great disappointment at the time. Later analyses revealed that by 1977 these were the chief items in the excess overall mortality risk among pill takers compared with controls, although it was simultaneously recognised that the higher rate of smoking among pill users seriously confounded the calculations of risk (Vessey et al

1977, Beral & Kay 1977). Mann and colleagues (Mann et al 1975, Mann & Inman 1975) had already revealed in case control studies the importance of other risk factors for myocardial infarction in pill users, such as age, smoking habit, obesity and predisposing disease conditions (diabetes mellitus, hypertension, familial hyperlipidaemia). Deaths were rare, however, and it was another 4 years of cohort observation before a reasonably large number could be studied. The effect of age on risk was found to be less; the effect of smoking still a very serious problem (Layde et al 1981). More detailed analysis of the effect of the progestogen dose on 'total arterial disease' could also be done in the RCGP study and the result showed a clear relationship with increased dose of both norethisterone and of levonorgestrel in combined pills (Kay 1982). Bradley et al (1978) from the Walnut Creek Study demonstrated the effect of different pill combinations on the levels of lipoprotein-bound cholesterol fractions in pill users. Kay was able to correlate the reduction in high density lipoprotein cholesterol (HDL-chol) with the dose-related effect of progestogens on the risk of total arterial disease in pill users.

Since this time, there has been a tendency to use the effect on HDL-cholesterol as an indicator of arterial risk when considering new types of contraceptive preparation. There is clearly room for logical error in this step and statements must be regarded cautiously. It has equally been made clear that, at the lower levels of the effective dose range of both components in the combined pill, there is very little risk indeed of circulatory adverse effects and little if any significant disturbance of lipoprotein levels attributable to the pill (Kay 1982).

Considering hormonal methods using progestogens only without an oestrogen component, there are no data linking any of these with hypertension, venous thromboembolism or arterial disorders, nor even the pill-induced migraine of bizarre symptomatology found with any combined formulation. It has to be added that there is a lack of organised research into the adverse effects of progestogen-only pills but on the other hand neither is there a background of case reports to suggest a need for large scale studies. It is generally believed that progestogen-only pills and other low-dose release methods such as vaginal rings have no serious adverse effects. The effect of progestogen-only pills on lipoprotein levels is slight (Briggs 1979). HDL-cholesterol may be reduced a little with higher dosage in the range but not sufficiently for a significant biological effect. With pills such as Microval (30 μg LNG) no significant change in HDL-cholesterol is detectable (Briggs & Briggs 1983).

Turning to depot progestogens, there have been large studies on side effects in Thailand and Southern Africa. There has also been a large multicentre WHO trial (Toppozada et al 1982). Cardiovascular adverse effects have not been reported. Unfortunately we lack data from the more affluent populations. Regarding the effect on HDL-cholesterol however, the evidence is much clearer. Both DMPA (Kremer et al 1980) and NETO (Fotherby et al 1982) cause a significant decrease in blood HDL-chol of the order of 20-25%. It is therefore surprising that there has not been any report of arterial effects.

Neoplasia

An association between liver tumours and use of the combined pill has been suspected for many years. There is an increased risk of benign hepatic adenoma in pill users and of the rare primary hepatoma, which remains extremely rare even in the pill taking population (Williams & Neuberger 1981). Benign tumours may present clinically with upper abdominal intra-peritoneal haemorrhage.

Lesions of the pituitary such as prolactin-secreting adenoma were once thought to be a risk from using combined pills. Carefully considered data do not now support any such conclusion (Wingrave et al 1980).

Intensive work has been carried out over the years to trace any association between pill use and carcinoma of the breast or genital tract. In the case of ovarian cancer (and benign cysts) and for endometrial carcinoma, the combined pill has been found to provide a protective effect. Endometrial cancer is uncommon in the pill-using age group.

The position with breast and cervical cancer is more complex. A number of investigators observing data from large scale studies have examined their results for such associations, but there are difficulties in clarifying the specific action of oral contraceptives in the background of other known risk factors. For example, the use of barrier methods is protective against cervical cancer but increased parity increases the risk. Suitable control groups and standardisation techniques have therefore to be found.

The Oxford FPA study has recently reported on 13 cases of invasive cervical cancer in pill users comparing these to IUD users as controls, in whom there were no cases (Vessey et al 1983). There was also a clear and significant increase in cervical intraepithelial neoplasia (CIN) in the pill group. Combining all these neoplastic changes, a significant increase with duration of pill use was demonstrable, whereas there was no clear change with duration in the control group of IUD users. It appears that the type of cancer concerned develops slowly and is preventable by regular cytological screening, with referral for appropriate and early treatment of women with CIN lesions. Other studies have not shown results similar to these but more evidence is awaited from, for example, the CDC Study.

Recent publications on breast cancer have shown some disturbing results. Pike and colleagues from Los Angeles looked at women taking oral contraceptives under 25 and developing breast cancer diagnosed by the age of 37, compared with a neighbourhood control group (Pike et al 1983). This was a retrospective case-control study in which those who had died could not be included. It depended on rather detailed recall of contraceptive formulations many years after actual use. There seemed to be a clear connection of risk with pill combinations of higher dosage, both of progestogen and of oestrogen. The relationship with lower oestrogen pills was less clear, but Pike developed a background hypothesis identifying high progestogen potency as the main risk factor. The scoring of potency was unfortunately based on an outmoded pharmacological method in which various combinations of progestogens with 100 μg of oestrogen were compared in the delay of menses test, a test relating to action on the endometrium (Greenblatt 1967). Some bizarre tables of 'progestogenic potency' were produced by extrapolation but these have attracted no credence among pharmacologists and specialist clinicians. More detailed and confirmatory evidence is awaited.

The Oxford Unit (McPherson et al 1983) have recently published preliminary results from a further case-control study connecting a breast cancer risk with use of the combined pill. In one analysis from the RCGP Study (Kay 1981) a significant risk appears in women who have been pill users diagnosed in the 30–34 age group but in no other. Interpretation of such an effect was felt to be difficult but in the light of Pike's later results this may be confirmatory. In the RCGP and Oxford-FPA Studies there is as yet no link with particular formulations.

It must be emphasised that in a number of other carefully organised and controlled studies (e.g. CDC 1983c, and see Kalache et al 1983) there is no evidence of a link with breast cancer. At present therefore, some doubt exists and confirmatory analyses are awaited.

As with cardiovascular risks, the effects are small and therefore hard to demonstrate and analyse. Much clearer are the protective effects of combined pill use on ovarian tumours and endometrial cancer. Weiss & Sayvetz (1980) showed a reduction of endometrial cancer risk in pill users of some 50% in a case-control study. This has since been confirmed in others. The effect appears to increase with duration of use and persists after the pill is stopped. Nine case-control studies show a protective effect of pill use on ovarian cancer (Vessey 1984); here again the effect is increased by duration of use and some studies show a persistent effect for at least 10 years after cessation of use (CDC 1983a).

The most serious current problem therefore for pill users is the question of breast cancer in young women. The effect is small but needs to be separated from confounding risk factors and the true extent identified. In the case of cervical cancer, the seriousness is mitigated by the possibility of effectively preventing the invasive lesion. The liver tumour risk remains but is a very rare factor to consider. Otherwise the reduction in ovarian and endometrial cancers from pill use is encouraging for users and prescribers.

A large multicenter study by the World Health Organisation in developing countries has shown no effect on the risk of breast cancer in users of DMPA (WHO Collaborative Study of Neoplasia and Steroid Contraceptives 1984). In this same study there was more concern with a doubling of the relative risk of cervical cancer in DMPA users, but only after 5 years of use. There was no trend with duration of use, however, to indicate a dose-related response and further analyses of these results are needed to assess their significance.

RISK FACTORS AND PILL PRESCRIBING

Previous sections illustrate that adverse effects of hormonal contraceptives are uncommon but there is a concentration of risk in various subpopulations of pill users. Mortality figures, for example, clearly define the interaction between age, smoking and pill use when considering circulatory conditions (Beral & Kay 1977, Layde et al 1981).

Mann's studies on myocardial infarction (MI) extended the concept of risk factors to chronic pathological conditions such as diabetes mellitus, essential hypertension, obesity and familial hyperlipidaemia. In his case-control study, all but one case of MI out of 60 were associated with other risk factors (Mann et al 1975). Kay has shown from mortality figures that, all other aspects being excluded from consideration, combined pills should not be prescribed for cigarette smokers (15 or more daily) over the age of 35 but that, for non-smokers, low dose pills can reasonably be continued into the early forties (Layde et al 1981). After 45 the mortality risk from pill use alone through cardiovascular conditions becomes unacceptable.

Table 17.4 Risk factors in pill prescribing

Cardiovascular:	
Older age group	
Smoking	
Obesity	
Diabetes	
Hypertension	
Familial hyperlipidaemia	
Neoplasia	
Cervix:	age, parity, smoking, multiple partners, early first coitus
Breast:	close family history, delayed first full-term pregnancy, early menarche

There are other conditions where risk factors arise from familial or constitutional conditions or more simply from the life style of the potential user. Cervical neoplasia risks are increased by early age of coital experience and by multiplicity of partners. Parity is also an important consideration, however, and the advantage of combined pills lies in their high effectiveness against pregnancy. With breast cancer delay between menarche and first childbirth is an important factor (Gray et al 1982) and so is a close family history of breast cancer (Kelsey 1979). Until more epidemiological information is available on breast cancer risks, the prescriber should maintain young people on pills with as low a dose of both components as possible. It may well seem relevant to question use of the combined pill in those young women, for example, whose mothers have had breast cancer and who are now delaying first pregnancy.

The effect on a woman of unwanted pregnancy needs to be brought into the risk-benefit equation. The protective effect against breast cancer of a younger first pregnancy is not conferred by a pre-viable abortion, induced or otherwise. If therefore a woman has decided against an early first childbirth under any circumstances, a low dose combined pill may still be the best option when all risks and benefits are taken into account. The easy availability or otherwise of safe and early pregnancy termination, its cost and acceptability, need to be considered if a less effective contraceptive is advised.

OTHER ADVERSE EFFECTS

Numerous laboratory studies have defined the action of hormonal contraceptives on carbohydrate metabolism. There is a shift in the glucose tolerance curve towards the diabetic (Wynn & Doar 1966). The extent of this is dose-related and studies on different populations give different results, possibly due to dietary differences. Such effects are reversible and indeed are insignificant with modern low-dose combined pills or triphasics (Briggs 1979, Spellacy 1982), but normality of blood glucose levels is achieved only by increased plasma insulin levels. Studies with depot progestogen injections give varying results (Spellacy et al 1972, Giwa-Osagie & Newton 1982). There is not a shred of evidence from longitudinal studies that clinical diabetes arises with a greater incidence in pill users than in others. In theory it is possible that the potential or 'pre-'diabetic is at risk of earlier manifestation, but there are no data supporting this contention.

Gallstones and cholecystitis were once considered to be an absolute excess risk in pill users. Further data over a long period from the RCGP study have shown, however, that the risk in incidence of gallbladder disease in the first 2½ years of use becomes a deficit by 7 years (Wingrave & Kay 1982). Evidently women susceptible to gallbladder disease develop this rather early on, but the overall proportion affected in the control group eventually catches up with the pill using group.

The effect on liver function has been intensively studied as the liver is the main seat of steroid metabolism apart from the hormonal target organs (for a brief review see McEwan 1983). Oestrogen is excreted in bile and reabsorbed from the gut. Blood levels are significantly reduced during the administration of broad spectrum antibiotics such as tetracyclines and ampicillins, with consequent escape from ovulatory control (Dossetor 1975, Bacon & Shenfield 1980). Changes in liver enzymes and excretion tests can be shown with older combinations (Sherlock 1969, Mowat & Arias 1969) but here again with the lower dose combined pills the effect is transient or absent (Dickenson et al 1980). It is advised that hormonal contraception is not given during disturbances of liver function, for example in an attack of acute infectious hepatitis, but there is no contraindication to resuming hormonal contraception once liver function has returned to normal (Eisalo et al 1971).

Combined pills not uncommonly appear to induce mild degrees of psychological depression, manifested by irritability or weepiness for no definable reason. This occurs at approximately the 5% level in any clinic population; rarely is the disturbance more severe. Alterations in the pyridoxine-dependent metabolic pathway of tryptophane to nicotinamide due to oestrogen have been well documented (Rose 1966). Some cases of depression can be postulated from this metabolic change. Giving large doses of oral B_6

reverses the biochemical abnormality and in a proportion of cases relieves the psychiatric symptoms (Adams et al 1973).

There is a large variety of discomforts affecting pill use, from acne or leg pains to cervical ectopy or mastodynia. These are not major threats to life or health. Usually manipulation of the combined pill formula is worth trying before abandoning the method.

With progestogen-only contraception, it is reiterated that there is no evidence of any serious adverse effects. Acceptability of these methods is profoundly affected by the tendency to disturbed menstrual patterns, varying from amenorrhoea to polymenorrhoea. With the depot injections, a significant number of amenorrhoeic women fail to ovulate again after stopping the medication. With DMPA such an effect may last up to 2 years. Statistical data show that fertility eventually returns (Pardthaisong et al 1980). In a developed society this effect may be less important as, if a pregnancy is desired, ovulation can be induced therapeutically. Where such techniques are not available the wisdom of using these contraceptive methods needs to be carefully considered and this effect discussed with the potential user. To some extent the post-medication anovulatory effect is seen also after combined pills in a small proportion of women (Vessey et al 1978) and in a greater proportion there may be some cycle irregularity for up to 3 months after stopping the pill. There is some controversy about whether so called 'post-pill amenorrhoea' is a specific action of combined pills or whether the regular withdrawal bleeds during administration have merely masked a potential pre-existing state of anovulatory amenorrhoea (Shearman 1968, 1971, Shearman & Turtle 1970, Marshall et al 1976).

Certainly amenorrhoea persisting for more than 6 months after stopping the pill warrants investigation for an underlying pathological cause, such as a prolactin-secreting pituitary adenoma, thyroid disorder, or primary ovarian failure.

CONCLUSION

The elucidation of the serious adverse effects of hormonal contraceptives has been put together piece by piece over a period of 15 years and is still continuing. These effects occur with subtlety and on a small scale in a large population of users. It has been possible by analysing the information from research studies to refine down prescribing policy using the principle of risk factors in sub-populations. As a result we can be reasonably confident that hormonal methods now have a high index of safety when used according to the recommendations.

The recent work on neoplasia, however, once again raises the inherent difficulty with systemic administration. There may be an adverse effect on a tissue or organ not immediately involved in the process of conception, for example, coronary arteries or mammary epithelium, in order to achieve the necessary concentration of the agent at the site of contraceptive action. The extent of degradation of steroids at the first pass through the liver entails that the dose administered must be relatively high for contraceptive success. Furthermore, the action of hepatic enzymes varies individually: some users will be exposed to higher blood and tissue levels of steroid than others to reach the same objective. The answer to this difficulty probably lies ultimately in the development of local administration ideally providing contraceptively active levels of the hormone analogues at the required site with small or unmeasurable spillover into the general circulation. This explains the development work on hormone releasing intrauterine devices, on vaginal rings and on the application of LH RH agonists to the olfactory or conjunctival epithelium. As long as administration is by injection, implant or intestine, some degree of adversity will always turn up. It is only by topical application at or very near to the site of action at a level of concentration no higher than necessary for contraceptive effectiveness, that some hope of eliminating adverse effects may be anticipated.

REFERENCES

Adams P W, Wynn V, Rose D P, Seed M, Folkard J, Strong R 1973 Effect of pyroxidine hydrochloride (vitamin B_6) upon depression associated with oral contraception. Lancet i: 897–904

Bacon J F, Shenfield G M 1980 Pregnancy attributable to interaction between tetracycline and oral contraceptives. British Medical Journal 1: 293

Beral V, Kay C R 1977 Mortality among oral-contraceptive users. Lancet ii: 727–731

Bergquist C. Nillius S J, Wide L 1979 Intranasal gonadotrophin-releasing hormone agonist as a contraceptive agent. Lancet ii: 215–216

Bickerstaff E R, Holmes J M 1967 Cerebral arterial insufficiency and oral contraceptives. British Medical Journal 1: 726–729

Boston Collaborative Drug Surveillance Programme 1973 Oral contraceptives and venous thromboembolic disease, surgically confirmed gall-bladder disease and breast tumours. Lancet i: 1399–1404

Bradley D D, Wingard J, Pettiti D B, Krauss R M, Ramcharan S 1978 Serum high-density lipoprotein cholesterol in women using oral contraceptives, estrogens and progestins. New England Journal of Medicine 299: 17–20

Briggs M H 1979 Biochemical basis for the selection of oral contraceptives. International Journal of Gynaecology and Obstetrics 16: 509–517

Briggs M, Briggs M 1983 Plasma lipids in women using progestogen-only oral contraceptives. British Journal of Obstetrics and Gynaecology 90: 549–552

Burkman R J 1981 Association between intrauterine device and pelvic inflammatory disease. Obstetrics and Gynaecology 57: 269–276

Burton F G, Skiens W E, Duncan G W 1979 Low-level progestogen-releasing vaginal contraceptive devices. Contraception 19: 507–516

Centres for Disease Control Cancer and Steroid Hormones Study 1983a Oral contraceptive use and risk of ovarian cancer. Journal of the American Medical Association 249: 1596–1599

Centres for Disease Control Cancer and Steroid Hormones Study 1983b Oral contraceptive use and the risk of endometrial cancer. Journal of the American Medical Association 249: 1600–1604

Centres for Disease Control Cancer and Steroid Hormones Study 1983c Long-term oral contraceptive use and the risk of breast cancer. Journal of the American Medical Association 249: 1591–1595

Dickerson J, Bressler R, Christian C D 1980 Liver function tests and low-dose oestrogen oral contraceptives. Contraception 22: 597–603

Doll R 1970 The long-term effects of oral contraceptives. Journal of Biosocial Science 2: 367–389

Dossetor E J 1975 Drug interaction with oral contraceptives. British Medical Journal 4: 467–468

Eisalo A, Konttinen O, Hietala O 1971 Oral contraceptives after liver disease. British Medical Journal 3: 561–562

Fotherby K, Trayner I, Howard G, Hamawi A, Elder M G 1982 Effect of injectable norethisterone oenanthate (Norigest) on blood lipid levels. Contraception 25: 435–446

Frank P, Kay C R 1978 Incidence of thyroid disease associated with oral contraceptives. British Medical Journal 2: 1531

Giwa-Osagie O F, Newton J R 1982 Injectable Norethisterone Enanthate contraception: absence of an effect on oral glucose tolerance. Contraceptive Delivery Systems 3: 61–62

Goldzieher J W, Dozier T S 1975 Oral contraceptives and thromboembolism: a reassessment. American Journal of Obstetrics and Gynaecology 123: 878

Gray G E, Pike M C, Hirayama T, Tellez J, Gerkins V, Brown J B, Casagrande J T, Henderson B E 1978 Diet and hormone profiles in teenage girls in four countries at different risk of breast cancer. Preventive Medicine 11: 108

Greenblatt R B 1967 Progestational agents in clinical practice. Medical Science 18: 37–49

Haspels A A, Andriesse R 1973 The effect of large doses of estrogens post coitum in 2000 women. European Journal of Obstetrics, Gynaecology and Reproductive Biology 3: 113

Inman W H W, Vessey M P 1968 Investigation of deaths from pulmonary, coronary and cerebral thrombosis and embolism. British Medical Journal 2: 193–199

Inman W H W, Vessey M P, Westerholm B, Engelund A 1970 Thromboembolic disease and the steroidal content of oral contraceptives. A report to the Committee on Safety of Drugs. British Medical Journal 2: 203–209

Irey N S, Marion W C, Taylor H B 1970 Vascular lesions in women taking oral contraceptives. Archives of Pathology 89: 1–8

Kalache A, McPherson K, Barlthrop K, Vessey M P 1983 Oral contraceptives and breast cancer. British Journal of Hospital Medicine 30: 278–283

Kay C 1974 Oral contraceptives and Health: an interim report from the Oral Contraception Study of the Royal College of General Practitioners. Pitman Medical, London

Kay C 1981 Breast cancer and oral contraceptives: findings in Royal College of General Practitioners Study. British Medical Journal 282: 2089–2093

Kay C R 1982 Progestogens and arterial disease — evidence from the Royal College of General Practitioners Study. American Journal of Obstetrics and Gynecology 142: 762–765

Kremer J, de Bruin H W A, Hindricks F R 1980 Serum high-density lipoprotein cholesterol levels in women using a contraceptive injection of depot-medroxyprogesterone acetate. Contraception 22: 359–367

Kelsey J L 1979 A review of the epidemiology of human breast cancer. Epidemiologic Reviews 1: 74–109

Layde P M, Beral V, Kay C R 1981 Further analyses of mortality in oral contraceptive users. Lancet i: 541–546

Lehtovirta P 1974a Haemodynamic effects of combined oestrogen/progestogen oral contraceptives. Journal of Obstetrics and Gynaecology of the British Commonwealth 81: 517–525

Lehtovirta P 1974b Peripheral haemodynamic effects of combined oestrogen/progestogen oral contraceptives. Journal of Obstetrics and Gynaecology of the British Commonwealth 81: 526–534

McEwan J 1983 Contraception for women with liver disease. British Journal of Family Planning 9: 57–59

McPherson K, Neil A, Vessey M P, Doll R 1983 Oral Contraceptives and breast cancer. Lancet ii: 1414–1415

Macrae K D 1980 Thrombosis and oral contraception. British Journal of Hospital Medicine 24: 438–442

Mann J I, Inman W H W 1975 Oral contraceptives and death from myocardial infarction. British Medical Journal 2: 245–248

Mann J I, Vessey M P, Thorogood M, Doll R 1975 Myocardial infarction in young women with special reference to oral contraceptive practice. British Medical Journal 2: 241–245

Marshall J C, Reed P I, Gordon H 1976 Luteinizing hormone secretion in patients presenting with post-oral contraceptive amenorrhoea: evidence for a hypothalamic feedback abnormality. Clinical Endocrinology 5: 131–143

Meade T W, Greenberg G, Thompson S G 1980 Progestogens and cardiovascular reactions associated with oral contraceptives and a comparison of the safety of 50 and 30 μg oestrogen preparations. British Medical Journal 280: 1157–1161

Meade T W 1982 Oral contraceptives, clotting factors and thrombosis. American Journal of Obstetrics and Gynecology 142: 758–761

Mowat A P, Arias A M 1969 Liver function and oral contraceptives. Journal of Reproductive Medicine 3: 19–29

Nilsson C G, Luukkainen T, Diaz J, Allonen H 1981 Intrauterine contraception with levonorgestrel: a comparative randomised performance study. Lancet i: 577–580

Pardthaisong T, Gray R H, McDaniel E B 1980 Return of fertility after discontinuation of depot medroxyprogesterone acetate and intrauterine devices in northern Thailand. Lancet i: 509–512

Pike M C, Henderson B E, Krailo M D, Duke A, Roy S 1983 Breast cancer in young women and use of oral contraceptives: possible modifying effect of formulation and age at use. Lancet ii: 926–930

Poller L, Thomson J M, Thomson W 1971 Oestrogen/progestogen oral contraception and blood clotting: a long term follow up. British Medical Journal 4: 648–650

Rose D P 1966 The influence of oestrogens on tryptophan metabolism in Man. Clinical Science 31: 265–272

Royal College of General Practitioners 1967 Oral contraception and thromboembolic disease. Journal of the College of General Practitioners 13: 267–269

RCGP Oral Contraception Study 1978 Reduction in incidence of rheumatoid arthritis associated with oral contraceptives. Lancet i: 569–571

Sagar S, Stamatakis J D, Thomas D P, Kakkar V V 1976 Oral contraceptives, antithrombin III activity and post-operative deep vein thrombosis. Lancet i: 509–511

Shearman R P 1968 Investigation and treatment of amenorrhoea developing after treatment with oral contraceptives. Lancet i: 325–326

Shearman R P 1971 Prolonged secondary amenorrhoea after oral contraceptive therapy: natural and unnatural history. Lancet ii: 64–66

Shearman R P, Turtle J R 1970 Secondary amenorrhoea with inappropriate lactation. American Journal of Obstetrics and Gynecology 106: 818

Sherlock S 1968 Diseases of the Liver and Biliary System. Blackwell Scientific Publications, Oxford

Snowden R 1977 The Progestasert and ectopic pregnancy. British Medical Journal 2: 1600

Spellacy W N 1982 Carbohydrate metabolism during treatment with estrogen, progestogen and low dose oral contraceptives. American Journal of Obstetrics and Gynecology 142: 732–734

Spellacy W N, McLeod G W, Buhi W C, Birk S A 1972 The effects of medroxyprogesterone acetate on carbohydrate metabolism; measurements of glucose, insulin and growth hormone after twelve months use. Fertility and Sterility 23: 239

Toppozada H K, Koetsawang S, Aimakhu V E, Khan T, Pretnar A, Chatterjee T K, Molitor-Peffer M P, Apelo R, Lichtenberg R, Crosignani P G, de Souza J C, Gomez-Rogers C, Haspels A A 1982 Multinational comparative clinical trial of long-acting injectable contraceptives: norethisterone enanthate given in two dosage regimes and depot medroxyprogesterone acetate: a preliminary report. Contraception 25: 1–10

Vessey M P 1980 Female hormones and vascular disease: an epidemiological overview. British Journal of Family Planning 6 (Suppl): 12

Vessey M P 1984 Cancer and the pill — some recent findings. Journal of Obstetrics and Gynaecology 4 (Suppl): S 52–S 56

Vessey M P, Inman W H W 1973 Speculations about mortality trends from venous thromboembolic disease in England and Wales and their relation to the pattern of oral contraceptive usage. Journal of Obstetrics and Gynaecology of the British Commonwealth 80: 562

Vessey M P, Doll R 1976 Evaluation of existing techniques. Is 'The Pill' safe enough to continue using. Proceedings of the Royal Society of London Series B. Biological Sciences 195: 69–80

Vessey M P, Doll R 1969 Investigation of relation between use of oral contraceptives and thromboembolic disease: a further report. British Medical Journal 2: 651–657

Vessey M P, Doll R, Sutton P M 1971 Investigation of the possible relationship between oral contraceptives and benign and malignant breast disease. Cancer 28: 1395

Vessey M P, Doll R, Peto R, Johnson B, Wiggins P 1976 A long-term follow up study of women using different methods of contraception — an interim report. Journal of Biosocial Science 8: 373–427

Vessey M P, McPherson K, Johnson B 1977 Mortality among women participating in the Oxford/Family Planning Association Contraceptive Study. Lancet ii: 731–757

Vessey M P, Wright N H, McPherson K, Wiggins P 1978 Fertility after stopping different methods of contraception. British Medical Journal 1: 265–267

Vessey M P, Lawless M, McPherson K, Yeates D 1983 Neoplasia of the cervix uteri and contraception: a possible adverse effect of the pill. Lancet ii: 930–934

Walnut Creek Contraceptive Drug Study 1974 A prospective study of the side effects of oral contraceptives. Ramchoran S (ed) Government Printing Office, Washington D C, Vol 1 DHEW Publication No (NIH) 74–562

Weiss N S, Sayvetz T A 1980 Incidence of endometrial cancer in relation to the use of oral contraceptives. New England Journal of Medicine 302: 551–554

Weström L, Bengtsson L P, Mardh P A 1976 The risk of pelvic inflammatory disease in women using intrauterine contraceptive devices as compared to non-users. Lancet ii: 221–224

WHO Collaborative Study of Neoplasia and Steroid Contraceptives 1984. Breast cancer, cervical cancer, and depot medrotyprogesterone acetate. Lancet letter ii: 1207–1208

Williams R, Neuberger J 1981 Occurrence, frequency and management of oral contraceptive associated liver tumours. British Journal of Family Planning 7: 35–41

Wingrave S J, Kay C R 1982 Oral contraceptives and gall bladder disease. Lancet ii: 957–959

Wingrave S J, Kay C R, Vessey M P 1980 Oral contraceptives and pituitary adenomas. British Medical Journal 280: 685–686

Woods J N 1967 Oral contraceptives and hypertension. Lancet ii: 653–654

Wynn V, Doar J W H 1966 Some effects of oral contraceptives on carbohydrate metabolism. Lancet ii: 715–719

Yuzpe A A, Lancee W J 1977 Ethinylestradiol and dl-norgestrel as a post-coital contraceptive. Fertility and sterility 28: 932–936

Dysmenorrhoea

INTRODUCTION

It is only over the last 20 years that dysmenorrhoea has been recognised by the medical profession as a problem. Prior to this, and for some even today, it is considered as a woman's 'lot' in life. However, with the changing role of women in society and the alteration in society's attitudes towards menstruation, serious scientific work is now being performed. In this chapter I would like to discuss the pathogenesis and treatment of dysmenorrhoea as well as suggest some future avenues for research.

DEFINITION

Dysmenorrhoea comes from the Greek word meaning difficult monthly flow, but is now usually taken to mean painful menstruation. It may occur secondary to an unrelated group of pelvic pathologies such as endometriosis, pelvic inflammatory disease, uterine abnormality and fibroids, or it may be ideopathic in origin. It is with the latter that this chapter will be principally concerned. Dysmenorrhoea is a symptom complex consisting of cramping lower abdominal pain, worst at the onset of the menses and often radiating to the back and legs; gastrointestinal, cardiovascular and neurological symptoms. It can cause severe incapacity lasting some days particularly if preceded by the premenstrual syndrome. Primary and secondary dysmenorrhoea do differ slightly in their symptomology, but it is often impossible to distinguish with accuracy between the two types on history and examination alone. Primary dysmenorrhoea is much commoner in young women in their teens and by definition is accompanied by a normal pelvic examination. For a definitive diagnosis laparoscopy must be performed as the presence of pathology in those thought to have primary dysmenorrhoea can influence the outcome of both treatment and the results of research.

INCIDENCE

The results of some of the epidemiological studies performed over the last fifty years to investigate the incidence of dysmenorrhoea are summarised in Table

18.1. The variable frequencies quoted indicate how difficult this is to estimate. Pain is a subjective symptom and cannot be assessed accurately by an outside observer. Different women will react to the same pain in different ways and the way each woman may perceive the pain will vary with altered circumstances.

Table 18.1 The frequency of dysmenorrhoea in young women

Study	Group	Mildly affected	Moderately affected	Severely affected
Miller (1930)	College students	47	17	3
McArthur (1957)	Schoolgirls			10
Svennerud (1959)	Students and workers	31		6
Widholm & Kantero (1971)	Schoolgirls	38	13	
Andersch & Milsom (1982)	19 year olds	72	15	8

For Refs 1–4 see Ref 5

Also, the definition and diagnosis are by no means absolute allowing different interpretations by the various workers. Severe dysmenorrhoea is usually defined as menstrual related pain requiring time off work or studies and occurs in 3–10% of young women. The studies mentioned in the table would also suggest that a majority of young women get some discomfort with their periods. It has been estimated that 2.6 million women in Great Britain alone are adversely affected by dysmenorrhoea (Anderson 1981) and it is a primary cause for women to visit their general practitioners (Richards 1979). This means that dysmenorrhoea has important social and economic consequences both in terms of loss of time from work or studies as well as decreased performance when present.

Much of the epidemiological work has been carried out in Scandinavia. Widholm has performed a number of valuable studies mainly involving the filling in of questionnaires by selected groups of women. In one of the earlier studies, he investigated 5000 girls between the ages of 10 and 20 years together with their mothers (Widholm 1979). He noted that dysmenorrhoea frequently started within 1 year of the menarche and in 40% of the young women was accompanied by pre-menstrual tension. A familial element may be present in that it was noted that girls who had mothers with dysmenorrhoea were more likely to suffer themselves. He also demonstrated that life style and occupation may influence the overall incidence as well as the prevalence of accompanying symptoms.

Recently an interesting study has been published from Gothenberg in Sweden (Andersch & Milsom 1982). This takes a random sample of 19 year olds from all social backgrounds. It indicates that the incidence of dysmenorrhoea is still very high and continues to be a problem in Western society.

PATHOGENESIS

There are many different theories as to why women suffer from dysmenorrhoea. The main theories which will be considered are:

1. Cervical obstruction.
2. Alterations in myometrial contractility.
3. Decreased uterine blood flow.
4. Hormones including the prostaglandins.
5. The presence of adrenergic nerves within the cervix.
6. Psychological.
7. More than one of these factors acting together.

Cervical obstruction

This theory was strongly advocated around the time of Hippocrates but probably has few advocates now. It is certainly true that cervical abnormalities and stenosis which prevents the flow of menstrual blood can cause dysmenorrhoea. However, hysterosalpingographic studies performed during the menses failed to show any difference in the tightness of the cervical canal in those with dysmenorrhoea (Asplund 1952) and also, the pain is often at its worst at the time when the bleeding is at its heaviest. Thus obstruction is unlikely to be important in the anatomically normal uterus.

Myometrial Contractility

The role of uterine hyperactivity in the causation of dysmenorrhoea has received attention in the literature since it was first suggested by Novac & Reynolds in 1932 (Wilson & Kurzrok 1940, Woodbury et al 1947, Filler & Hall 1970, Lundstrom et al 1976, Csapo et al 1977, Andersson & Ulmsten 1978, Akerlund 1979). However, there is no real agreement on the type of hyperactivity which occurs. It may be due to irregular dysrhythmic contractions or simply elevated uterine tone (Filler & Hall 1970). Akerlund feels that high amplitude peaks which have been shown to accompany the severe pain are responsible (Akerlund et al 1976) but the problem with many of these studies is that the groups of women with dysmenorrhoea and the control groups are small in size and unmatched making interpretation of the results difficult. In a recent study carried out in 13 women with primary dysmenorrhoea and 11 matched controls (Lumsden & Baird 1985), high amplitude peaks were found in both those with and without pain (Fig. 18.1). No significant difference between the two groups was detected for amplitude, duration or resting pressure although they tended to be greater in those with dysmenorrhoea than in those without and was maximal at the time of greatest pain. However uterine work, estimated by measuring the area under the curve which is the work performed by a hollow viscous (Csapo & Sauvage 1968, Kenedi 1981), was greater in those with dysmenorrhoea.

Blood flow

Recent studies performed in Sweden indicate that blood flow may also be of importance in the aetiology of primary dysmenorrhoea. This is extremely

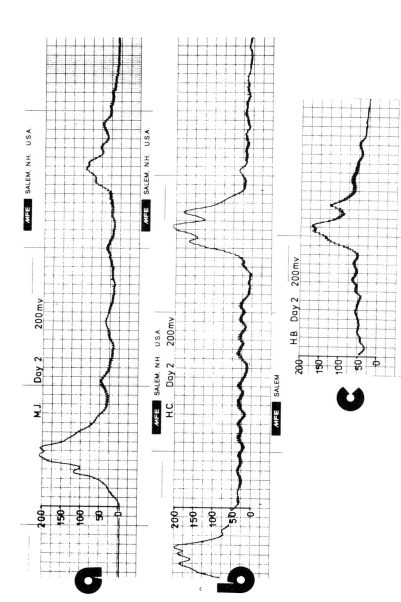

Fig. 18.1 (a) (b) were made on day 2 of the menses in subjects with dysmenorrhoea and (c) was made from a member of the control group. The pressure was measured in mmHg and each small square is equivalent to 5 seconds. Note the presence of uterine artery pulsation in the control tracing (c) which is absent from the tracings accompanied by pain. (These tracings were made in the subjects 1, 2 and A referred to in Fig. 18.3)

difficult to measure in the human female *in vivo*, but Akerlund succeeded in inserting a thermister probe into the uterus to measure endometrial blood flow (Akerlund et al 1976). He demonstrated that during exacerbations of the pain, blood flow was decreased and was accompanied by pain. Unfortunately, I am not aware of any studies of myometrial blood flow in a similar subject group. However, using highly sensitive methods for measuring uterine contractility it is possible to see the uterine artery pulsations (Fig. 18.1). In the subject with dysmenorrhoea (a) the pulsation disappears whereas it remains throughout the peak in the control subjects. Although this finding could not be quantitated, it is frequently observed during intrauterine pressure measurements.

Prostaglandins and primary dysmenorrhoea

The idea that prostaglandins may be involved in dysmenorrhoea was first suggested by Pickles during the 1960s (Pickles et al 1965). He extracted a smooth muscle stimulant from menstrual fluid which was identified as a mixture of prostaglandins. Since this time much evidence has been put forward to confirm that prostaglandins are indeed involved although their mechanism of action is not clear. In view of the oxytocic properties of many of the prostaglandins, it is hardly surprising that it has been suggested that these potent agents are involved in the increase in uterine contractility associated with dysmenorrhoea. Prostaglandin $(PG)F_{2\alpha}$ is a potent myometrial stimulant *in vitro* (Bygdeman 1964). When administered *in vivo* it causes an increase in contractility which is consistently accompanied by dysmenorrhoea — like pain (Fig. 18.2) (Lundstrom 1977, Lumsden — unpublished observation) and even, on occasions, menstrual bleeding (Karim et al 1971). $PGF_{2\alpha}$ has now been measured in endometrium (Singh 1975, Pulkkinen & Csapo 1978) menstrual fluid (Pickles et al 1965, Chan & Hill 1978, Pulkkinen & Csapo 1978, Lumsden et al 1983a) and endometrial jet washings (Halbert et al 1975) and is found to be present in significantly greater amounts in those suffering from dysmenorrhoea.

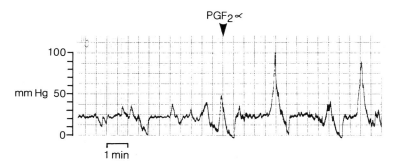

Fig. 18.2 This illustrates the increase in intra-uterine pressure produced by an infusion into the uterus of 5 μg/min $PGF_{2\alpha}$ on day 18 of the menstrual cycle. The patient also complained of pain identical to that of the dysmenorrhoea she experienced on day 1 of the menses

PGE_2 is also present in greater amounts in the menstrual fluid of those with dysmenorrhoea (Lumsden et al 1983a) but its effect on uterine contractility are not as well defined as those of $PGF_{2\alpha}$. During the menses a pharmacological dose may lead to relaxation (Martin & Bygdeman 1965) and the effects are further complicated by the fact that it may not have the same action on pieces of muscle taken from varying positions in the uterine wall (Wilhelmsson 1981). Prostacyclin (PGI_2) which is probably a myometrial relaxant (Omini et al 1978, Wilhelmsson et al 1981, Lye & Challis 1982) appears to be present in endometrium (Smith et al 1981) and menstrual fluid (Lumsden et al 1983a) only in very small amounts. Its effects on the human uterus *in vivo* will be discussed further, later in this chapter.

The prostaglandins also have potent effect on the peripheral vascular system. $PGF_{2\alpha}$ is a powerful vasoconstrictor and PGI_2 is one of the most potent vasodilators known. As a group there are therefore many ways that they could be involved in dysmenorrhoea and these are summarised in Table 18.2.

The steroid hormones

Primary dysmenorrhoea occurs almost exclusively in ovulatory menstrual cycles although there is evidence to suggest that anovulatory cycles soon after the menarche may be associated with pain (Widholm 1979). It is well known that the abolition of ovulation with the oral contraceptive pill will often dramatically improve dysmenorrhoea.

Table 18.2 Evidence for the involvement of prostaglandins in dysmenorrhoea

1. $PGF_{2\alpha}$ and PGE_2 are present in menstruating endometrium and menstrual fluid in high concentrations.
2. $PGF_{2\alpha}$ stimulates myometrial contractility both *in vivo* and *in vitro*.
3. $PGF_{2\alpha}$ is a vasoconstrictor.
4. $PGE_{2\alpha}$ can increase the sensitivity of nerve endings.
5. Prostaglandin synthetase inhibitors relieve dysmenorrhoea, decrease menstrual fluid prostaglandin concentrations and decrease uterine contractility.

Before the maximum synthetic capacity of the endometrium to produce prostaglandins can be expressed, ovulation is necessary. Concentrations of prostaglandins are higher during the secretory than the proliferative phase of the cycle (Downie et al 1974, Maathius & Kelly 1978) and a period of progesterone priming appears to be necessary for maximum synthetic capacity (Abel & Baird 1980). The control of $PGF_{2\alpha}$ and PGE_2 concentrations appears to differ in that whereas $PGF_{2\alpha}$ production is under steroid hormone control, that of PGE_2 is not (Downie et al 1974). The mechanism of this control is not clear. Oestrogen appears to be involved in the synthesis of the enzymes necessary to produce prostaglandins, but the nature of the priming role of progesterone is unknown although increasing availability of the prostaglandin precurser arachidonic acid is a possibility.

Steroid hormones also affect the pattern of contractility of the human uterus (Cibils 1967, Bengtssen & Theobald 1967). During the follicular phase, frequent contractions of small amplitude are apparent. Wilson & Kurzrok (1938) also demonstrated that high doses of oestrogen relieve the pain of dysmenorrhoea and decrease uterine contractility, the latter feature also having been demonstrated in ovariectomised rats (Downing et al 1978). A small series of tracings (n = 5) carried out within 24 hours of the midcycle luteinising hormone surge demonstrated very little activity at this time (Lumsden — unpublished observation) whereas during the secretory phase, contractions of longer duration and higher amplitude are seen. This pattern is also seen with gestagen administration (Bengtssen 1970). However, maximum activity is always seen when the steroid hormone levels drop at the onset of menstruation.

No consistent abnormality in steroid hormone production has been conclusively demonstrated in those with dysmenorrhoea. An unconfirmed study has demonstrated low urinary progesterone and oestradiol concentrations (Bell & Loraine 1976), although clinically, the presence of dysmenorrhoea is often used as an indicator of a well functioning ovulatory mechanism. Although progesterone appears necessary for its presence, a progesterone secreting IUCD which continuously releases small amounts of hormone is associated with relief of the problem (Troburgh & Guderian 1978).

The sensory nervous system

The uterus has features in common with cardiac muscle in that the adrenergic and cholinergic nerves supplying the uterus modify rather than initiate contractions. Total transection of the cord abolishes activity for a short time only (Shabanagh et al 1964) and lumbar sympathectomy, a well established method for treating dysmenorrhoea (Jacobs et al 1963, Ingersoll and Meigs 1948) does not appear to affect subsequent reproductive function. The sensory nerves of the uterus run with the autonomic nerves and cutting the latter may promote vasodilatation as well as interrupting the sensory supply. Some recent work has investigated the presence of short adrenergic neurones in the myometrium of the guinea pig (Sjoberg 1979). These nerves are destroyed during pregnancy and fail to regenerate to any extent. This is an interesting observation as primary dysmenorrhoea tends to be relieved by the birth of a child.

Psychological factors

When reading the literature, one often gets the impression that psychological and physical causes for dysmenorrhoea are mutually exclusive. A psychological cause alone for dysmenorrhoea would seem unlikely in view of the evidence already discussed. Also some very successful remedies are available and it seems unlikely that complex psychological problems (for review see Cox & Santerro 1981) would disappear by simply taking tablets. It is more likely that psychological factors modify the pain. A severe, recurring pain can easily cause depression and anxiety in a woman of any age particularly when it impairs performance. Surely any psychological problems must be present before the menarche and after the dysmenorrhoea is treated, although it is certainly true that in a minority of cases the 'supra-tentorial' element is most important.

Vasopressin

Vasopressin is a powerful stimulant of the non-pregnant uterus particularly at the onset of menstruation (Coutinho & Lopes 1968, Åkerlund & Anderssen 1976). It also causes a decrease in myometrial blood flow, both properties which might lead to pain. On day 1 of the menses, plasma concentrations of vasopressin are higher in those with dysmenorrhoea than those without (Åkerlund et al 1979), although it has been suggested that this increase is in response to the pain rather than its cause. However, levels are not decreased when the pain of dysmenorrhoea is relieved by prostaglandin synthetase inhibitors (Stromberg et al 1981) and the stimulatory effect of Vasopressin is now not thought to be mediated by prostaglandins (Stromberg et al 1983). Its possible mechanism of action has not as yet been clarified.

A POSSIBLE AETIOLOGY FOR DYSMENORRHOEA?

As with so many problems in medicine, it is possible that there is more than one cause for primary dysmenorrhoea. I have been considering a number of possible aetiologies for dysmenorrhoea, but it may be that they contribute by acting in some sort of sequence. If one looks at a nulliparous, teenage girl with regular ovulatory menstrual cycles, the concentration of $PGF_{2\alpha}$ in menstrual fluid is likely to be high (above 300 ng/ml fluid on day 1 of the menses), on the days of maximal pain (Fig. 18.3). It is possible that these high levels are produced by the degenerating mass of endometrium and the absorbed $PGF_{2\alpha}$ increases the myometrial contractility. $PGF_{2\alpha}$ is known to correlate with the work performed by the uterus (Lumsden et al 1983b) and also causes vasoconstriction. When infused into the uterus, $PGF_{2\alpha}$ increases activity (Fig. 18.2) in a dose-dependent fashion and the menstrual fluid concentrations tend to correlate with the severity of the pain (Fig. 18.4). These factors would worsen ischaemia and further increase PG production thus causing a viscious cycle. Although PGE_2 is present in menstrual fluid in high concentrations, it does not appear to be related to myometrial activity (Lumsden et al 1983b) but may act through another mechanism. But is there a role for PGI_2, the most potent vasodilator known? Intra uterine infusion tends to decrease activity and relieve pain although this is not due to blocking effect on $PGF_{2\alpha}$ receptors. Large doses (5 $\mu g/min$) are required but systemic effects are not noticed. It would thus seem that there may be a local vasodilatory effect within the uterus (Lumsden & Baird — in preparation).

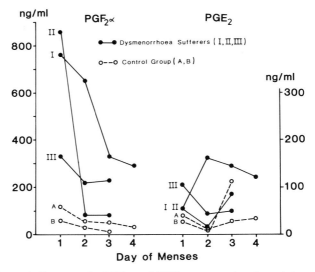

Fig. 18.3 This graph illustrates the $PGF_{2\alpha}$ and PGE_2 concentrations in ng/ml menstrual fluid of five subjects, three with dysmenorrhoea and two controls. Levels of $PGF_{2\alpha}$ consistently fall during the menses. PGE_2 declines between days 1 and 2 but then frequently rises between days 2 and 3. Prostaglandin concentration is therefore greatest on the days of maximum pain

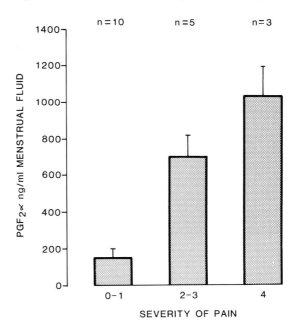

Fig. 18.4 $PGF_{2\alpha}$ tended to correlate with the severity of the pain on day 1 of the menses. The grading of the pain was 0 = no pain, 1 = mild pain, 2 = moderate, 3 = severe and 4 = very severe. One of the dysmenorrhoea group experienced unusually mild pain and the control group experienced mild pain at the worst

There is no evidence as yet to suggest that prostaglandins act as a link in a chain. However, the stimulatory effects of prostaglandins may be increased by increasing calcium transport across the cell membrane (Carsten 1973). Prostaglandins also affect the formation of cyclic AMP, the levels of which are increased in the oestrogen dominated rat uterus by PGI_2 and PGE_2 (Harbon 1982). An increase in cyclic AMP leads to relaxation of the muscle by altering phosphorylation of the myosin light chain as well as the uptake of calcium into the sarcoplasmic reticulum. It is therefore possible that PGs act either through other cell mediators or are themselves affected by diverse influences such as the adrenergic nervous system or posterior pituitary hormones (Hedqvist 1970, Clarke et al 1977). Prostaglandin cell surface receptors have been identified within myometrium (Wakeling & Wyngarden 1974, Bauknecht et al 1981) which may explain how prostaglandin production by endometrium could affect myometrium. The varied effects of the prostaglandins on myometrial contractility may be explained in terms of their effects on calcium or cyclic AMP. However, it will take much further work to elucidate finally the mechanism of action.

THE TREATMENT OF PRIMARY DYSMENORRHOEA

Diagnosis of primary dysmenorrhoea is usually made on history and examination alone and treatment instituted immediately. Medical treatments are normally tried as a first line although surgical treatments are available. Two effective methods are prostaglandin synthetase inhibitors and the oral contraceptive pill, the choice often depending on the contraceptive requirements of the patient in question or the presence of a contraindication to the use of a particular drug.

Prostaglandin synthetase inhibitors

It was only 10 years ago that non-steroidal anti-inflammatory agents (NSAIAs) were first suggested for the treatment of primary dysmenorrhoea (Schwartz 1974). Since then they have contributed greatly to our understanding of the aetiology and treatment of the problem. These drugs inhibit the synthesis of prostaglandins as well as having a direct analgesic effect and are successful in about 75% of patients with primary dysmenorrhoea (Dingfelder 1981). There are five groups of NSAIAs which depend on the acid from which they are derived. All groups are effective apart from the benzoic acid derivatives (aspirin). The reason for this is not known although it may be due to inadequate levels within the uterus itself.

The NSAIAs decrease the concentrations of PGs within menstrual fluid (Chan & Dawood 1980) although it has been recently suggested that with some drugs, e.g. Ibuprofen, $PGF_{2\alpha}$ may be preferentially affected (Chan et al 1983). They also decrease uterine contractility at the same time as providing pain relief (Lumström et al 1976, Smith & Powell 1982). It is unclear why only 75%

respond, although other aetiological mechanisms are a possibility. Side-effects with the NSAIAs include gastric irritation, central nervous system effects, allergic and blood disorders, although these are unusual when the drugs are taken on an intermittent basis as in dysmenorrhoea. However, gastric ulceration and a history of allergy to aspirin are contraindications to their use which should also be considered carefully in an asthma sufferer. It should be noted that Leukotrienes are also produced from arachidonic acid, the prostaglandin precursor and that the synthesis of these powerful smooth muscle stimulents (Sirois et al 1981) is unaffected by the NSAIAs. It is therefore possible that they play a role in some cases of dysmenorrhoea.

The oral contraceptive pill

This is successful in treating dysmenorrhoea most likely due to its inhibitory effect on ovulation. There is therefore no secretory phase rise in endometrial PG concentration and the volume of endometrium is also very small leading to low menstrual fluid levels (Chan & Dawood 1980) and decreased uterine activity (Hendricks 1966, Cibils 1967, Filler & Hall 1970). This group of drugs is very useful in those desiring contraception and may also be used in combination with a NSAIA if necessary.

Calcium antagonists

This group of drugs is useful if the above methods fail or are inappropriate. They inhibit both calcium influx into the cell as well as the release of intracellular stores. A dose of 30–80 mg daily of nifedepine will relieve pain and decrease uterine contractility (Anderssen & Ulmsten 1979) but side-effects are common. These include headache, hypotension, bradycardia and constipation although the extent of these side-effects depends on which drug is used. They are not widely prescribed in Great Britain although I have found a much lower dose of nifedepine (15–30 mg daily during the menses) is often effective with few side-effects.

B-receptor stimulants

The use of terbutaline to increase endometrial blood flow was mentioned earlier (Akerlund et al 1976). Other members of the group have been investigated (Hansan & Secher 1975, Nesheim & Walloe 1976) and are effective in relieving dysmenorrhoea. However, the incidence of unpleasant side-effects is so high that they have no use at the moment in clinical practice.

Progestogens

The 'progestasert' intra-uterine contraceptive device has been shown to relieve dysmenorrhoea and lower menstrual fluid prostaglandins (Troburgh &

Guderian 1978). However, they have little use in practice as they are associated with a very high risk of ectopic pregnancy.

THE SURGICAL TREATMENT OF PRIMARY DYSMENORRHOEA

Although cervical stenosis is not thought to be a contributory factor to primary dysmenorrhoea, dilatation and curettage of the uterus has been used as a treatment for many years. Its value is debatable particularly as adequate dilation may lead to future cervical incompetence. It may act by promoting blood flow or by the disruption of sensory nerves from the cervix. In general it is more often used in the investigation and treatment of secondary dysmenorrhoea.

The nerve supply to and from the uterus may be interrupted by pre-sacral neurectomy or division of the uterosacral ligaments. Advocates claim a very high success rate (Ingersoll & Meigs 1948, Jacobs et al 1963), but the complications of major abdominal surgery mean that these operations are now performed rarely.

PSYCHOTHERAPY

Psychotherapy is part of every treatment for dysmenorrhoea. All sufferers need reassurance and also to be taken seriously. Many teenage girls are grateful not to be told that they must live with it until they have a baby — an approach which is still remarkably prevalent. Professional psychiatric advice may be required on occasions although it is usually obvious when the underlying problem is psychological rather than organic.

It is very important that if conventional methods of treatment fail, e.g. a trial with an NSAIA and the oral contraceptive pill, that further investigations are performed such as laparoscopy. Although pelvic pathology is rare in young women, it does occur.

SECONDARY DYSMENORRHOEA

Dysmenorrhoea occurring as the result of disease (Table 18.3) is also a problem although much less is known about its aetiology as it is a less well defined entity than primary dysmenorrhoea. Frequently it affects an older age group and causes pain with different characteristics (Moos 1968, Chan 1972) although clinicians will often find exceptions to the rule. Secondary dysmenorrhoea is normally considered to be period-associated pain occurring in the presence of pathology, or pain which has its onset after regular menstruation has been established for some years. Pelvic examination is frequently abnormal due to the presence of pathology, e.g. uterine abnormality, chronic pelvic infection, endometriosis, uterine fibroids, cervical stenosis or adenomyosis. However, the final diagnosis is often made after laparoscopy or laparotomy.

Table 18.3 The causes of secondary dysmenorrhoea

Congenital abnormalities
    Congenital abnormalities of the uterus, e.g.
    1. redundant uterine horn
    2. imperforate hymen
    3. cryptomenorrhoea
Acquired uterine abnormalities
    Uterine fibroids
    Endometrial Polyps
    Adenomyosis
Infection
    Pelvic inflammatory disease
Foreign bodies
    Intra-uterine contraceptive device
Endometriosis
    Cervical stenosis following surgery, e.g. cone biopsy

The actual cause of the pain in many cases of secondary dysmenorrhoea is not clear. Studies on prostaglandin concentrations in pathological tissues are sparse. Willman & Collins (1976) demonstrated high prostaglandin levels in a variety of pathologies but this study was on small numbers and has not been repeated. Recently in Edinburgh, in work as yet unpublished, we demonstrated that tissue collected from uteri affected with adenomyosis contain greater concentrations of prostaglandins than uteri with normal histology. Dysmenorrhoea was present in over 60% of these women and it may be that prostaglandins are involved in a final common pathway. Also, if endometriosis is induced in rabbits then the peritoneal fluid contains elevated levels of $PGF_{2\alpha}$ (Schenken & Asch 1980). However, this only occurs if haemorrhage is present (Sondheimer & Flikinger 1982). Thus, apart from cervical stenosis where the cause is obvious, the exact aetiology in other types of pathology is unknown. It is possible that the presence of uterine abnormalities, e.g. adenomyomas or fibroids lead to irregularities of uterine contractility resulting in pain. However, the role of prostaglandins in secondary dysmenorrhoea is disputed by the fact that the NSAIAs are not generally effective.

Treatment is aimed at the cause rather than the symptom and reference should be made to standard gynaecological texts, the type of treatment often depending on the severity, age and parity of the patient.

There is thus the need for much further research to establish why the same symptom should occur with such diverse pathologies.

CONCLUSION

Much is now known about the aetiology of primary dysmenorrhoea, a problem which can be successfully solved for millions of women. Although prostaglandins are almost certainly involved, their mechanism of action has yet to be finally elucidated. In fact, the control of myometrial contractility in general is a fascinating subject, the surface of which has barely been scratched.

The measurement of myometrial blood flow *in vivo* would contribute much useful information and may be possible with the development of sophisticated ultrasound techniques. Also the role of lipoxygenase products requires investigation. It is hoped that by studying menstrual problems that we may learn more about the control of normal menstruation and also develop more treatments for their relief.

REFERENCES

Abel M H, Baird D T 1980 The effect of 17β estradiol and progesterone on prostaglandin production by human endometrium maintained in organ culture. Endocrinology 106: 1599–1606

Abel M H, Kelly R W 1979 Differential production of prostaglandins within the human uterus. Prostaglandins 18: 821–828

Akerlund M 1979 Pathophysiology of dysmenorrhoea. Acta Obstetrica Gynecologica Scandinavica 87: 27–32

Akerlund M, Anderssen K E 1976 Vasopressin response and terbutaline inhibition of the uterus. Obstetrics and Gynaecology 48: 528–536

Akerlund M, Anderssen K, Ingemarssen I 1976 Effects of terbutaline on myometrial activity, uterine blood flow and lower abdominal pain in women with primary dysmenorrhoea. British Journal of Obstetrics and Gynaecology 83: 673–678

Akerlund M, Stromberg P, Forsling M L 1979 Primary dysmenorrhoea and vasopressin. British Journal of Obstetrics and Gynaecology 86: 484–487

Andersch B, Milsom I 1982 An epidemiologic study of young women with dysmenorrhoea Am J Obstet Gynecol 144: 655–660

Anderson A 1981 The role of prostaglandin synthetase inhibitors in gynaecology. The Practitioner 225: 1460–1470

Anderssen K E, Ulmsten U 1978 Effects of Nifedepine on myometrial activity and lower abdominal pain in women with primary dysmenorrhoea. British Journal of Obstetrics and Gynaecology 85: 142–148

Asplund J 1952 The uterine cervix and isthmus under normal and pathological conditions. Acta Radiologica (Suppl) 91: 1–76

Bauknecht T, Krane B, Rechenbaeh U, Zahradnik H P 1981 Distribution of prostaglandin E_2 and prostaglandin $F_{2\alpha}$ receptors in human myometrium. Acta Endocrinologica 98: 446–450

Bell E T, Loraine J A 1966 Hormone excretion patterns in patients with dysmenorrhoea. Lancet ii: 519–521

Bengtsson L P 1970 Studies on the effect of gestagen on myometrial in vivo activity in non-pregnant women. Acta Obstetrica Gynecologica Scandinavica (Suppl) 49: 5–12

Bengtsson L, Theobald G W 1966 The effect of oestrogens and gestagen on the non-pregnant human uterus. British Journal of Obstetrics and Gynaecology 73: 273–281

Bygdeman M 1964 The effect of different prostaglandins on the human myometrium in vitro. Acta Physiologica Scandinavica 242: 1 (Suppl) 63

Carsten M W 1973 Prostaglandins and cellular calcium transport in the pregnant human uterus. American Journal of Obstetrics and Gynecology 117: 824–832

Chan D P C 1972 Differential diagnosis of dysmenorrhoea. Medical Journal of Australia 2: 321

Chan W Y, Yusoff Dawood M 1980 Prostaglandin levels in menstrual fluid of non-dysmenorrheic and of dysmenorrheic subjects with and without oral contraceptive or Ibuprofen therapy. Advances in Prostaglandin and Thromboxane Research 8: 1443–1447

Chan W Y, Hill J C 1978 Determination of menstrual prostaglandin levels in non-dysmenorrheic and dysmenorrheic subjects. Prostaglandins 15: 365–375

Chan W Y, Fuchs F, Powell A M 1983 Prostaglandins in primary dysmenorrhoea and the effects of naproxen sodium and ibuprofen in dysmenorrheic therapy. Abstract No. 18 International Symposium on Premenstrual Tension and Dysmenorrhoea, Kiawah Island, USA

Cibils L A 1967 Contractility of the non-pregnant human uterus. Obstetrics and Gynaecology 30: 441–461

Clarke K E, Farley D B, Van Orden D E, Brody M J 1977 Role of endogenous prostaglandins in regulation of uterine blood flow and adrenergic neurotrammission. American Journal of Obstetrics and Gynecology 127: 455–461

Coutinho E M, Lopes A C V 1968 Response of the non-pregnant uterus to vasopressin as an index of ovarian function. American Journal of Obstetrics and Gynecology 102: 479–489

Cox D J, Santirocco L L, 1981 Psychological and behavioral factors in dysmenorrhoea. In: Dawood M Y (ed) Dysmenorrhoea, p. 75–93. Williams and Wilkins, Baltimore

Csapo A, Sauvage V 1968 The evolution of uterine activity during human pregnancy. Acta Obstetrica Gynaecologica Scandinavica 47: 181–212

Csapo A, Pulkkinen M O, Henzl M R 1977 The effect of naproxen sodium on the intrauterine pressure and menstrual pain of dysmenorrheic patients. Prostaglandins 13: 193–199

Dingfelder J R 1981 Primary dysmenorrhoea treatment with prostaglandin inhibitors: a review. American Journal of Obstetrics and Gynecology. 140: 874–879

Downie J, Poyser N L, Wunderlich M 1974 Levels of prostaglandins in human endometrium during the normal menstrual cycle. Journal of Physiology 236: 465–472

Downing S J, Lye S, Bradshaw J M, Porter D G 1978 Rat myometrial activity in vivo; effects of oestadiol — 17β and progesterone in relation to the concentration of cytoplasmic progesterone receptors. Journal of Endocrinology 78: 103–117

Filler W, Hall W 1970 Dysmenorrhoea and its therapy: a uterine contractility study. American Journal of Obstetrics and Gynecology 106: 104–109

Halbert D R, Demers L M, Fontana V, Jones D 1975 Prostaglandin levels in patients with dysmenorrhoea before and after indomethacin therapy. Prostaglandins 10: 1047–1056

Hansen M K, Secher N J 1975 Beta-receptor stimulation in essential dysmenorrhoea. American Journal of Obstetrics and Gynecology 121: 566

Harbon S 1982 Modulation of cAMP content of the rat myometrium β adrenergic and PGE_2 stimulation and desensitization. Contribution to the VIth F.R.E.S.E.R.H. International Symposium on Uterine Contractility. Brussels

Hedqvist L, Stajarne, Wennmalm A 1970 Inhibition by prostaglandin E_2 of sympathetic neurotransmission in the rabbit heart. Acta Physiologica Scandinavica 79: 139–141

Hendricks C H 1966 Inherant motility patterns and response characteristics in the non-pregnant human uterus. American Journal of Obstetrics and Gynecology 96: 824–843

Ingersoll F M, Meigs J W 1948 Presacral neurectomy for dysmenorrhoea. New England Journal of Medicine 238: 357

Jacobs W M, Conner J S, Rogers S F 1963 Presacral neurectomy. American Journal of Obstetrics and Gynecology 85: 437

Karim S M, Hillier K, Somers K, Trussel R R 1971 The effects of prostaglandins E_2 and $F_{2\alpha}$ administered by different routes on uterine activity and the cardiovascular system in pregnant and non-pregnant women. Journal of Obstetrics and Gynaecology of the British Commonwealth 78: 172–179

Kenedi R M 1981 Human body biomechanics. In: A Textbook of Biomedical Engineering, p. 22. Blackie, Glasgow

Lumsden M A, Baird D T (In press) Intrauterine pressure changes in primary dysmenorrhoea. Acta Obstetrica and Gynaecologica Scandinavica

Lumsden M A, Kelly R W, Baird D T 1983a Primary Dysmenorrhoea: the importance of both prostaglandins E_2 and $F_{2\alpha}$. British Journal of Obstetrics and Gynecology 90: 1135–1140

Lumsden M A, Kelly R W, Baird D T 1983b Is prostaglandin $F_{2\alpha}$ involved in the increased myometrial contractility of primary dysmenorrhoea? Prostaglandins 25: 683–692

Lumsden M A, Kelly R W, Abel M H, Baird D T 1983c The possible role of prostaglandins in the menstrual abnormalities associated with adenomyosis (In preparation)

Lundstrom V 1977 The myometrial response of intrauterine administration of $PGF_{2\alpha}$ and PGE_2 in dysmenorrheic women. Acta Obstetrica and Gynaecologica Scandinavica 56: 167–172

Lundstrom V, Green K, Wiqvist N 1976 Prostaglandins, indomethacin and dysmenorrhoea. Prostaglandins 11: 893–904

Lye S R, Challis J R 1982 Inhibition by prostacyclins of myometrial activity in vivo in non-pregnant ovariectomised sheep. Journal of Reproduction and Fertility 66: 311–315

Maathius J B, Kelly R W 1978 Concentrations of prostaglandins $F_{2\alpha}$ and E_2 in the endometrium throughout the human menstrual cycle, after the administration of clomiphene or an oestrogen-progestergen pill and in early pregnancy. Journal of Endocrinology 77: 362–371

Martin J N, Bygdeman M 1975 The effect of locally administered PGE_2 on the contractility of the non-pregnant human uterus in vivo. Prostaglandins 10: 258–265

Moos R H 1968 The development of a menstrual distress questionnaire. Psychosomatic Medicine 30: 853

Nesheim B I, Walloe L 1976 The use of isoxsuprine in essential dysmenorrhoea. A controlled clinical study. Acta Obstetrica and Gynaecologica Scandinavica 55: 315

Novac E, Reynolds B R 1932 The cause of primary dysmenorrhoea with special reference to hormonal factors. Journal of the American Medical Association 99: 1466–1472

Omini C, Pasargiklian R, Folco G C, Funo M, Berts F 1978 Pharmacological activity of PGI_2 and its metabolite 6-oxo-$PGF_{1\alpha}$ on human uterus and fallopian tubes. Prostaglandins 15: 1045–1054

Pickles V R, Hall W J, Best F A, Smith G N 1965 Prostaglandins in endometrium and menstrual fluid from normal and dysmenorrheic subjects. British Journal of Obstetrics and Gynaecology 72: 185–192

Pulkkinen M O, Csapo A I 1978 The effect of ibuprofen on the intrauterine pressure and menstrual pain of dysmenorrheic patients. Prostaglandins 15: 1055–1062

Richards D H 1979 A general practice view of functional disorders associated with menstruation. Research and Clinical Forums 1: 39–45

Schenken R S, Asch R H 1980 Surgical induction of endometriosis in the rabbit: effects on fertility and concentrations of peritoneal fluid prostaglandins. Fertility and Sterility 34: 581–587

Schwartz A, Zor U, Lindner H R, Naor S 1974 Primary dysmenorrhoea. Alleviation by an inhibition of prostaglandin synthesis and action. Obstetrics and Gynaecology 44: 709–712

Shabanah E H, Toth A, Maughan G B 1964 The role of the autonomic nervous system in uterine contractility and blood flow: the interaction between neurohormones and sex hormones in the intact and isolated uterus. American Journal of Obstetrics and Gynecology 89: 841–859

Singh E J, Baccarini I M, Zuspan F P 1975 Levels of prostaglandins $F_{2\alpha}$ and E_2 in human endometrium during menstrual cycle. American Journal of Obstetrics and Gynecology 121: 1003–1006

Sirois P, Borgeat P, Jeanson A 1981 Comparative effects of leukotriene B_2, prostaglandins I_2 and E_2, 6-oxo-$PGF_{1\alpha}$, thromboxane B_2 and histamine on selected smooth muscle preparations. Journal of Pharmacy and Pharmacology 33: 466

Sjoberg N O 1979 Dysmenorrhoea and uterine neurotransmitters. Acta Obstetrica and Gynaecologica Scandinavica 87 (Suppl): 57–59

Smith R, Powell J 1982 Intrauterine pressure changes during dysmenorrhoea therapy. American Journal of Obstetrics and Gynecology 143: 286–289

Smith S K, Abel M H, Kelly R W, Baird D T 1981 Prostaglandin synthesis in the endometrium of women with ovular dysfunctional uterine bleeding. British Journal of Obstetrics and Gynaecology 88: 434–442

Sondheimer S J, Flickinger G 1982 Prostaglandin $F_{2\alpha}$ in the peritoneal fluid of patients with endometriosis. International Journal of Fertility 27: 73–75

Stromberg P, Forsling M L, Kindehl H 1983 Involvement of prostaglandins in vasopressin stimulation of the uterus. British Journal of Obstetrics and Gynaecology 90: 332–337

Trobough G, Guderian A 1978 The effect of exogenous intrauterine progesterone on the amount of $PGF_{2\alpha}$ content of menstrual blood in dysmenorrheic women. Journal of Reproductive Medicine 21: 153–158

Wakeling A E, Wyngarden L J 1974 Prostaglandin receptors in the human, monkey and hampster uterus. Endocrinology 95: 55–64

Widholm O 1979 Dysmenorrhoea during adolescence. Acta Obstetrica and Gynaecologica Scandinavica 87 (Suppl): 61–66

Wilhelmsson L 1981 Biological actions of prostaglandins on different tissues within the non-pregnant human uterus. MD Thesis, Goteberg, p. 10

Wilhelmsson L, Wikland M, Wiqvist N 1981 PGH_2, PXA_2 and PGI_2 have potent and differentiated actions on human uterine contractility. Prostaglandins 21: 227–286

Willman E A, Collins W P, Clayton S G 1976 Studies in the involvement of prostaglandins in uterine symptomatology and pathology. British Journal of Obstetrics and Gynaecology 83: 337–341

Wilson L, Kurzrok R 1940 Uterine contractility in functional dysmenorrhoea. Endocrinology 27: 23–28

Woodbury R A, Torpin R, Child G P, Watson H, Jarber M 1947 Physiology and its relation to pelvic pain. Journal of the American Medical Association 134: 1081–1085

Menorrhagia

INTRODUCTION

A change in the volume or pattern of menstrual bleeding is one of the commonest causes of concern for health in women. This concern is heightened not only by the many myths and taboos which surround the subject of menstruation (Snow & Johnson 1977) but also by the well orchestrated campaigns for the early detection of gynaecological malignancy.

This anxiety with abnormal menstruation is especially a problem of the 20th century. Previously late menarche, early menopause and prolonged periods of childbearing and lactational amenorrhoea reduced the number of menses experienced by women in their lifetime. The reduction of family size, by the widespread use of contraception and sterilisation has resulted in an approximately tenfold increase in the number of periods that women experience during their reproductive life (Short 1976). Although initially restricted to the Western World, this demographic change in the pattern of family life is now well established in Third World countries (Kendall 1979).

There is little doubt that women find menstruation a source of discomfort and inconvenience, and this view is aggravated by the changing role of women within society in which a more active role in occupations outside of the household is being pursued. Modern contraceptive practices and the widespread use of sterilisation further add to the problem as many women will not have experienced a spontaneous ovulatory menstrual cycle for around 10 years prior to and during their childbearing years.

The controversy about the effect of sterilisation on menorrhagia remains unanswered as a large prospective, objective long-term study on menstrual loss before and after this procedure is still awaited. However, Kasonde & Bonnar (1976) showed that there was no change in menstrual blood loss (MBL) in 15 women at 6 months and 10 women at 12 months following sterilisation.

WHAT IS MENORRHAGIA?

Before considering the mechanisms of menstruation and the possible ways in which they can be manipulated it is important to have a clear view as to the parameters of normal menstrual blood loss (MBL).

Many methods have been used to measure MBL but the presently preferred technique involves the determination of the concentration of haemoglobin in menstrual fluid by its conversion to alkaline haematin (Hallberg et al 1966, Newton et al 1977). Most studies refer to small numbers of selected patients but two large scale population studies undertaken with 476 women in Gothenberg (Hallberg et al 1966) and 348 women in Northumberland (Cole et al 1971) remain the basis for the characterisation of normal MBL (see Fig. 19.1).

The distribution of menstrual blood loss is positively skewed, the mean and median MBL, being 43 and 30 ml (Hallberg et al 1966) and 38 and 28 ml (Cole et al 1971) respectively. In the former study the skewness was significantly reduced by the exclusion of women who complained of abnormal menstruation or those who had abnormal haematological parameters. One hundred and eighty three women remained in this normal group and the average MBL was 33 ml. The 95th centile for MBL was found to be 76.4 ml.

Another way of determining an upper limit of normal for MBL is to relate the menstrual loss to various haematological indices. Excessive menstrual bleeding is the commonest cause of iron deficiency anaemia in the United Kingdom (for a review see Cohen & Gibor 1980), affecting 20–25% of the fertile female population (Rybo 1966a, Kilpatrick 1979) and 1.6 million women will have either iron storage deficiency or actual anaemia (Fairhurst et al 1977). It can be calculated that on a normal Western diet a state of negative iron balance will arise if the MBL exceeds about 50–60 ml per month (Rybo 1966a, Smith 1982) and indeed 67% of women whose loss is greater than 80 ml have actual anaemia (Hallberg et al 1966).

On the basis of these findings the upper limit of normal for MBL appears to lie between 60 and 80 ml and losses in excess of 80 ml can be considered pathological.

MECHANISMS OF MENSTRUATION

Changes in the volume or pattern of menstrual blood loss may arise because of local factors such as endometrial polyps, fibroids, malignancy, infection or pregnancy and rarely systemic factors such as bleeding disorders. In the majority of patients no obvious pathology can be found at dilatation and curettage (D & C) (Mackenzie & Bibby 1978) and these cases are described as dysfunctional uterine bleeding (Novak & Woodruff 1974) or 'essential menorrhagia'. As treatment of the preceding disorders is usually self-evident and because the latter group constitute the majority of cases, discussion in this chapter will be restricted to this topic.

Knowledge of the mechanisms which initiate and control menstrual bleeding are central to our understanding of the pathology of excessive menstrual blood loss. Unfortunately this understanding is still unclear but four principal factors have been identified which appear to be involved in the mechanism of menstruation.

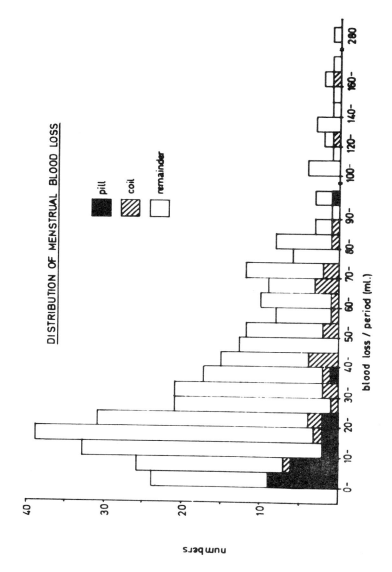

Fig. 19.1 Distribution of menstrual blood loss in a population of 348 women (from Cole et al 1971)

Vascular theory

The most celebrated work on the changes of the vasculature in the endometrium at the time of menstruation is that of Markee (1940), whose studies done almost 50 years ago remain the basis of the vascular theory of menstruation. Much emphasis has been placed on the significance of the spiralling of the end-arterioles which supply the endometrium, as these changes only occur in species such as man, anthropoid apes, and platyrrhine and catarrhyne monkeys which have regular menstrual bleeding. However, probably of more importance was the observation that bleeding was always preceded by vasoconstriction of the spiral arterioles which resulted in local ischaemia. Seventy per cent of the subsequent bleeding arose from transient vasodilatation of the same vessels. A much smaller volume of bleeding arose from ruptured venules and capillaries.

Haemostasis

If menstrual blood was to clot as peripheral blood then man would be at a grave evolutionary disadvantage as menarche would result in extensive formation of intra-uterine adhesions and infertility. Haemostatic plug formation is the primary mechanism controlling bleeding from transected vessels in the body and this is achieved by the deposition of a platelet plug which is reinforced by fibrin (Sixma & Wester 1977). One of the fascinating aspects of menstruation is that menstrual blood does not clot (Scommegna et al 1980) and the endometrium has a high fibrinolytic activity (Albrechtsen 1956). Menstrual blood contains platelets which fail to aggregate in response to pro-aggregatory agents such as ADP and collagen (Rees et al 1983), contains no fibrinogen and reduced amounts of coagulation factors compared to peripheral blood (Hahn 1980). It does contain fibrin (Sheppard et al 1983) and fibrin degradation products confirming the potent fibrinolytic activity within the uterus. This fibrinolytic activity is enhanced in women with dysfunctional uterine bleeding (Bonnar et al 1983).

Christiaens et al (1980) found a reduced formation of haemostatic plugs in endometrium obtained within 20 hours of the onset of menstruation. Normally these plugs would be situated both in and outside of the ruptured vessel like a mushroom but in the endometrial vessels they are situated only within the vessel. After the first 24 hours of bleeding there is complete absence of these plugs and the vessels are found to be gaping but not bleeding or constricted.

Lysosomal theory

Lysosomes are intra-cellular granules that contain large numbers of enzymes which initiate cellular digestion, hydrolise the ground substance of the endometrium and promote the degradation of collagen fibres (for a review see Shaw & Roche 1980). Lysosomes increase in endometrium in the luteal phase

(Wood 1973). It is suggested that the release of autolytic enzymes on withdrawal of the ovarian steroids, promotes the regression of the endometrium in the premenstrual period (Henzl et al 1972). Phospholipase A_2, an enzyme important in prostaglandin synthesis, is present in lysosomes and its significance will be discussed later.

Tissue regeneration

Regeneration of the endometrium begins within 48 hours of the onset of menstrual bleeding (Ferenczy 1976, Nogales-Ortiz et al 1978). As most bleeding occurs in the first 3 days of menses (Haynes et al 1977) it is difficult to see how such a process would stop arteriolar bleeding although prolonged menses may be influenced by the effects of regeneration. It is most likely that all of these mechanisms are involved in the process of menstruation but it remains unclear which is the local trigger which begins menstrual bleeding and the relative importance of each of these mechanisms in controlling the bleeding once it has begun.

THE ENDOCRINOLOGICAL BASIS OF MENORRHAGIA

Ovulatory menorrhagia

It has long been asserted that the majority of cases of menorrhagia are associated with anovulatory menstrual cycles but detailed analyses of large numbers of patients with objectively assessed MBL have not been done. Haynes et al (1979) found no difference in the levels of FSH, LH, 17β-oestradiol or progesterone throughout the cycle of 27 women with a heavy menstrual loss (i.e. >80 ml) compared to 13 women with a light loss (i.e. <80 ml). Furthermore 50–80% of histological specimens obtained at dilatation and curettage of women complaining of menorrhagia show no abnormality (Smith 1982). In the presence of regular menstrual cycles, even in the perimenopausal years, there is a high incidence of ovulatory menstrual cycles (Metcalf 1979). Eighty and 78% of women aged 40 to 44 and 45 to 49 respectively had three consecutive ovulatory cycles and the incidence of ovulatory cycles in 139 women aged 40 to 55 where menstrual length was between 21 to 35 days was 93%.

It is, therefore, likely that most menstrual bleeding occurs because of the withdrawal of progesterone support from an endometrium primed by 17β-oestradiol and this applies to both heavy and light menstrual blood loss. A crude distinction between ovulatory and anovulatory menstrual cycles may be misleading. Menstruation is only part of the reproductive cycle, its function being to prepare the endometrium for the implantation of the ovum in the next cycle. Subtle changes of progesterone synthesis and/or its action on the endometrium have been implicated in the aetiology of infertility (Jones 1976, DiZerega & Hodgen 1981). Similarly, the onset of menstrual bleeding occurs in the presence of a wide variability of plasma levels of progesterone (Godfrey et al 1979). In cycles of normal overall length but with a short luteal phase, for example, menstruation arises in the presence of higher levels of progesterone than in cycles of normal luteal phase length (Smith et al 1984a) and these cycles are not restricted to the infertile population (Smith et al 1984b). Abnormalities of the luteal phase have been implicated in between 15 and 25% of cases of ovulatory menorrhagia on the grounds of irregular shedding or under-development of the endometrium on histological examination (Holstrom & McLennan 1947, Murthy et al 1970).

Further work is required to define more clearly the hormone profiles of these cycles and to determine the relationship between peripheral levels of steroid and their action on the uterus.

Anovulatory menorrhagia

The increased variability of menstrual cycle length at the two extremes of reproductive life (Treloar et al 1967, Vollman 1977) are due in part to an increased number of anovulatory cycles (Doring 1969). Only 62% of women aged between 20 and 24 years ovulated consecutively over 3 months compared to 91% of women aged over 30 years (Metcalf & Mackenzie 1980). In the early years, failure of ovulation appears to be due to an absence or impairment of the positive feedback mechanisms of oestrogen (Van Look et al 1978). In the perimenopausal years when the classical condition of cystic glandular hyperplasia is found most commonly (Fraser & Baird 1972), inadequate follicular development in the presence of raised FSH and LH levels seems to be the cause of the anovulation (Van Look et al 1977, Sexton et al 1981).

As most cases of menorrhagia arise in the absence of gross ovarian dysfunction, the search for local agents in the uterus which may influence menstrual bleeding has been increased.

PROSTAGLANDINS AND MENSTRUATION

There are several factors which point to the involvement of prostaglandins in the mechanism of menstruation. They are present in high concentration in endometrium and myometrium (Ramwell et al 1980), they have actions on vascular smooth muscle which are consistent with a role in menstruation (Armstrong et al 1980), their synthesis by endometrium is fundamentally dependent on ovarian steroids (Abel & Baird 1980, Smith et al 1984c), instillation of prostaglandins into the uterine cavity reduces endometrial blood flow in the rhesus monkey (Einer-Jenson 1973) and induces bleeding in the human (Wiquist et al 1971, Toppozada et al 1980) and as will be described, inhibition of their synthesis reduces menstrual blood loss (Anderson et al 1976, Fraser et al 1981).

Prostaglandins are not stored in tissues but result from the rapid metabolism of a precursor, arachidonic acid (Bito 1975). This substance is stored with membrane-bound phospholipids and the rate limiting step in the synthesis of prostaglandins is the release of free arachidonic acid from these stores, a reaction catalysed by phospholipase enzymes which are present in high concentration in lysosomes.

Prostaglandins and normal menstruation

During the luteal phase of the cycle, the capacity of endometrium to synthesise prostaglandins is increased by accumulation of endogenous precursor and by a raised activity of the enzymes which convert the arachidonic acid precursor to the primary prostaglandins (Baird et al 1982). In the presence of high levels of progesterone minimal amounts of prostaglandins are released but with the withdrawal of 17β-oestradiol and progesterone during regression of the corpus luteum, the full potential of the tissue to synthesise prostaglandins becomes apparent. The principal prostaglandin synthesised by secretory endometrium taken from women with a normal volume of MBL is $PGF_{2\alpha}$, followed by PGE_2 and PGD_2 (Smith et al 1981a) (see Fig. 19.2). Prostacyclin, released by endothelial cells and a potent anti-aggregator of platelets is synthesised more readily in the myometrium but this synthesis is enhanced by endometrium (Abel & Kelly 1979).

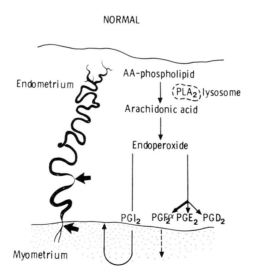

Fig. 19.2 Schematic representation of the possible events occurring in the endometrium on withdrawal of progesterone from a 17β-oestradiol primed endometrium. Arachidonic Acid (AA) stored in the phospholipids is released by the action of phospholipase (PLA_2). Free arachidonic acid is metabolised to various prostaglandins of which $PGF_{2\alpha}$ is the principal one. This prostaglandin may induce vasoconstriction of the spiral arterioles whilst prostacyclin (PGI_2) inhibits platelet aggregation

Prostaglandins and abnormal menstruation

The relative ability of endometrium to synthesise different prostaglandins could be important as some, for example $PGF_{2\alpha}$ may promote vasoconstriction whilst others, for example prostacyclin, PGE_2 and PGD_2 induce vasodilatation and have potent actions on platelet aggregation (Armstrong et al 1978).

Secretory endometrium taken from women with heavy periods in the presence of added precursor has a greater capacity to synthesise PGE_2 and PGD_2 at the expense of $PGF_{2\alpha}$ than endometrium taken from women with light periods (Smith et al 1981a), and may also enhance the synthesis of prostacyclin from the myometrium (Smith et al 1981b). This differential activity of the endometrium seems to arise from an increased availability of precursor (Kelly 1984, personal communication) (see Fig. 19.3).

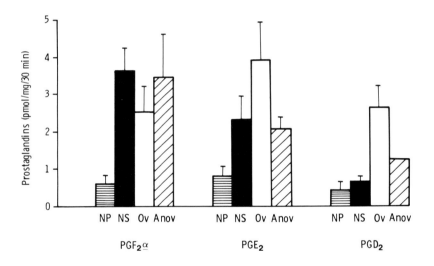

Fig. 19.3 Amounts of prostaglandins synthesised by endometrium in vitro in the presence of added arachidonic acid. Values given are the mean and standard error of the mean. NP = normal proliferative; NS = normal secretory; n = 6 and 15 respectively, measured menstrual blood loss <50 ml; Ov = ovulatory dysfunctional uterine bleeding, i.e. secretory endometrium; n = 14, MBL >50 ml; Anov = anovulatory dysfunctional uterine bleeding n = 11, MBL >50 ml

In anovulatory menstrual cycles characterised by heavy MBL the endometrium lacks the ability to synthesise $PGF_{2\alpha}$ probably as a consequence of the reduced availability of precursor (Smith et al 1982). This finding may explain the clinical observation that menses which follow an anovulatory cycle are usually painless, as persistent proliferative endometrium lacks the ability to synthesise $PGF_{2\alpha}$ which is found in high levels in menstrual fluid of women with dysmenorrhoea (Lumsden et al 1983).

ALTERED HAEMOSTASIS AND MENSTRUATION

Menstrual blood contains fibrin and fibrin degradation products, low levels of coagulation factors and platelets and no fibrinogen, all indicating potent fibrinolytic activity in the endometrial cavity.

Fibrinolytic activity in utero is greatly increased in women with menorrhagia (Bonnar et al 1983) probably as a consequence of raised levels of plasminogen activator which is derived from the endometrium (Rybo 1966b).

The actual mechanisms by which the prostaglandins influence vascular and haemostatic mechanisms remain unclear, but are likely to be central to the understanding of the mechanisms of menstruation.

TREATMENT

Diagnosis

As outlined previously, excessive menstrual bleeding may arise in the presence of pregnancy, local infection and as a consequence of gynaecological malignancy. These causes must, of course, be excluded before a diagnosis of dysfunctional uterine bleeding can be made, and this is usually achieved with the aid of a dilatation and curettage.

Dilatation and curettage

Dilatation of the cervix and curettage of the uterine cavity (D & C) should be considered as a diagnostic not a therapeutic procedure. Occasionally removal of an endometrial polyp may alleviate heavy bleeding but polyps are only found in about 2% of cases (Mackenzie et al 1978). Menstrual blood loss after D & C is reduced in the first post-operative cycle (Haynes et al 1977) and patients should be seen 2–3 months after the operation to reassess their MBL. The usual rationale for the procedure is to exclude the presence of malignancy. However, this is a rare event in women before the menopause, Mackenzie et al (1978) failing to demonstrate a single case in 624 women who complained of menstrual disturbance. The overall rate of detection of endometrial carcinoma for D & C lies between 0.7 and 6.5% (Carey 1968, Mackenzie et al 1978). In the latter study all cases of carcinoma were found in women with post-menopausal bleeding and it was calculated that the predicted frequency of endometrial carcinoma in women below the age of 36 was 1/100 000 per year.

Grimes (1982) has reviewed the reported efficacy and associated complications between D & C and out-patient Vabra aspiration in five large case studies undertaken between 1958 and 1979 which included 13 598 D & C and 5 851 Vabra procedures (Table 19.1). Infection, haemorrhage and perforation were more common in D & Cs than when undertaking Vabra aspiration. Even allowing for cases of failed Vabra aspiration the efficiency of diagnosis with the Vabra was compatible with the D & C. In the light of these findings and the very low incidence of carcinoma in young women, Vabra

Table 19.1 Events per 1000 procedures

	D & C	Vabra
Haemorrhage	4	0
Infection	3–5	0–4
Perforation	6–13	0–4
Major Operation	0.3–5	0
Adequacy	0.77–0.94	0.85–0.99
Polyps	Unknown	0.80
Carcinoma	Unknown	0.96

Taken from Grimes (1982)

aspiration has been suggested as the preferred technique for investigation of menstrual disturbance in women below the age of 40 (Grimes 1982).

Medical treatment

Non-steroidal ani-inflammatory drugs (NSAID)

NSAIDs act by inhibiting the cyclo-oxygenase enzyme which is situated in the microsomal fraction of the cell. This reduces the availability of endoperoxide for subsequent conversion to other prostaglandins. It should be remembered that different NSAIDs give different responses not only in the degree of enzyme inhibition but also with respect to different organs (Flower & Vane 1974). Ibuprofen, for example, reduces $PGF_{2\alpha}$ release from the uterus to a greater degree than PGE, whereas Naproxen suppresses both equally (Chan 1983).

Clinical experience. Anderson et al (1976) gave mefenamic acid to five women and flufenamic acid to one woman with menorrhagia and demonstrated a mean reduction of MBL from 119±10 ml to 60 ± 7 ml. Fraser et al (1981) studied the effect of mefenamic acid 500 mg three times daily on 69 women with menorrhagia. There was a 28% reduction of mean MBL and 78% of the women had a reduction of MBL. The largest reduction occurred in women with the heavier losses and there was no reduction of loss in 14 women whose pre-treatment MBL was below 35 ml. In one case the MBL increased from 33 to 115 ml whilst on treatment. The duration of the loss was reduced in this study although this was not the case in the presence of an IUCD (Guillebaud et al 1979).

Naproxen also reduces MBL (Rybo et al 1981) but this probably does not occur with acetylsalicylic acid or paracetamol (Petrusson et al 1977).

The advantage of the use of these agents is that they are only taken at the time of menstruation. Side-effects with longer term use may include nausea, vomiting, dyspepsia, diarrhoea, headache, skin rashes and very rarely auto-haemolytic anaemia (Prescott 1975).

Danazol

The mode of action of danazol in reducing MBL is unclear. The effect of danazol on menstrual pattern is dose-related. At 400 mg and above more than 80% of patients are amenorrhoeic, but at 200 mg daily the picture is less clear. Young & Blackmore (1977) demonstrated amenorrhoea in 45% of women after 2 months treatment but Chimbira et al (1980) using a similar dose found that 15 of 18 women retained regular menstruation during 3 months therapy. At doses 200–800 mg danazol blunts or prevents the mid-cycle surge of FSH and LH (Greenblatt et al 1971) and van Dijk et al (1979) demonstrated anovulation in 21/21 patients receiving 200 mg a day of danazol.

In this latter study, 12 women were oligomenorrhoeic, six amenorrhoeic and three had regular cycles. Danazol induces atrophy of the endometrium and this may involve not only a systemic effect but also a local one, as danazol competes for 17β-oestradiol and progesterone receptor sites in the uterus (Jenkin 1980).

These systemic and local effects would be expected to inhibit prostaglandin synthesis but a direct effect on haematological parameters seems unlikely (Chimbira et al 1979). It is not clear how the induction of atrophy of the endometrium induces a reduction of MBL.

Clinical experience. Chimbira et al (1980) gave 200 mg of danazol daily to 18 patients over a 3 month period. The mean pre-treatment MBL over two cycles was 183 ± 25 ml. There was a slight reduction of MBL during the first treatment cycle but this reached statistical significance by the second (38 ± 11 ml) and third treatment cycles (26 ± 9 ml). Menstrual loss did not return to pre-treatment levels until the third month after treatment. The average duration of menstrual bleeding was reduced from 7 to 5 days. Danazol at a dose of 100 mg also reduced MBL but resulted in an increased incidence of irregular menstrual bleeding. No effect on MBL was found when treatment was given in either the follicular or luteal phase of the cycle alone.

The disadvantage of this treatment is that it requires daily medication. Side-effects include acne, fluid retention, weight gain (mean increase 2.3 kg), mild hirsutism, skin rashes and muscle cramps.

Anti-fibrinolytic agents

Anti-fibrinolytic agents probably act by reducing the enhanced fibrinolytic activity found in the uterus in women with excessive MBL (Bonnar et al 1983).

Clinical experience. Nilsson & Rybo (1971) treated 172 women with epsilon-amino-caproic acid and 85 patients with tranexamic acid. All women had been shown to have an MBL above 80 ml. The average reduction of MBL was 47 and 54% respectively. Ninety of the women on EACA complained of side-effects which included nausea, dizziness, diarrhoea, headache and abdominal pain. Systemic fibrinolytic activity is slightly reduced by these agents and intracranial thromboses have been reported (Rydin & Lundberg 1976, Agnelli et al 1983).

Oral contraceptives

Few studies have investigated the mode of action of oral contraceptives in reducing MBL. Oral contraceptives induce hypoplasia of the endometrium and total synthesis of prostaglandins by endometrium is reduced by these agents (Chan 1983).

Clinical experience. Various preparations of combined synthetic steroids reduce MBL (Nilson & Rybo 1971) by on average about 50% of pre-treatment values but there are few contemporary studies with low dose preparations in view of the contraindications to their use over the age of 35.

Gestagens

Perhaps the most widely used regimes for the treatment of menorrhagia are cyclical gestagens, e.g. norethisterone. The rationale for their use was to oppose the action of oestrogens on endometrium in anovulatory cycles. Surprisingly there are few, if any, studies which objectively assess the efficacy of this treatment in ovulatory or anovulatory cycles, although the situation is presently under review.

Other agents

Ethamsylate, a drug which probably reduces capillary fragility, reduces MBL by about 50% of pre-treatment values (Harrison & Campbell 1976).

Surgical Treatment

The definitive treatment of menorrhagia is removal of the uterus. Clearly this operation can only be undertaken on women who have finished their family. In view of the effective agents reviewed above an attempt at medical management is usually tried first but if unsuccessful then hysterectomy is performed. There is little doubt that in many cases, hysterectomy is considered by the patient and doctor to be a satisfactory solution to the problems of menstruation.

Various surgical techniques for ablating the endometrium have been tried (Chamberlain 1981) and present interest centres on the use of the laser for photovaporisation of the endometrium (Goldrath et al 1981).

CONCLUSION

A feature of life for women who limit the size of their families by the use of contraception and sterilisation is an increased incidence of menstruation with all of the attendant consequences. It seems unreasonable that in the long term the response to this problem should be the surgical removal of the uterus from about one-fifth of womankind. It is only by a greater understanding of the mechanisms which initiate and control menstrual bleeding that alternative approaches to this common problem may be sought.

ACKNOWLEDGMENTS

I would like to thank Professor D T Baird and Drs M H Abel and R W Kelly without whom the studies into the role of prostaglandins in menorrhagia would not have been possible.

REFERENCES

Abel M H, Kelly R W 1979 Differential production of prostaglandins within the human uterus. Prostaglandins 18: 821–828

Abel M H, Baird D T 1980 The effect of 17β-estradiol and progesterone on prostaglandin production by human endometrium maintained in organ culture. Endocrinology 160: 1599–1606

Agnelli G, Gresele P, De Cunto M, Gallai V, Nenci G G 1982 Tranexamic acid, intrauterine contraceptive devices and fatal cerebral arterial thrombosis. Case Report. British Journal of Obstetrics and Gynaecology 89: 681–682

Albrechtsen O K 1956 The fibrinolytic activity of the human endometrium. Acta Endocrinologica 23: 219–229

Anderson A B M, Haynes P J, Guillebaud J, Turnbull A C 1976 Reduction of menstrual blood loss by prostaglandin synthetase inhibition. Lancet i: 774–776

Armstrong J M, Dusting G J, Moncada S, Vane J R 1978 Cardiovascular action of prostacyclin (PGI_2) a metabolite of arachidonic acid which is synthesized by blood vessels. Circulation Research 43: (Suppl) 112–119

Baird D T, Abel M H, Kelly R W, Smith S K 1982 Endocrinology of dysfunctional uterine bleeding: The role of endometrial prostaglandins. In: Crosignani P G, Rubin B L (eds) Proceedings of the Serono Clinical Colloquia on Reproduction 2, pp 399–417. Academic Press, London

Bito L Z 1975 Are prostaglandins intracellular, transcellular or extracellular autoacids? Prostaglandins 9: 851–855

Bonnar J, Sheppard B L, Dockerey C J 1983 The haemostatic system and dysfunctional uterine bleeding. Research and Clinical Forums 5: 27–36

Carey E 1968 In: Barter R H, Brennan G, Newman W, Merill K W The place of curettage in the diagnosis of carcinoma of the endometrium. American Journal of Obstetrics and Gynecology 100: 696–702

Chamberlain G 1981 Dysfunctional uterine bleeding. Clinics in Obstetrics and Gynaecology 8: 93–101

Chan W Y 1983 Prostaglandins and nonsteroidal anti inflammatory drugs in dysmenorrhoea. Annual Reviews of Pharmacology and Toxicology 23: 131–149

Chimbira T H, Cope E, Anderson A B M, Bolton F G 1979 The effect of danazol on menorrhagia, coagulation mechanisms, haematological indices and body weight. British Journal of Obstetrics and Gynaecology 86: 46–50

Chimbira T H, Anderson A B M, Naish C, Cope E, Turnbull A C 1980 Reduction of menstrual blood loss by danazol in unexplained menorrhagia: lack of effect of placebo. British Journal of Obstetrics and Gynaecology 87: 1152–1158

Christiaens G C M L, Sixma J J, Haspels A A 1980 Morphology of haemostasis in menstrual endometrium. British Journal of Obstetrics and Gynaecology 87: 425–439

Cohen B J B, Gibor Y 1980 Anaemia and menstrual blood loss. Obstetrical and Gynecological Survey 35: 597–618

Cole S K, Billewicz W Z, Thomson A M 1971 Sources of variation in menstrual blood loss. Journal of Obstetrics and Gynaecology of the British Commonwealth 78: 933–939

Di Zerega G S, Hodgen G D 1981 Luteal phase dysfunction infertility: a sequel to aberrant folliculogenesis. Fertility and Sterility 35: 489–499

Doring G K 1969 The incidence of anovular cycles in women. Journal of Reproduction and Fertility 6: (Suppl) 77–81

Einer-Jensen N 1973 Decreased endometrial blood flow and plasma progesterone level after instillation of 10 μg $PGF_{2\alpha}$ into the lumen of uteri of rhesus monkey. Prostaglandins 4: 517–522

Fairhurst E, Pale T L, Fidge B D 1977 A comparison of anaemia and storage iron deficiency in working women. Proceedings of the Nutrition Society 36: 98A

Ferenczy A 1976 Studies on the cytodynamics of human endometrial regeneration. I. Scanning electron microscopy. American Journal of Obstetrics and Gynecology 124: 64–74

Flower R J, Vane J R 1974 Inhibition of prostaglandin synthesis. Biochemistry and Pharmacology 23: 1439–1450

Fraser I S, Baird D T 1972 Endometrial cystic glandular hyperplasia in adolescent girls. Journal of Obstetrics and Gynaecology of the British Commonwealth 79: 1009–1015

Fraser I S, Pearse L, Shearman R P, Elliot P M, McIlveen J, Markham R 1981 Efficacy of mefenamic acid in patients with a complaint of menorrhagia. Obstetrics and Gynecology 58: 543–551

Godfrey K A, Aspillaga M O, Taylor A, Lind T 1981 The relation of circulating progesterone and oestradiol concentrations to the onset of menstruation. British Journal of Obstetrics and Gynaecology 88: 899–903

Goldrath M H, Fuller T A, Segal S 1981 Laser photovaporization of endometrium for the treatment of menorrhagia. American Journal of Obstetrics and Gynecology 140: 14–19

Greenblatt R B, Dmowski W P, Mahesh V E, Scholar H F L 1971 Clinical studies with an antigonadotrophin — danazol. Fertility and Sterility 22: 102–112

Grimes D A 1982 Diagnostic dilation and curettage: a re-appraisal. Americal Journal of Obstetrics and Gynecology 142: 1–6

Guillebaud J, Anderson A B M, Turnbull A C 1978 Reduction by mefenamic acid of increased menstrual blood loss associated with intra-uterine contraception. British Journal of Obstetrics and Gynaecology 85: 53–62

Hahn L 1980 Composition of menstrual blood. In: Diczfalusy E, Fraser I S, Webb F T C (eds) WHO Symposium on Endometrial Blood and Steroidal Contraception. Pitman Press, England

Hallberg L, Hogdahl A M, Nilsson L, Rybo G 1966 Menstrual blood loss — a population study. Acta Obstetrica et Gynaecologica Scandinavica 45: 320–351

Harrison R F, Campbell S 1976 A double blind trial of ethamsylate in the treatment of primary and intrauterine-device menorrhagia. Lancet ii: 283–285

Haynes P J, Hodgson H, Anderson A B M, Turnbull A C 1977 Measurement of menstrual blood loss in patients complaining of menorrhagia 84: 763–768

Haynes P J, Anderson A B M, Turnbull A C 1979 Patterns of menstrual blood loss in menorrhagia. Research and Clinical Forums 1: 73–78

Henzl M R, Smith R E, Boost G, Tyler E T 1972 Lysosomal concept of menstrual bleeding in humans. Journal of Clinical Endocrinology and Metabolism 34: 860–875

Holstrom E G, McLennan C E 1947 Menorrhagia associated with irregular shedding of endometrium; clinical and experimental study. American Journal of Obstetrics and Gynecology 53: 727–748

Jenkin G 1980 Review: the mechanism of action in danazol, a novel steroid derivative. Australia and New Zealand Journal of Obstetrics and Gynaecology 20: 113–118

Jones G S 1976 The luteal phase defect. Fertility and Sterility 27: 351–356

Kasonde J M, Bonnar J 1976 Effect of sterilization on menstrual blood loss. British Journal of Obstetrics and Gynaecology 83: 572–575

Kendall M 1979 The world fertility survey: Current status and findings. Population Reports of the Johns Hopkins University Series M 3

Kilpatrick G S 1970 Prevalence of anaemia in the United Kingdom. In: Hallberg L, Harworth H G, Vannot A (eds) Iron deficiency: Pathogenesis, Clinical Aspects, Therapy pp 441–445. Academic Press, New York

Lumsden M A, Kelly R W, Baird D T 1983 Primary dysmenorrhoea: the importance of both prostaglandins E_2 and $F_{2\alpha}$. British Journal of Obstetrics and Gynaecology 90: 1135–1140

Mackenzie J Z, Bibby J G 1978 Critical assessment of dilatation and curettage in 1029 women. Lancet ii: 566–569

Markee J E 1940 Menstruation in intraocular endometrial transplants in the rhesus monkey. Contributions to Embryology Carnegie Institute 28: 219–308

Metcalf M G 1979 Incidence of ovulatory cycles in women approaching the menopause. Journal of Biosocial Sciences 11: 39–48

Metcalf M G, Mackenzie J A 1980 Incidence of ovulation in young women. Journal of Biosocial Sciences 12: 345–352

Murthy Y S, Arronet G H, Parekh M C 1970 Luteal phase inadequacy. Its significance in infertility. Obstetrics and Gynecology 36: 758–761

Newton J, Barnard G, Collins W 1977 A rapid method for measuring menstrual blood loss using automatic extraction. Contraception 16: 269–282

Nilsson L, Rybo G 1971 Treatment of menorrhagia. American Journal of Obstetrics and Gynecology 110: 713–719

Nogales-Ortiz F, Puerta J, Nogales F F 1978 Normal menstrual cycle. Chronology and mechanisms of endometrial desquamation. Obstetrics and Gynecology 51: 259–264

Novak E R, Woodruff J D 1974 In: Novak's Gynecologic and Obstetric Pathology, p. 175. W B Saunders, Philadelphia

Petrussen B, Hahn L, Korsan-Bengtsen K, Hallberg L 1977 Influence of acetylsalicylic acid and paracetamol on menstrual blood loss. Haemostasis 6: 266–268

Prescott L F 1975 Anti-inflammatory analgesics and drugs used in the treatment of rheumatoid arthritis. In: Dukes M N G (ed) Meylers Side-effects of Drugs. Excerpta Medica 8: 207

Ramwell P W, Foegh M, Loeb R, Leovey E M 1980 Synthesis and metabolism of prostaglandins, prostacyclin and thromboxanes: the arachidonic acid cascade. Seminars in Perinatology 4: 3–13

Rees M C P, Anderson A B M, Demers L M, Turnbull A C 1983 A functional study of platelets in menstrual blood. British Journal of Obstetrics and Gynaecology. Submitted.

Rybo G 1966a Clinical and experimental studies on menstrual blood loss. Acta Obstetrica et Gynaecologica Scandinavica 45 (Suppl): 1–23

Rybo G 1966b Menstrual blood loss in relation to parity and menstrual pattern. Acta Obstetrica et Gynaecologica Scandinavica 45 (Suppl): 25–45

Rybo G, Nilsson S, Sikstrom B, Nygren K G 1981 Naproxen in menorrhagia. Lancet i: 608–609

Rydin E, Lundberg P O 1976 Tranexamic acid and intracranial thrombosis. Lancet ii: 49

Scommegna A, Vorys N, Givens J R 1980 Menstrual dysfunction. In: Gold J J, Josimovich J B (eds) Gynecologic Endocrinology, pp 290–326. Harper and Row, New York

Sexton L, Lenton E A, Cooke I D 1980 Age related changes in the menstrual cycle of older women. Presented at the Society for the Study of Fertility, Oxford

Shaw S T, Roche P C 1980 Menstruation. In: Finn C A (ed) Oxford reviews of Reproductive Biology, Vol. II, pp 41–96. Clarendon Press, Oxford

Sheppard B L, Dockeray C J, Bonnar J 1983 An ultrastructural study of menstrual blood in normal menstruation and dysfunctional uterine bleeding. British Journal of Obstetrics and Gynaecology 90: 259–265

Short R V 1976 The evolution of human reproduction. Proceedings of the Royal Society of London 195: 3–24

Sixma J J, Wester J 1977 The hemostatic plug. Seminars in Hematology 14: 265–299

Smith S K, Abel M H, Kelly R W, Baird D T 1981a Prostaglandin synthesis in the endometrium of women with ovular dysfunctional uterine bleeding. British Journal of Obstetrics and Gynaecology 88: 434–442

Smith S K, Abel M H, Kelly R W, Baird D T 1981b A role for prostacyclin (PGI$_2$) in excessive menstrual bleeding. Lancet i: 522–524

Smith S K 1982 Physiological and pharmacological aspects of prostaglandins in the female reproductive tract p. 59. MD Thesis, University of London

Smith S K, Abel M H, Kelly R W, Baird D T 1982 The synthesis of prostaglandins from persistent proliferative endometrium. Journal of Clinical Endocrinology and Metabolism 55: 284–289

Smith S K, Lenton E A, Cooke I D 1984a Premenstrual levels of 17β oestradiol and progesterone in plasma in cycles of short and normal luteal phase length. Clinical Reproduction and Fertility. In press.

Smith S K, Lenton E A, Landgren B M, Cooke I D 1984b. The short luteal phase and infertility. British Journal of Obstetrics and Gynaecology. Submitted.

Smith S K, Abel M H, Baird D T 1984c Effects of 17β-estradiol and progesterone on the levels of prostaglandins F$_{2\alpha}$ and E in human endometrium. Prostaglandins. In press.

Snow L F, Johnson S M 1977 Modern day menstrual folklore — some clinical implications. Journal of the American Medical Association 237: 2736–2739

Toppozada M, El-Attar A, El-Ayyat M A, Khamis Y 1980 Management of uterine bleeding by PGs or their synthesis inhibition. Advances in Prostaglandins and Thromboxanes Research 8: 1459–1463

Treloar A E, Boynton R E, Behn B G, Brown D W 1967 Variation of the human menstrual cycle through reproductive life. International Journal of Fertility 12: 77–126

Van Dijk J G, Frohlich M, Brand E C, Van Hall E V 1979 The treatment of unexplained infertility with danazol. Fertility and Sterility 31: 481–485

Van Look P F A, Lothian H, Hunter W M, Michie E A, Baird D T 1977 Hypothalamic-pituitary-ovarian function in perimenopausal women. Clinical Endocrinology 7: 13–31

Van Look P F A, Hunter W M, Fraser I S, Baird D T 1978 Impaired estrogen-induced luteinizing hormone release in young women with anovulatory dysfunctional uterine bleeding. Journal of Clinical Endocrinology and Metabolism 46: 816–823

Vollman R F 1977 The menstrual cycle. In: Friedman E A (ed) Major Problems in Obstetrics and Gynaecology, 7. W B Saunders, Philadelphia

Wiquist N, Bygdeman M, Kirton K 1971 Non-steroidal infertility agents in the female. In: Diczfalusy E, Borell B (eds) Nobel Symposium 15, Control of Human Fertility, p. 137

Wood J C 1973 Lysosomes of the uterus. In: Bishop M W H (ed) Advances in Reproductive Physiology, No. 6, pp 221–230. Elek Science, London

Young M D, Blackmore W P 1977 The use of danazol in the management of endometriosis. Journal of International Medical Research 5: 86–91

Sexually transmitted diseases

In the United Kingdom the incidence of the statutory venereal diseases — syphilis, gonorrhoea and chancroid — has remained fairly static for the past 5 years. The numbers of new cases of these diseases reported in the UK in 1981 (the last year for which complete data are available) were 4,211, 58,301 and 100 respectively (Sexually Transmitted Disease Surveillance 1981). Now only some 12% of patients who attend sexually transmitted diseases (STD) clinics, suffer from venereal disease.

However, there has been a significant increase in the numbers of patients who attend STD clinics with viral infections. This has been particularly marked in the case of genital herpes which showed an increase of 12.1% in the numbers of attendances over those in 1980. Genital warts showed a 5.3% increase in the same period.

The greatest increase in numbers of cases has occurred with non-specific genital infection, perhaps a misnomer as *Chlamydia trachomatis* is associated with the majority of such infections. Probably related to this has been the increased incidence of pelvic inflammatory disease in young women. These issues have been addressed in a previous volume of the series.

The numbers of patients who attend STD clinics with 'other conditions requiring treatment' has also increased dramatically over the past few years. Within this category are patients suffering from pelvic inflammatory disease, vaginitis (or vaginosis) caused by organisms other than *Trichomonas vaginalis* and *Candida spp*, dermatological diseases of the genitals and gynaecological problems.

Although precise data are difficult to obtain, the prevalence of the venereal diseases is high in developing countries and can lead to considerable mortality and morbidity amongst neonates and their mothers. In the developed countries of the world, the emergence of 'third generation' sexually transmitted diseases is becoming apparent. These diseases include carcinoma of the uterine cervix and the acquired immune deficiency syndrome (AIDS).

In this chapter recent developments in the field of sexually transmitted diseases will be discussed. Serological tests for syphilis have remained essentially unaltered for the past decade and will not be considered here. For a review of treponemal serology, the reader is referred to Notowicz & Menke

(1981). Although there have been important advances in the understanding of the immunobiology of the gonococcus, the most significant development in the past 8 years has been the emergence and worldwide spread of β-lactamase producing *Neisseria gonorrhoeae*. The increasing incidence of genital herpes, its implication in the aetiology cf cervical cancer, its consequences in pregnancy, its treatment and prospects for prophylaxis necessitate its inclusion within this chapter. Recent studies on the association of human papillomavirus with cervical carcinoma dictate discussion here.

β-LACTAMASE PRODUCING *NEISSERIA GONORRHOEAE*

Although the global prevalence of isolates of *N.gonorrhoeae* with reduced sensitivity to penicillin and other antimicrobial agents has been increasing for three decades, as a result of indiscriminate use of antibiotics, it was only in 1976 that β-lactamase (penicillinase) producing strains of the organism (PPNG) were isolated from clinical material (Phillips 1976, Ashford et al 1976).

Prior to 1976 the genes for antibiotic resistance were considered to be chromosomal and not carried on plasmids (Biswas et al 1976). Among PPNG, resistance is encoded for by two distinct types of plasmid — a 3.2 megadalton plasmid ('African' plasmid) which was initially linked with West Africa (Perine et al 1977) and a 4.4 megadalton plasmid ('Asian' plasmid) associated with isolates from the Far East (Embden et al 1980). In addition PPNG may carry a self-transferable 24.5 megadalton plasmid which can mobilise the 3.2 and 4.4 megadalton plasmids to other gonococci or to *Escherichia coli* (Roberts & Falkow 1977, Embden et al 1981). There appears to be a strong correlation between plasmid pattern and auxotype. In Amsterdam Ansink-Schipper et al (1984) found that the majority (91%) of PPNG isolates which harboured the 3.2 M dal plasmid were non-requiring inhibited by phenylalanine whereas 67% of isolates carrying the 4.4 M dal plasmid were proline requiring.

Epidemiology

Epidemiological data suggest that in the mid-1970s there were two separate endemic zones of infection — in South East Asia and in West Africa (Johnston et al 1981). During the early phase of spread of the infection in developed countries PPNG were imported from these endemic areas (Percival et al 1976, Phillips 1976). However, the numbers of cases of gonorrhoea associated with PPNG increased exponentially and the indigenous spread of these organisms has become an important factor in the epidemiology of the infection (Nayyar et al 1980, Jaffe et al 1981, McCutchan et al 1982, Thin et al 1983).

The prevalence of PPNG infections varies geographically. For example, in many areas of the Far East 30–60% of isolates are PPNG; in Amsterdam 18% of cases of gonorrhoea are caused by PPNG (Ansink-Schipper et al 1984) and in London clinics, 4% of isolates are PPNG (Thin et al 1983).

Treatment of infection caused by β-lactamase producing Neisseria gonorrhoeae

Uncomplicated infection

Table 20.1 indicates the principal antimicrobial agents which have been used in the treatment of women with gonorrhoea associated with PPNG. Although spectinomycin has been valuable in the treatment of these infections PPNG resistant to this drug have been isolated (Ashford et al 1981, Easmon et al 1982) and are increasing in prevalence (Ison et al 1983).

At present the most valuable drugs for the treatment of PPNG infection are the newer cephalosporins. The World Health Organisation (1982) recommend treatment with cefotaxime 1.0 g or cefoxitin 2.0 g by intramuscular injection, both preceded by the oral administration of 1.0 g probenecid; treatment with ceftriaxone 250 mg by intramuscular injection is also recommended. Similar recommendations have been proposed by the Centers for Disease Control, Atlanta USA (1982). The cephalosporins are expensive and in SE Asia, kanamycin in a single 1 g intramuscular injection has been used successfully in the treatment of PPNG infections (Rajan et al 1979). The toxicity of the latter drug should be borne in mind and must be avoided in pregnancy.

The combination of amoxycillin (3.0 g) with the β-lactamase inhibitor clavulanic acid (250 mg) in a single oral preparation has theoretical advantages over injectable forms of treatment for gonorrhoea. However, although the combination has proved useful in the treatment of men with gonococcal urethritis (Latif et al 1984), experience in the treatment of women with PPNG infection is limited. Further studies are necessary before conclusions can be drawn regarding treatment efficacy. Pharyngeal infections with N.gonorrhoeae are difficult to treat; WHO (1982) recommend treatment of pharyngeal gonorrhoea caused by PPNG with cotrimoxazole (trimethoprin 80 mg, sulphamethoxazole 400 mg) 10 tablets daily as a single oral dose for 5 days.

Complicated infections

β-lactamase producing strains of N.gonorrhoeae resemble non PPNG strains in their ability to produce pelvic inflammatory disease (PID) and disseminated gonococcal infection. Treatment schedules are based on somewhat limited experience in the management of these complications. CDC (1982) recommend treatment of acute PID associated with PPNG with cefoxitin 2.0 g by intravenous injection four times per day for at least 4 days. Third generation cephalosporins are likely to be effective alternatives. As acute gonococcal PID is likely to be associated with chlamydial and anaerobic infection, it is probably useful to add to the treatment regimen a tetracycline, for example doxycycline 100 mg by mouth or if necessary intravenously every 12 hours for 10 to 14 days, and metronidazole 1 g by mouth or intravenously every 12 hours.

Table 20.1 Treatment of uncomplicated anogenital gonorrhoea in women caused by β-lactamase producing *Neisseria gonorrhoeae*

Antimicrobial agent	Dosage	Cure rate (%)	Reference	Comments
Spectinomycin	2 g as single intramuscular injection	52/52 (100)	Tupasi et al (1983)	Resistance emerging
Cefuroxime	1.5 g by intramuscular injection preceded by 1 g probenecid by mouth	58/59 (98.3)	Tupasi et al (1983)	Reduce dose in renal impairment
Cefotaxime	500 mg by intramuscular injection	40/41 (97.6)	Rajan et al (1980)	
	1 g by intramuscular injection Preceded by probenecid 1 g by mouth	34/34 (100.0)	de Koning (1983)	
Cefaclor	3 g by mouth	27/27 (100.0)	Tupasi et al (1982)	
Rosoxacin	300 mg by mouth	18/18 (100.0)	Calubiran et al (1982)	Dizziness and vertigo common
Thiamphenicol	2.5 g by mouth	57/58 (98.3)	Tupasi et al (1983)	Contraindicated in pregnancy
Gentamicin	280 mg by intramuscular injection	80/83 (96.4)	Tan et al (1980)	Contraindicated in pregnancy. Can produce vestibular damage and reversible nephrotoxicity

Gonococcal arthritis has responded well to treatment with cefoxitin 2 g intravenously every 6 hours for 3 weeks, or to spectinomycin 4 g by intramuscular injection followed by 2 g daily for 3–5 days (Rinaldi et al 1982).

Gonococcal ophthalmia neonatorum

Cefotaxime 100 mg per kg of body weight per day in three divided doses for 7 days has proved useful in the treatment of gonococcal ophthalmia (Doreiswamy et al 1983). Kanamycin as a single intramuscular dose of 0.5 g has also been used in treatment of gonococcal ophthalmia (Thirumoorthy et al 1982). Dunlop et al (1980) successfully treated two neonates with cefuroxime in an intramuscular dosage of 100 mg/kg/day in three divided doses for seven days.

Follow-up and contact tracing

Material from previously infected sites should be cultured for *N.gonorrhoeae*. Ideally, two sets of negative results obtained 1 week apart should be obtained before cure is assumed. Tracing of primary and secondary contacts is of immense importance in preventing the spread of the gonococcus.

GENITAL HERPES

The increasing incidence of this disease amongst sexually active young people has attracted much attention in the mass media. The acquisition of herpes simplex virus Type I appears to afford some protection against infection with HSV2, the type most commonly associated with genital disease. However, the increasing number of individuals reaching early adult life with no HSV1 antibody may partly explain the increasing number of patients with genital herpes.

Aetiology

Herpes simplex virus (HSV) is a DNA containing virus of which two types, 1 and 2, occur in humans. These types were originally differentiated by differences in the size of the pocks produced on the chorio-allantoic membrane of hen's eggs, by the presence or absence of filaments in the nuclei of tissue culture cells, by the different cytopathic effect produced in baby hamster kidney cells (Smith et al 1973), by quantal neutralisation tests and by immunofluorescence. More recently, restriction-endonuclease analysis of DNA has been shown to be unambiguous in the differentiation of the two types (Lonsdale 1979). Restriction enzyme analysis of the DNA of HSV isolated from genital lesions has shown differences between viruses isolated from different individuals (Chaney et al 1983). Although some studies have been undertaken (Buchman et al 1979) further work is planned to investigate the usefulness of this technique in epidemiological studies. Classically, HSV1 and

2 have been associated with oral and genital herpes respectively. However, in Edinburgh some 30% of isolates for women with genital herpes are type 1 HSV; 16% of isolates from infected men are HSV type 1 (Peutherer et al 1981).

Pathogenesis

This has been reviewed by Wildy et al (1982).

Before considering the pathogenesis, immunology and clinical features of genital herpes, it is useful to set out the terminology used (Wildy et al 1982):

Primary infection	— an acute infection which may remain localised or become generalised. An initial infection is the first clinically apparent one occurring in an individual who has serum herpes antibodies.
Latency	— there is recovery from the primary infection, but virus remains dormant in the ganglia cells.
Reactivation	— virus can be 'reawakened' from the neuronal cells either spontaneously or as a result of external stimuli.
Recrudescence	— Reactivated virus passes to a peripheral site and, a peripheral lesion develops. Virus can be cultured from the site.
Recurrence	— Reactivated virus passes to the peripheral site and, although there is probably multiplication of virus there is no peripheral lesion. Virus can be cultured from the site.

Virus from the site of initial infection is transported within the axon cylinder to the neurones of the sensory ganglia (and, possibly to those of the central nervous system), where latency is established. Following reactivation, the virus in some, as yet undetermined, form is transported in the reverse direction. The nature of latency has not been closely defined. It is postulated that virus remains static in some unknown form within neurones and is occasionally reactivated. Translocated virus infects epidermal cells which in turn, after multiplication, infect nerve endings.

Reactivation of virus has followed nerve section, u.v. treatment, burning with solid CO_2 and hair plucking.

In man recrudescence of HSV has followed pyrexia, exposure to sunlight and trauma.

Immunology of herpes simplex virus infection

This subject is well reviewed by Wildy et al (1982). Most experimental studies on the immunology of HSV have used guinea-pig, mouse and rabbit models; the interpretation of the data obtained and its relevance to human genital infection should be treated with caution until further studies have been completed.

Patients undergoing recrudescence of herpes labialis (type 1 HSV) have impaired cell-mediated immunity. Their T-cells fail to produce macrophage inhibition factor in response to herpes, but not other antigens (Shillitoe et al 1977). Similar observations were made by Donnenberg et al (1980) working with guinea-pigs. This may represent a reduced proportion of lymphokine secreting T-cells or an increased number of suppressor cells, resulting in defective clearance of virus. In mice delayed type hypersensitivity (DTH) is found on day 4 of infection and remains inducible for life. DTH can be transferred to syngeneic animals only within the first 10 days of infection. B-cells appear in the draining lymph nodes which suppress the expression of DTH when transferred to immune mice. Their appearance may explain why DTH transfer is restricted to the first 10 days of infection. If DTH is suppressed, there will be failure of localisation of antiviral cells at the site of infection with reactivated virus and result in recrudescence. Neutralising antibody is detectable after the fifth day of infection. Cytotoxic T cells appear within a few days of infection, peak in numbers about 7 days and are not detectable 12 days post infection. T memory cells appear by about 8 days post infection and are detectable for life.

These findings have no relevance to the control of latency or reactivation: the immunological mechanism involved in that control are ill-understood.

Epidemiology

In most cases, genital herpes is acquired through sexual contact with an infected partner, who may have recurrent disease in the absence of clinical features of herpes. Serological studies support the role of sexual contact in the epidemiology of HSV2 infection. With the exception of young babies with maternally-derived antibody, the prevalence of HSV2 serum antibodies which are rarely found in prepubertal children in developed countries increases from the age of 14. Although the serum of only 3% of nurses contained HSV2 antibody, this was found in 100% of prostitutes (Nahmias & Roizmann 1973). Interestingly there are geographical differences in the prevalence of HSV2 serum antibodies: in Nigeria Sogbetun et al (1979) demonstrated HSV2 antibody in the sera of 11% of children between the ages of 3 and 5 years.

Association of HSV2 and cervical carcinoma

The higher prevalence of HSV antibodies (subject reviewed by Skinner 1981) in the sera of women with cervical carcinoma has led workers to consider an aetiological role for HSV2. However, HSV-specific DNA has not been clearly demonstrated in biopsies of cervical cancers and it is probable that other factors play a role in the causation of cervical malignancy (see section on Human papillomavirus).

Clinical features

Primary infection

After a prepatent period which is difficult to determine with precision, the patient complains of tingling and burning in the ano-genital skin. Vesicles rapidly develop on an erythematous base; these vesicles rupture forming shallow, tender ulcers which may coalesce. In the female the area affected is often extensive involving the labia majora, labia minora, introitus, urethral orifice, vagina, cervix, perineum and anal margin. The inguinal lymph nodes are enlarged and tender. Features of the viraemia include pyrexia, malaise, headache and cervical and axillary lymph node enlargement.

As a result of sacral radioculomyelitis, paraesthesiae of the buttocks and thighs, urinary hesitancy or retention and constipation may result (Smith & Gordon 1981).

Within 12 days of the appearance of symptoms the lesions crust and heal (median time to healing 14 days; range 7 to 29 days (Mindel et al 1982)), without scarring; new lesions develop for up to 16 days and virus is excreted from those for more than 21 days (median duration of viral shedding 8.5 days (Mindel et al 1982) from the start of the disease).

Rarely, disseminated herpes complicates genital infection. In general, this has occurred in immuno-compromised individuals but has been described in patients with no obvious immunosuppression (Juel-Jensen & MacCallum 1972) and in pregnant women (Anderson & Nicholls 1972).

Recrudescence and recurrence

Sixty per cent and 14% of patients with HSV2 and HSV1 infections respectively develop recrudescent lesions within 6 months of the initial episode (Reeves et al 1981); 64% of primary and 56% of initial infections will have recurred within that time.

In general, the clinical features are less severe than during primary or initial infection. Guinan et al (1981) reported on the natural history of recrudescent genital herpes in 27 women. They found that the majority (82%) of women have prodromal symptoms in the form of tenderness, burning, itching or tingling at the site of the subsequent lesions. The mean healing time (8.0 days) is shorter than that reported in primary infection. Pain was experienced mainly during the first 2 days of the episode and then decreased rapidly in intensity. The mean duration of viral shedding was significantly shorter (4.8 days) than in primary infection; all lesions cultured after day 10 were negative.

Asymptomatic shedding of HSV (recurrence) from the cervix or vulva occurs and was demonstrated in 2 of 6 women who had previous genital HSV infection (Rattray et al 1978).

Genital Herpes in pregnant women

Although there have been several reports on the intra-uterine acquisition of HSV (South et al 1969, Komorous et al 1977), the major problem facing obstetricians is transmission of the virus to the child during vaginal delivery.

Neonatal herpes is an uncommon disease in the United Kingdom, only some 66 cases having been reported to the Communicable Disease Surveillance Centre between 1973 and 1979. The condition occurs more frequently in the USA where, amongst women in the lower social classes, one child per 7500 deliveries develops neonatal herpes (Nahmias et al 1970). The majority (about 75%) of infections are associated with HSV2.

There is little doubt that the majority of neonatal infections are acquired at the time of delivery (Nahmias et al 1970) and are more likely to develop in children born to mothers with primary genital herpes at term than in those with recrudescent lesions (Nahmias et al 1971). However, although HSV antibody which is present in the sera of mothers with recrudescence or recurrence of their disease, crosses the placenta and may protect against generalised disease in the neonate (Nahmias & Visintine 1976) it affords little protection against the acquisition of infection localised to the brain, eyes or skin (Amstey et al 1976).

The mortality rate of generalised herpes of the neonate approaches 90% and almost half of the survivors have neurological sequelae (Nahmias et al 1975). In neonates with disease localised to the CNS, the mortality rate is under 50% but about 80% have permanent sequelae; only 30% of infants with localised disease of the eyes, skin or mouth develop sequelae.

It is clear that about 40% of infants born to mothers with primary genital herpes at term will develop neonatal herpes if they are delivered vaginally (Nahmias et al 1971). However, this risk is substantially reduced if the child is delivered by Caesarian section before, or certainly within 4 hours of membrane rupture. After that time, the risk of neonatal disease is the same as that of children born per vaginam (Nahmias et al 1975). The obstetrical management of women with clinically apparent primary herpes and with less certainty, recrudescent lesions at term is therefore, clear.

However, shedding of HSV has been shown to be asymptomatic in over 40% of pregnant women (Nahmias et al 1971). Although 13% and 20% of mothers of children who developed neonatal herpes gave a past history of genital herpes or were sexual contacts of infected men respectively, 50% of these women were unaware of their HSV infection or exposure to risk (Whitley et al 1980). Short of screening all pregnant women for excretion of HSV, little can be done to identify the latter group of women. When there is a past history of genital herpes or history of contact with an infected partner, weekly viral cultures of the cervical material in the third trimester has been postulated (Amstey et al 1979) and women who are excreting virus at term should be delivered by Caesarean section.

As the incidence of neonatal herpes in the United Kingdom is small, Marshall & Peckham (1983) feel that Caesarean section is not indicated in women who give a past history of genital herpes and whose cultures for HSV are negative or unknown, or in women who are sexual contacts of infected men.

Although the maternal genital tract is the most important source of HSV infection for the neonate, infection from other infants and adults has been described (Francis et al 1975) as has infection during internal fetal scalp-monitoring (Parvey & Ch'ien 1980).

Treatment of pregnant women with primary genital herpes with acyclovir in the prevention of neonatal herpes remains to be evaluated.

Although the main risk during pregnancy is infection of the child at term, severe maternal disease resulting from dissemination of the virus is rare (Anderson & Nicholls 1972, Young et al 1976).

Treatment

The introduction in 1982 into clinical practice of acyclovir marked a significant advance in the treatment of primary genital herpes and is now the drug of choice for use in primary infection.

Acyclovir is an acyclic nucleoside guanosine which inhibits DNA synthesis. Thymidine kinase produced by HSV catalyses the phosphorylation of the drug which is otherwise inactive. As host cell enzymes are ineffective in the phosphorylation of acyclovir (Centifanto & Kaufman 1979) non-infected cells are not affected. Viral DNA polymerase is also inhibited by acyclovir (Elion et al 1977). Acyclovir is also active against varicella-zoster virus, but less so against cytomegalovirus (Elion et al 1977). The drug is eliminated unchanged by glomerular filtration or tubular secretion.

Initial experience with acyclovir, given intravenously within 7 days of onset of symptoms, to patients with initial episode genital herpes was encouraging. Mindel et al (1982) studied 15 patients with primary and initial disease and compared the results with 15 patients given placebo. They found that median healing time for all lesions was significantly shorter in the acyclovir treated group (7 days) than in the placebo group (14 days). Although there was no significant difference between the two groups in the median healing times of external lesions, internal lesions in the female showed a shorter healing time than the external. New lesion formation was reduced: none developed after the second day in the control group, but continued to appear for up to 15 days in the placebo group. Vesicles persisted longer in placebo-treated patients (16 days vs 8 days in acyclovir group). However, in women the duration of symptoms was not significantly affected. Viral shedding ceased within 5 days of the institution of therapy, compared with the control patients whose lesions showed virus for up to 20 days.

Nilsen et al (1982) reported similar results in the treatment of initial genital herpes with acyclovir given orally in a dosage of 200 mg five times per day for 5 days. Significant side-effects were not reported by either group.

Unfortunately, there is no significant difference in the delaying or recrudescence rate of genital herpes between patients with primary or initial disease treated with acyclovir or with placebo (Corey et al 1983).

Although oral acyclovir treatment, initiated within 48 hours of the appearance of recrudescent lesions, reduces significantly, by comparison with placebo therapy, the duration of viral shedding (from a median of 2 days to 1 day), the time to healing of lesions (from 6 days to 5 days), and new lesion formulation (from 19% to 2%) (Nilsen et al 1982), the value of therapy for recrudescent disease remains to be proven. The drug is expensive and its use does not produce the marked improvement associated with the treatment of initial genital herpes.

Topical acyclovir ointment (5% w/w) applied five times per day for up to 10 days, is available and its use in initial genital herpes has been described by Corey et al (1982) and Thin et al (1983). By comparison with the placebo-treated group the duration of viral shedding from external lesions is reduced (from a median of 7 days to 2), but there is little difference in the duration of virus excretion from all lesions, internal and external, in women. The duration of vesicles is reduced for a median of 2 days to 1 day; the time to complete healing of all lesions is shortened (15.5 days to 7 days); and after initiation of treatment new lesion formation is significantly reduced (from 57% to 9%). Although the duration of pain is not reduced significantly, the duration of all symptoms is markedly shortened (from 10 to 6 days).

Although there is a significant reduction in the median duration of viral shedding from lesions treated with topical acyclovir as against placebo, virus can be cultured from lesions for up to 12 days. By contrast viral shedding ceases within 5 days of initiation of oral or intravenous acyclovir. In some patients new lesion formation occurs for up to 7 days of the start of topical acyclovir: this contrasts markedly with experience in oral or systemic therapy which prevents and rapidly reduces new lesion formation. For this reason oral, or in some cases, intravenous acyclovir should be the form selected for the treatment of primary or initial genital herpes. Experience with acyclovir cream is limited but the results of application of this preparation in initial genital herpes are awaited with interest.

Acyclovir has been used widely in the treatment of extensive anogenital herpes in immunodeficient individuals (Meyers et al 1982) and has proved useful in the protection of bone marrow transplant patients against HSV infection (Prentice 1983).

Acyclovir treatment is safe, the only notable side-effect of intravenous therapy is pain at the injection site if there has been extravasation of the drug into the tissues. Transient elevation of plasma urea and/or creatinine levels have been described (Keeney et al 1982) following an intravenous injection of acyclovir. This is thought to represent crystal formation in the renal tubules and can be avoided by slow infusion and adequate hydration of the patient. Care should be exercised if the drug is used in combination with nephrotoxic drugs. The elimination of acyclovir in patients with renal failure is greatly reduced, and the dosage should be modified (Laskin et al 1982, de Miranda & Blum 1983).

No fetal toxicity or teratogenic effects have been found in rabbits, rats and mice. At doses of 250 $\mu g/ml$ of acyclovir, chromosomal damage in cultured human lymphocytes has been demonstrated: these effects were not found with doses of 125 $\mu g/ml$. As the latter level represents some 500 times the HSV ID$_{50}$, the use of the drug in pregnancy appears safe (Brigden & Whiteman 1983).

Acquired resistance to acyclovir has been described and is reviewed by Field (1983). One type of mutant which can be selected in *in vitro* experiments lacks the ability to induce thymidine kinase. Such mutants have been isolated from immunocompromised patients (Burns et al 1982, Schipper et al 1982). As these strains of HSV have been shown to be attenuated when compared with the parent strains (Field & Wildy 1978), the clinical relevance of these is unknown. In the laboratory, resistance to acyclovir and sometimes to related nucleoside analogue inhibitors can be induced by another mechanism involving a change in the substrate specificity of either thymidine kinase or DNA-polymerase (Crumpacker et al 1982). These variants are virulent in mice (Field et al 1982). To date acquired resistance of HSV to acyclovir is uncommon (McLaren et al 1982), but careful monitoring of the sensitivity of HSV isolates is needed to detect the development of resistance to the drug.

Idoxuridine applied topically to herpetic lesions was used widely prior to the introduction of acyclovir. Its use in genital herpes is no longer indicated.

Povidone iodine paint (Betadine, Napp Laboratories) applied to the lesions three times per day is useful in the management of minor recrudescent herpetic lesions.

Prophylaxis

Several studies have shown that vaccination with live or inactivated type 2 virus or type 1 vaccine offers some degree of protection against latent HSV2 infection of nerve ganglia (McKendall 1977, Walz et al 1977, Hilleman et al 1981). Skinner et al 1982 have prepared a vaccine containing glycosylated polypeptides and have shown that some 90% of 60 subjects developed neutralising antibody against HSV1 when given two subcutaneous inoculations of vaccine, the injections being separated by 1 month. After a short term follow-up of these subjects none had contracted genital herpes. The same workers (Woodman et al 1983) found that 31% of 22 patients who were vaccinated after a primary HSV infection developed eight recrudescent episodes; by contrast, there were 51 recrudescent episodes in 85% of 20 subjects who had not been vaccinated.

Further studies to confirm these findings are urgently needed.

ANOGENITAL WARTS

The number of patients with anogenital warts who attend STD clinics in the UK is increasing. In 1977, 26 063 cases were reported from the UK clinics to the Department of Health and Social Security; the number had increased to 33 480 in 1981 (Sexually Transmitted Diseases Surveillance 1981). Of importance is the association with genital malignancy.

Aetiology

Human warts are caused by the human papilloma virus (HPV) a small DNA virus which has not been propagated *in vitro*. Although it has been known for more than a decade that there are antigenic differences between the HPV demonstrated in anogenital warts and those at other sites (Almeida et al 1970), it has only been within the past 5 years that the heterogeneity of HPV has become evident. DNA which has been cloned from HPV isolates has been analysed by restriction enzyme digestion and nucleic acid hybridisation. On the basis of such experiments, 18 subtypes of HPV have been identified. Types 6 and 11 are associated with genital warts (Gissman et al 1982, 1983). However, all papillomaviruses from humans, cattle, deer, horses and dogs share at least one capsid antigenic determinant and a broadly cross-reactive antiserum containing antibodies against these determinants can be prepared (Jenson et al 1980). These antisera have proved useful in epidemiological studies (Baird 1983) and in the identification of HPV antigens in tissue sections (Woodruff et al 1980).

Pathology

Condylomata acuminata show marked acanthosis and papillomatosis. The individual processes have connective tissue cores which often contain tortuous capillaries and a mild chronic inflammatory cell infiltrate. Within the superficial layers of the epithelium are found koilocytes — cells with marked cytoplasmic vacuolation; the nuclei of some, but not all, of these cells can be shown by electron microscopy and by immunoperoxidase methods to contain HPV virus and antigen, respectively (Ferenczy et al 1981). The vacuolation seen in koilocytes is a cytopathic effect of HPV infection; these cells are degenerating and are shed from the epithelium. Dysplasia of the basal layers of the epithelium is not common.

Although koilocytes and dyskeratotic cells may be identified in Papanicolaou smears of the cervix of women with cervical condylomata acuminata and 'flat koilocytosis' (see below) cells resembling those shed from dysplastic lesions are commonly found (Coleman 1979, Meisels et al 1981). HPV infection may produce non-condylomatous lesions of the cervix. The terminology of these lesions which may be associated with dysplasia is confusing but is well reviewed by Fletcher (1983). These lesions (flat condyloma, 'atypical condyloma', flat koilocytosis) consist of thickened epithelium which is only slightly elevated above the surrounding tissue and does not show the digitation characteristic of condylomata acuminata. Koilocytes, accompanied by occasional dyskeratotic cells, are found in the superficial layers of the epithelium; HPV virus and antigen can be demonstrated within the nuclei of some of these cells (Meisels et al 1981). Changes indistinguishable from dysplasia of varying degree are commonly associated with these lesions. It may be that these 'dysplastic' cells are early non-koilocytic and pre-koilocytic stages of HPV infection which regress when infection is terminated (Fletcher & Norval 1983). On the other hand these cells may be dysplastic but the association with HPV may be coincidental. However, it is quite probable that HPV induces transformation of the basal layer of the cervical epithelium into dysplasia in multiple foci. Interestingly, HPV infection was found associated with cervical intra epithelial neoplasia in 14 of 22 cases studied by McCance et al (1983) HPV6 was found in 59% of cases; another type of HPV, for example type 11 may have been associated with the other cases.

Association of human papillomavirus infection and malignancy

An association between HPV and genital malignancy has been suggested for several reasons:-

1. Condylomata acuminata may precede or co-exist with squamous carcinoma of the vulva (Shafeek et al 1979).
2. HPV is associated with other malignancies in man and other animals.

About a third of patients with the planar skin warts of the hereditary skin disease epidermodysplasia verruciformis (EV) develop squamous cell carcinoma of the skin (Lutzner 1978). Types 3 and 5 HPV are the principal subtypes found in these warts, but only patients infected with type 5 develop skin malignancies (Ostrow et al 1982). There is an increased incidence of warts and cutaneous malignancy in patients who are immunosuppressed after renal transplantation (Koranda et al 1974); HPV 5 has been demonstrated in the benign and malignant lesions of one such patient (Lutzner et al 1983).

Bovine papillomavirus type 5 DNA has been demonstrated in alimentary tract carcinomas in cattle (Campo et al 1980). Using DNA hybridisation methods with ^{32}P HPV-EV as probe, Zachow et al (1982) demonstrated HPV-DNA in biopsies from four of eight women with vulval squamous cell carcinoma. HPV-DNA has been found in premalignant lesions of the genitals. Zachow et al (1982) detected HPV-DNA in biopsies from a woman with Bowenoid papules of the vulva and Ikenberg et al (1983) demonstrated DNA homologous with HPV16 DNA in four of five patients with genital Bowen's disease and in eight of 10 individuals with Bowenoid papules; HPV-DNA was not detected in normal genital tissue. Green et al (1982) also found HPV-EV related DNA in women with Bowen's disease of the vulva and in two of 31 cases of cervical cancer. DNA homologous to probes with DNA-HPV 11 was found in three of 20 biopsies from women with cervical carcinoma (Gissman et al 1983). Recently Dürst et al (1983) detected HPV16 DNA in 11 of 18 biopsies of cervical carcinoma. HPV16 DNA has also been demonstrated in tissue from verrucous carcinomas (Gissmann et al 1982).

It is clear that different types of HPV may be found in genital squamous cell carcinomas. In Germany, HPV of some sub type was found in 72% of cervical carcinomas (Dürst et al 1983). Geographical differences in the prevalence of papillomavirus DNA in cervical carcinoma are also apparent. Dürst et al (1983) found HPV-DNA in only 34.8% of these cancers in Kenya and Brazil.

The occurrence of HPV-DNA in biopsies of malignant and premalignant lesions of the genitalia does not prove that HPV is causative. However, it may at least play a role in carcinogenesis. Carcinoma of the alimentary tract of cattle (associated with bovine papilloma virus type 5) requires interaction between virus and carcinogens present in bracken (Jarrett et al 1978) and the malignant transformation of Shope-papillomavirus papillomas is aided by chemical carcinogens (Rous & Friedwald, 1944). Zur Hausen (1982) postulates that human genital cancer may arise in a similar fashion through synergism between HPV and a previous initiating viral infection, possibly HSV. Although attractive this hypothesis remains to be established.

Clinical features

In order of frequency, condylomata acuminata are found on the posterior part of the introitus, on the labia minora and clitoris, on the labia majora, on the perineum, within the vagina, in the perianal region, at the urethral meatus and on the cervix (Oriel 1971). During pregnancy and in immunocompromised patients, these condylomata are often extensive, but regress after delivery or restoration of immune-competence. Untreated, warts may remain unaltered for months or even years, but may regress rapidly. The immunological mechanisms which determine the outcome of the lesions are not understood.

Wart virus infection may be associated with non-condylomatous lesions of the cervix ('flat koilocytosis' which are not visible to the naked eye). At colposcopy these lesions are acetowhite, there is mosaicism and punctation in the transformation zone, and there are often satellite lesions (Meisels et al 1981). Although condylomatous lesions of the cervix only occur in about 6% of women with anogenital warts (Oriel 1971), Walker et al (1983a) found cytological or coloscopic evidence of 'flat koilocytosis' in 28% of 50 women with vulval warts. Although conclusions cannot be drawn from studies on small numbers of patients, the latter authors found little regression in the cervical lesions associated with wart virus infection (Walker et al 1983b).

Treatment of anogenital warts

There is no specific treatment for anogenital warts. The topical application of podophyllin, whose active ingredient is podophyllotoxin, is widely used in the management of women with anogenital warts. The use of this agent should be avoided in pregnancy as abortion and peripheral neuropathy has followed systemic absorption of topically-applied podophyllin (Clark & Parsonage 1957, Stoehr et al 1978). As a severe inflammatory reaction may follow its application to vaginal warts, podophyllin should be avoided in lesions of this site and of the cervix.

Podophyllotoxin has been purified from both species of *Podophyllum* and has been used as an 0.5–8% w/v ethanolic solution in the treatment of penile warts (von Krogh 1981). Twice or thrice daily application of a 10% w/s solution for 3 days was found to be effective in the eradiction of the warts in almost 50% of cases. The author considered that the risk of systemic absorption of drug was much less than when podophyllin is used.

Cryotherapy and electrocautery are widely used in the treatment of anogenital warts; the results of treatment by either method are similar (Simmons 1981).

Treatment with the carbon dioxide laser is effective and has the advantage that vaginal and cervical warts are easily managed (Calkins et al 1982). Although general anaesthesia is seldom necessary patients with vulval and perianal lesions usually require local anaesthesia.

In skilled hands, submucous resection of vulval, perianal and anal warts produces excellent results: there is little post-operative pain and scarring is minimal (Gollock et al 1982). As treatment necessitates admission to hospital, this procedure should be reserved for extensive lesions and warts which have failed to respond to other forms of treatment.

As the extensive hyperplastic warts found in pregnant women generally resolve spontaneously within 6 weeks of delivery, treatment is generally not indicated. Podophyllin is contraindicated in pregnancy and as there is pelvic congestion, surgical methods of treatment are hazardous.

Immunotherapy for warts has contributed little to the management of warts. Attempted BCG immunotherapy (Malison & Salkin 1981) and the use of autologous vaccine (Malison et al 1982) were unsuccessful in the treatment of condylomata acuminata.

In the future, therapy with intralesional interferon may be useful; such studies are in progress.

As genital warts may be associated with other sexually transmissible diseases (Kinghorn 1978), the appropriate microbiological tests to exclude these should be undertaken and contact tracing of sexual partners should be instituted.

JUVENILE LARYNGEAL PAPILLOMAS

Juvenile laryngeal papillomas have been shown to be associated with HPV. Although virus particles resembling HPV have been reported rarely in the nuclei of the epithelial cells of these neoplasms (Boyle 1973). Costa et al 1981 using an immunoperoxidase method, have documented papillomavirus antigen in the nuclei of cells from about 50% of cases of juvenile laryngeal papillomas. There seems little doubt that they are acquired during passage through the birth canal of an infected mother. DNA homologous with that from HPV6 and HPV11 has been found in biopsies of these papillomas (Mounts et al 1982,

Gissmann et al 1983). Malignant transformation of these lesions has been observed in patients treated by radiation (Kleinasser 1958).

REFERENCES

Introduction

Anon 1981 Sexually transmitted disease surveillance 1981. British Medical Journal 286: 1500–1501
Notowicz A, Menke H E 1981 Routine diagnostic procedures in treponemal disease. In: Harris J R W (ed.) Recent Advances in Sexually Transmitted Diseases, No. 2, pp 93–100. Churchill Livingstone, Edinburgh

β-lactamase producing *Neisseria gonorrhoeae*

Ansink-Schipper M C, Huikeshoven M H, Woudstra R K, Klingeren Bvan, Koning G A J de, Tio D, Schoonhoven F J, Coutinho R A 1984 Epidemiology of PPNG infection in Amsterdam: analysis of auxanographic typing and plasmid characterisation. British Journal of Venereal Diseases 1976 60: 23–28
Ashford W A, Golash R G, Hemming V G 1976 Penicillinase-producing Neisseria gonorrhoeae. Lancet ii: 657–658
Ashford W A, Potts D W, Adams H J U, English J C, Johnson S R, Thornsberry C, Jaffe H W 1981 Spectinomycin resistant penicillinase-producing Neisseria gonorrhoeae. Lancet ii: 1035–1037
Biswas G, Comer S, Sparling P F 1976 Chromosomal location of antibiotic resistance genes in Neisseria gonorrhoeae. Journal of Bacteriology 125: 1207–1212
Calubiran O V, Crisologo-Vizconde L B, Tupasi T E, Torres C A, Limson B M 1982 Treatment of uncomplicated gonorrhoea in women: comparison of rosoxacin and spectinomycin. British Journal of Venereal Diseases 58: 231–235
Centers for Disease Control 1982 Sexually transmitted diseases treatment guidelines 1982. Morbidity and Mortality Weekly Report 31
Doreiswamy B, Hammerschlag M R, Pringle G F, du Boucher L 1983 Ophthalmia neonatorum caused by β-lactamase producing Neisseria gonorrhoeae. Journal of the American Medical Association 250: 790–791
Dunlop E M C, Rodin P, Seth A D, Kolator B 1980 Ophthalmia neonatorum due to beta-lactamase-producing gonococci. British Medical Journal i: 483
Easmon C S F, Ison C A, Bellinger C M, Harris J W 1982 Emergence of resistance after spectinomycin treatment for gonorrhoea due to β-lactamase-producing strain of Neisseria gonorrhoeae. British Medical Journal 284: 1604–1605
van Embden J D A, van Klingeren B, Dessens-Kroon M, van Wijngaarden L J 1980 Penicillinase-producing Neisseria gonorrhoeae in the Netherlands: epidemiology and genetic and molecular characteristics of their plasmids. Antimicrobial Agents Chemotherapy 18: 789–797
van Embden J D A, van Klingeren B, Dessens-Kroon M, van Wijngaarden L J 1981 Emergence in the Netherlands of penicillinase-producing gonococci carrying 'African' plasmid in combination with transfer plasmid. Lancet i: 938
Ison C A, Littleton K, Shannon K P, Easmon C S F, Phillips I 1983 Spectinomycin resistant gonococci. British Medical Journal 287: 1827–1829
Jaffe H W, Biddle J W, Johnson S R, Weisner P 1981 Infection due to penicillinase-producing Neisseria gonorrhoeae in the United States from 1976 to 1980. Journal of Infectious Diseases 144: 191–197
Johnston N A, Kolator B, Seth A D 1981 A Survey of β-lactamase producing gonococcal isolates reported in the United Kingdom 1979-1980. The present trend. Lancet i: 263–264
de Koning G A J, Tio D, van den Hoek J A R, van Klingeren B 1983 Single dose of cefotaxime in the treatment of infection due to penicillinase producing strains of Neisseria gonorrhoeae. British Journal of Venereal Diseases 59: 100–102

Latif A S, Sithole J, Bvumbe S, Gumbo B, Kawemba M, Summers R S 1984 Treating gonococcal urethritis in men: oral amoxycillin potentiated by clavulanate compared with intramuscular procaine penicillin. British Journal of Venereal Diseases 60: 29-30

McCutchan J A, Adler M W, Berrie J R H 1982 Penicillinase-producing Neisseria gonorrhoeae in Great Britain 1979-1981; alarming increase in incidence and recent development of endemic transmission. British Medical Journal 285: 337-340

Nayyar K C, Noble R C, Michel M F, Stolz E. Gonorrhoea in Rotterdam caused by penicillinase-producing gonococci. British Journal of Venereal Diseases 56: 244-248

Percival A, Corkill J A, Arya O P, Rowlands J, Alergant C D, Rees E, Annels E H 1976 Penicillinase producing gonococci in Liverpool. Lancet ii: 1379-1382

Perine P L, Thornsberry C, Schalla W, Biddle J, Siegel M S, Wong K-H, Thompson S E 1977 Evidence for two distinct types of penicillinase-producing Neisseria gonorrhoeae. Lancet ii: 993-995

Phillips I 1976 β-lactamase producing penicillin-resistant gonococcus. Lancet ii: 656-657

Rajan V S, Pang R, Tan N J, Sng E H 1979 Kanamycin in the treatment of penicillinase-producing gonococcal infections. Asian Journal of Infectious Diseases 3: 37-39

Rajan V S, Sng E H, Pang R, Tan N J, Thirumoorthy T, Yeo K L 1980 HR756: A new cephalosporin in the treatment of gonorrhoea caused by ordinary and penicillinase producing strains of Neisseria gonorrhoeae. British Journal of Venereal Diseases 1982 56: 255-258

Rinaldi R Z, Harrison W O, Fan P T 1982 Penicillin resistant gonococcal arthritis. A report of 4 cases. Annals of Internal Medicine 97: 43-45

Roberts M, Falkow S 1977 Conjugal transfer of R plasmids in Neisseria gonorrhoeae. Nature 266: 630-631

Tan N J, Rajan V S, Pang R, Sng E H 1980 Gentamicin in the treatment of infections due to penicillinase-producing gonococci. British Journal of Venereal Diseases 56: 394-396

Thin R N, Barlow D, Eykyn S, Phillips I 1983 Imported penicillinase-producing Neisseria gonorrhoeae becomes endemic in London. British Journal of Venereal Diseases 59: 364-368

Thirumorthy T, Rajan V S, Hoh C L 1982 Penicillinase-producing Neisseria gonorrhoeae ophthalmia neonatorum in Singapore. British Journal of Venereal Diseases 58: 308-310

Tupasi T E, Calubiran O V, Torres C A 1982 Single oral dose of cefaclor for the treatment of infections with penicillinase producing strains of Neisseria gonorrhoeae. British Journal of Venereal Diseases 58: 176-179

Tupasi T E, Crisologo L B, Torres C A, Calubiran O V, Jesus I D 1983 Cefuroxime, thiamphenicol, spectinomycin and penicillin G in uncomplicated infections due to penicillinase producing strains of Neisseria gonorrhoeae. British Journal of Venereal Diseases 59: 172-175

World Health Organisation 1982 Current treatments in the control of sexually transmitted diseases. Report of a WHO Consultative Group, Geneva

Genital Herpes

Amstey M S, Lewin E B, Meyer M R 1976 Herpesvirus infection in the newborn. Obstetrics and Gynecology 47: 335-341

Amstey M S, Monif G R G, Nahmias A J, Josey W E 1979 Caesarean section and genital herpesvirus infection (Editorial). Obstetrics and Gynecology 53: 641-642

Anderson J M, Nicholls N W N 1972 Herpes encephalitis in pregnancy. British Medical Journal i: 632

Brigden D, Whiteman P 1983 The mechanism of action pharmocokinetics and toxicity of acyclovir — a review. Journal of Infection 6 (Suppl. 1): 3-9

Buchman T G, Roizman B, Nahmias A J 1979 Demonstration of exogenous genital reinfection with herpes simplex virus Type 2 by restriction endonuclease fingerprinting of viral DNA. Journal of Infectious Diseases 140: 295-304

Burns W H, Saral R, Santos G W, Laskin O L, Lietman P S, McLaren C, Barry D W 1982 Isolation and characterization of resistant herpes simplex virus after acyclovir therapy. Lancet i: 421-425

Centifanto Y M, Kaufman H E 1979 9-(2-hydroxyethoxy-methyl) guanine as an inhibitor of herpes simplex virus replication. Chemotherapy 25: 279-281

Chaney S M J, Warren K G, Ketlyls J, Zbitnue A, Subak-Sharpe J H 1983 A comparative analysis of restriction enzyme digests of the DNA of herpes simplex virus collected from genital and facial lesions. Journal of General Virology 64: 357–371

Corey L, Nahmias A J, Guinan M E, Benedetti J K, Critchlow C W, Holmes K K 1982 A trial of topical acyclovir in genital herpes simplex virus infections. New England Journal of Medicine 306: 1313–1319

Corey L, Benedetti J, Critchlow C, Mertz G, Douglas J, Fife K, Fahnlander A, Remington M L, Winter C, Dragavon J 1983 Treatment of primary first episode genital herpes simplex virus infections with acyclovir: results of topical intravenous and oral therapy. Journal of Antimicrobial Chemotherapy 12 (Suppl. B): 79–88

Crumpacker C S, Schnipper L E, Chartrand P, Knopf K W 1982 Genetic mechanisms of resistance to acyclovir in herpes simplex virus. American Journal of Medicine 73: 361–368

Donnenberg A D, Bell R B, Aurelian L 1980 Immunity to herpes simplex virus type 2. Development of virus specific lymphoproliferative and LIF responses in HSV-2 infected guinea pigs. Cellular Immunology 56: 526–539

Elion G B, Furman P A, Fyfe J A, de Miranda P, Beauchamp L, Schaeffer H J 1977 Selectivity of action of an antiherpetic agent, 9-(2-hydroxyethoxy-methyl) guanine. Proceedings of the National Academy of Sciences of the USA 74: 5716–5720

Field H J, Wildy P 1978 The pathogenicity of thymidine kinase deficient mutants of herpes simplex virus in mice. Journal of Hygiene 81: 267–277

Field H J, Larder B A, Darby G 1982 Isolation and characterization of acyclovir-resistant strains of herpes simplex virus. American Journal of Medicine 73: 369–371

Field H J 1983 Acquired resistance to acyclovir: laboratory phenomenon or clinical problem. Journal of Infection 6 (Suppl. 1): 11–14

Francis D P, Herrmann K L, MacMahon J H, Cahavigny K H, Sanderlin M S 1975 Nosocomial and maternally acquired herpes virus hominis infections. American Journal of Diseases of Children 129: 889–893

Guinan M E, MacCalman J, Kern E M, Overall J C, Spruance S L 1981 The course of untreated recurrent genital herpes simplex infection in 27 women. New England Journal of Medicine 304: 759–763

Hilleman R M, Larson V M, Lehman E D, Salerno R A, Conrad P G, McLean A A 1981 Subunit herpes simplex viruses vaccine. In: Nahmias A J, Dowdle W R, Shinazi R F (eds) The Human Herpes Viruses, pp 503–506. Elsevier, New York

Juel-Jensen B E, MacCallum F O 1972 Herpes simplex varicalla and zoster. Clinical Manifestations and Treatment, p. 69. William Heinemann, London

Keeney R E, Kirk L E, Brigden D 1982 Acyclovir tolerance in humans. American Journal of Medicine 73: 176–181

Komorous J M, Wheeler P E, Briggamann R A 1977 Intrauterine herpes simplex infection. Archives of Dermatology 113: 918–922

Laskin O L, Longstreth J A, Whelton A, Krasny H C, Keeney R E, Roccoll, Lietman P S 1982 Effect of renal failure on the pharmacokinetics of acyclovir. American Journal of Medicine 73: 197–201

Lonsdale D M 1979 A rapid technique for distinguishing herpes simplex virus type 1 from type 2 by restriction-enzyme technology. Lancet i: 849–857

McKendall R R 1977 Efficacy of herpes simplex virus type 1 immunization in protecting against acute and latent infection by herpes simplex virus type 2 in mice. Infection and Immunity 16: 717–719

McLaren C, Sibrack C D, Barry D W 1982 Spectrum of sensitivity to acyclovir of herpes simplex virus clinical isolates. American Journal of Medicine 73: 376–379

Marshall W C, Peckham C S 1983 The management of herpes simplex in pregnant women and neonates. Journal of Infection 6 (Suppl. 1): 23–29

Meyers J D, Wude J C, Mitchell C D, Saral R, Lietman P S, Durack D T, Levin M J, Segreti A C, Balfour H H 1982 Multicenter collaborative trial of intravenous acyclovir for treatment of mucocutaneous herpes simplex virus infection in the immunosuppressed host. American Journal of Medicine 73: 229–235

Mindel A, Adler M W, Sutherland S, Fiddian A P Intravenous acyclovir treatment for primary genital herpes. Lancet i: 697–700

de Miranda P, Blum M R 1983 Pharmacokinetics of acyclovir after intravenous and oral administration. Journal of Antimicrobial Chemotherapy 12 (Suppl. B): 29–37

Nahmias A J, Alford C A, Korones J B 1970 Infections of the newborn with herpesvirus hominis. Advances in Pediatrics 17: 185–226

Nahmias A J, Josey W E, Naib Z M, Freeman M G, Fernandez R J, Wheeler J H 1971 Perinatal risk associated with maternal genital herpes simplex virus infection. American Journal of Obstetrics and Gynecology 110: 825–834

Nahmias A J, Roizmann B 1973 Infection with herpes simplex viruses 1 and 2. New England Journal of Medicine 289: 781–789

Nahmias A J, Visintine A M, Reimer C D, Del Buonos I, Shore S L, Starr S E 1975 Herpes simplex virus infection of the fetus and newborn. In: Krugman S, Gershon A A (eds) Infections of the Fetus and Newborn Infant, pp 63–77. A R Liss, New York

Nahmias A, Visintine A 1976 Herpes simplex infection. In: Remington J, Klein J (eds) Infectious Diseases of the Fetus and Newborn Infant pp 156–190. W B Saunders, Philadelphia

Nilsen A E, Aasen J, Halsos A M, Kinge B R, Tjøtta E A L, Wilkstrom K, Fiddian A P 1982 Efficacy of oral acyclovir in the treatment of initial and recurrent genital herpes. Lancet ii: 571–573

Parvey L S, Ch'ien L 1980 Neonatal herpes simplex virus introduced by fetal monitor scalp electrodes. Pediatrics 65: 1150–1153

Peutherer J F, Smith I W, Robertson D H H 1981 Association of herpes simplex virus types 1 and 2 with clinical sites of infection. In: Nahmias A J, Dowdle W R, Schinazi R (eds) The Human Herpesviruses p. 595. Elsevier, New York

Prentice H G 1983 Use of acyclovir for prophylaxis of herpes infection in severely immunocompromised patients. Journal of Antimicrobial Chemotherapy 12 (Suppl. B): 153–159

Rattray M C, Corey L, Reeves W C, Vontver L A, Holmes K K 1978 Recurrent genital herpes among women: symptomatic v asymptomatic viral shedding. British Journal of Venereal Diseases 54: 262–265

Reeves W S, Corey L, Adams H G, Vontver L A, Holmes K K 1981 Risk of recurrence after first episode of genital herpes. Relation to HSV type and antibody response. New England Journal of Medicine 305: 315–319

Schipper L E, Crumpacker C S, Marlowe S I, Kowalsky P, Hershey B J, Levin M J 1982 Drug resistant herpes simplex virus in vitro and after acyclovir treatment in an immunocompromised patient. American Journal of Medicine 73: 387–392

Shillitoe E J, Wilton J M A, Lehner T 1977 Sequential changes to herpes simplex virus after recurrent herpetic infection in humans. Infection and Immunity 18: 130–137

Skinner G 1981 Sero-epidemiological evidence of association between type 2 herpes simplex virus infection and carcinoma of the uterine cervix. In: Jordan J A, Sharp F, Singer A (eds) Preclinical Neoplasia of the Cervix, pp 47–56. Royal College of Obstetricians and Gynaecologists, London

Skinner G R B, Woodman C B J, Hartley C E, Buchan A, Fuller A, Durham J, Synnott M, Clay J C, Melling J, Wiblin C, Wilkins J 1982 Prepartion and immunogenicity of vaccine Ac NFU$_1$(S) MRC towards the prevention of herpes genitalis. British Journal of Venereal Diseases 58: 381–386

Smith D H, Gordon Y B 1981 Neurogenic bladder after vaginal herpes infection. Lancet i: 837

Smith I W, Peutherer J F, Robertson D H H 1973 Characterization of genital strains of Herpesvirus hominis. British Journal of Venereal Diseases 49: 385–390

Sogbetun A O, Montefiore D, Anong C W 1979 Herpesvirus hominis antibodies among children and young adults in Ibadan. British Journal of Venereal Diseases 55: 44–47

South M A, Tompkins W A F, Morris C R, Rawles W E 1969 Congenital malformations of the central nervous system associated with genital (type 2) herpesvirus. Journal of Pediatrics 75: 13–18

Thin R N, Nabarro J M, Parker J D, Fiddian A P 1983 Topical acyclovir in the treatment of initial herpes. British Journal of Venereal Diseases 59: 116–119

Walz M A, Price R W, Hayashi K, Katz B J, Notkins A L 1977 Effect of immunization in acute and latent infection of vaginal-uterine tissue with herpes simplex virus types 1 and 2. Journal of Infectious Diseases 135: 744–752

Whitley R J, Nahmias A J, Soong S J, Galasso G G, Fleming C L, Alford C A 1980 Vidarabine therapy of neonatal herpes simplex virus infection. Pediatrics 66: 495–501

Wildy P, Field H J, Nash A A 1982 Classical herpes latency revisited. In: Mahy B W J, Minson A C, Darby G K (eds) Virus Persistence, pp 133–167. Cambridge University Press, Cambridge

Woodman C B J, Buchan A, Fuller A, Hartley C, Skinner G R B, Stocker D, Sugrue D, Clay J C, Wilkins G, Wiblin C, Melling J 1983 Efficacy of vaccine Ac NFU₁(S⁻) MRC5 given after an initial clinical episode in the prevention of herpes genitalis. British Journal of Venereal Diseases 59: 311–313

Young E J, Killam A P, Greene J F 1976 Disseminated herpesvirus infection. Association with primary genital herpes in pregnancy. Journal of the American Medical Association 235: 2731–2733

Anogenital warts

Almeida J D, Oriel J D, Stannard L M 1970 Wart viruses. British Journal of Dermatology 83: 698–701

Baird P J 1983 Serological evidence for the association of papillomavirus and cervical neoplasia. Lancet ii: 17–18

Boyle W F 1973 Electron microscopic identification of polyvina virus in laryngeal papilloma Laryngoscope 83: 1102–1108

Calkins J W, Masterson B J, Magrina J F, Capen C V 1982 Management of condyloma acuminatum with the carbon dioxide laser. Obstetrics and Gynecology 59: 105–108

Campo M S, Moar M H, Jarrett W F H, Laird L M 1980 A new papillomavirus associated with alimentary cancer in cattle. Nature 286: 180–182

Clark A N G, Parsonage M J 1957 A case of podophillum poisoning with involvement of the nervous system. British Medical Journal ii: 1155–1157

Coleman D V 1979 Cytological diagnosis of virus infected cells in Papanicolaou smears and its application in clinical practice. Journal of Clinical Pathology 32: 1075–1089

Costa J, Howley P M, Bowling M C, Howard R, Bauer N C 1981 Presence of human papilloma viral antigens in juvenile multiple laryngeal papilloma. American Journal of Clinical Pathology 75: 194–197

Durst M, Gissmann L, Ikenberg H, zur Hausen H 1983 A papillomavirus DNA from a cervical carcinoma and its prevalence in cancer biopsy samples from different geographic regions. Proceedings of the National Academy of Sciences 80: 3812–3815

Ferenczy A, Braun L, Shah K V 1981 Human papillomavirus (HPV) in condylomatous lesions of the cervix. American Journal of Surgical Pathology 5: 661–670

Fletcher S 1983 Histopathology of papilloma virus infection of the cervix uteri: the history, taxonomy, nomenclature and reporting of koilocytic dysplasias. Journal of Clinical Pathology 36: 616–624

Fletcher S, Norval M 1983 On the nature of the deep cellular disturbances in human papilloma virus infection of the squamour cervical epithelium. Lancet ii: 546–549

Gissmann L, DeVilliers E-M, zur Hausen H 1982 Analysis of human genital warts (condylomata acuminata) and other genital tumours for human papillomavirus type 6 DNA. International Journal of Cancer 29: 143–146

Gissmann L, Wolnik L, Ikenberg H, Koldovsky U, Schnürch H G, zur Hausen H 1983 Human papillomavirus types 6 and 11 DNA sequences in genital and laryngeal papillomas and in some cervical cancers. Proceedings of the National Academy of Sciences 80: 560–563

Gollock J M, Slatford K, Hunter J M 1982 Scissor excision of anogenital warts. British Journal of Venereal Diseases 58: 400–401

Green M, Brackmann K H, Sanders P R, Loewenstein P M, Freel J H, Eisinger M, Switlyk S A 1982 Isolation of a human papillomavirus from a patient with epidermodysplasia verruciformis: presence of related viral DNA genomes in human urogenital tumour. Proceedings of the National Academy of Sciences 79: 4437–4441

Ikenberg H, Gissmann L, Gross G, Grussendorf-Conen E I, zur Hausen H 1983 Human papillomavirus type 16 related DNA in genital Bowen's disease and Bowenoid papules. International Journal of Cancer 32: 563–565

Jarrett W E, McNeill P, Grimshaw W, Selman I, McIntyre W 1978 High incidence area of cattle cancer with a possible interaction between an environmental carcinogen and a papilloma virus. Nature 274: 215–217

Jenson A B, Rosenthal J R, Olson C, Pass F, Lancaster W D, Shah K 1980 Immunological relatedness of papillomavirus from different species. Journal of the National Cancer Institute 64: 495–498

Kinghorn G R 1978 Genital warts: incidence of associated genital infection. British Journal of Dermatology 99: 405–409

Kleinasser O 1958 Uber die gut — und bosartigen Formen der Kehlkopf-papilloma und deren histologisches und Klinisches Bild. Archiv fur Ohren-, Nasen-, und Kehl kopfheilkunde 174: 44–69

Koranda F C, Dehmel E M, Khan G, Penn I 1974 Cutaneous complications in immunosuppressed renal homograft recipients. Journal of the American Medical Association 229: 419–422

von Krogh G 1982 Penile condylomata acuminata: an experimental model for evaluation of topical self treatment with 0.5–1.0% ethanolic preparation of podophyllotoxin for three days. Sexually Transmitted Diseases 8: 179–187

Lutzner M A 1978 Epidermodysplasia verruciformis: an autosomal recessive disease characterised by viral warts and skin cancer. A model for viral oncogenesis. Bulletin of Cancer 65: 169–182

Lutzner M A, Orth G, Dutronquay V, Ducasse M F, Kreis H, Crosnier J 1983 Detection of human papillomavirus type 5 DNA in skin cancers of an immuno-suppressed renal allograft recipient. Lancet ii: 422–424

McCance D J, Walker P G, Dyson J L, Coleman D V, Singer A 1983 Presence of human papillomavirus DNA sequences in cervical intraepithelial neoplasia. British Medical Journal 287: 784–788

Malison M D, Salkin D 1981 Attempted BCG immunotherapy for condyloma acuminata. British Journal of Venereal Diseases 57: 148

Malison M D, Morris R, Jones L W 1982 Autogenous vaccine therapy for condyloma acuminatum: a double blind controlled study. British Journal of Venereal Diseases 58: 62–65

Meisels A, Roy M, Fortier M, Morin C, Casas-Cordero M, Shah V K, Turgeon H 1981 Human papillomavirus infection of the cervix. The atypical condyloma. Acta cytologica 25: 7–16

Mounts P, Shah K V, Kashima H 1982 Viral etiology of juvenile — and adult — onset squamous papilloma of the larynx. Proceedings of the National Academy of Sciences 79: 5425–5429

Oriel J D 1971 Natural history of genital warts. British Journal of Venereal Diseases 47: 1–13

Ostrow R S, Bender M, Nimwa M, Seki T, Kawashima M, Pass F, Faras A J 1982 Human papillomavirus DNA in cutaneous primary and metastasized squamous cell carcinoma from patients with epidermodysplasia verucciformis. Proceedings of the National Academy of Sciences 79: 1634–1638

Rous P, Friedwald W F 1944 The effect of chemical carcinogens on virus induced rabbit carcinomas. Journal of Experimental Medicine 79: 511–537

Shafeek M A, Osman M I, Hussein M A 1979 Carcinoma of the vulva arising in condylomata acuminata. Obstetrics and Gynecology 54: 120–123

Simmons P D, Langlet F, Thin R B T 1981 Cryotherapy versus electrocautery in the treatment of genital warts. British Journal of Venereal Diseases 57: 273–274

Stoehr G P, Peterson A C, Taylor W J 1978 Systemic complications of local podophyllin therapy. Annals of Internal Medicine 89: 362–363

Walker P G, Colley N V, Grugg C, Tejerina A, Oriel J D 1983a Abnormalities of the interne cervix of women with vulval warts: a preliminary communication. British Journal of Venereal Diseases 59: 120–123

Walker P G, Singer A, Dyson J L, Oriel J D 1983b Natural history of cervical epithelial abnormalities in patients with vulval warts: a colposcopic study. British Journal of Venereal Diseases 59: 327–329

Woodruff J D, Braun L, Cavalieri R, Gupta P, Pass F, Shah K V 1980 Immunologic identification of papillomavirus antigen in condyloma tissues from the female genital tract. Obstetrics and Gynecology 56: 727–732

Zachow K R, Ostrow R S, Bender M, Watts S, Okagaki T, Pass F, Faras A J 1982 Detection of human papillomavirus DNA in anogenital neoplasias. Nature 300: 771–773
zur Hausen H 1982 Human genital cancer: synergism between two virus infections or synergism between a virus infection and initiating events. Lancet ii: 1370–1372

The climacteric

Unlike the ageing male, in whom sex steroid production changes little, the ageing female is subjected to a major endocrine insult by a marked decline in gonadal function which usually occurs either late in the fourth or early in the fifth decade of life. Partial gonadal failure gives rise to the climacteric, the 2 to 3 year transitional phase during which reproduction ceases and which, when complete, leads to the postmenopause. The endocrine changes associated with the climacteric and postmenopause attracted little interest and were of minimal clinical consequence as recently as 50 years ago because the mean female life expectancy in the United Kingdom at this time was approximately 61 years. Therefore, the postmenopausal population was small.

Today, however, the mean female life expectancy approaches 83 years and the postmenopausal population numbers 9.6 million, comprising 18% of the total population of the United Kingdom. The special problems posed by large numbers of climacteric and postmenopausal women in terms of morbidity, mortality and utilisation of health resources are thus a relatively recent development and our knowledge of them remains incomplete.

Major advances have, however, been made in the understanding of the short and long-term sequelae of oestrogen-deprivation. The main purpose of this article is to review the clinical consequences of ovarian failure and to discuss the benefits and hazards of the treatments used to combat them. The pathophysiological and endocrine aspects of oestrogen deficiency have been presented and reviewed elsewhere (Studd et al 1977a, Upton 1982, Whitehead 1983), and are only briefly referred to here.

Consequences of ovarian failure

The climacteric has only one constant feature — the menopause or last menstrual bleed — and unscheduled bleeding per vaginam must be regarded as abnormal and demands appropriate investigation. In certain women, the climacteric is associated with the development of various physical and psychological symptoms often referred to collectively as the 'Menopausal Syndrome'. Additionally, it is related to the onset of a reduction in bone mass relative to bone volume and with the development of what are currently believed to be adverse changes in blood lipid and lipoprotein concentrations. The clinical consequences of these latter events, although not arising until much later in the postmenopause, still stem at least in part from oestrogen-deficiency.

MENOPAUSAL SYNDROME

Vasomotor instability

Hot flushes and night sweats are widely accepted as resulting from oestrogen lack. They are the most typical acute symptoms and often develop early during the climacteric when menstruation, albeit irregular, is still occurring. Flushes and sweats are experienced by between 50 and 75% of climacteric and immediately postmenopausal women (McKinley & Jeffreys 1974), and although self-limiting to a degree last longer than 5 years in approximately 20–25% of women (Thompson et al 1973).

Although hot flushes have been present from time immemorial, only one large-scale study has attempted to document the resultant morbidity and subjective experience (Voda 1981), and the first report detailing the physiological effects of flushing episodes did not appear until 1975 (Molnar 1975). In her series of observations on 929 hot flushes, Voda (1981) reported that 49% were described as mild but fairly noticeable, 39% were moderate lasting up to 2 or 3 minutes and 12% were severe and associated with profuse sweating. The magnitude of the changes in peripheral and central body temperature during flushing/sweating episodes recorded in one post-menopausal subject during a 90 minute period are illustrated in Fig. 21.1 (Molnar 1975). Central body temperature measured either within the rectum or at the tympanic membrane declined by 0.6°C to 0.7°C whereas finger and toe temperature rose by approximately 5°C. Similar data on peripheral temperature changes using thermocouple methodology have been reported by Sturdee et al (1978b) and by Meldrum et al (1979, 1980). Flushing episodes are also associated with marked increases in heart rate of up to 20 beats per minute, fluctuations in baseline electrocardiographic recordings, a decrease in skin resistance and peripheral vasodilatation (Sturdee et al 1978b, Meldrum et al 1979, 1980).

Application of this type of methodology in conjunction with continuous EEG monitoring has shown a highly significant correlation between nocturnal flushing and sweating with episodes of wakefulness (Erlik et al 1981). In this series, 47 hot flushes and sweats were observed in 9 subjects during sleep and 45 were associated with a waking episode. Thus, oestrogen-deficient women can be subject to chronic and repeated interruptions of normal sleep rhythms and the extent to which these affect mental processes and well-being remains to be elucidated but is likely to be considerable.

The physiological changes observed during flushing and sweating episodes are, for the most part, a normal pattern of responses to an increase in central

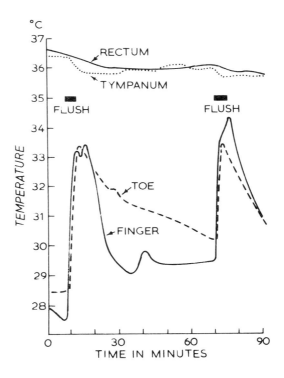

Fig. 21.1 Changes in peripheral (toe and finger) and central (rectum and tympanum) temperatures during episodes of flushing in a postmenopausal woman (adapted from Molnar (1975) and reproduced with permission)

body temperature. However, the core temperature of climacteric and postmenopausal women is not elevated and thus the temperature-regulating centre appears to be responding in a normal manner but to an inappropriate stimulus. The source of these stimuli remains to be identified but is almost certainly within the hypothalamus. The cause of these stimuli also requires elucidation and detailed discussion of the possible aetiological mechanisms is beyond the scope of this review but can be found elsewhere (Upton 1982, Lightman 1982). Suffice it to say that it has been proposed that peripheral oestradiol-17β deficiency results in a reduction in the hypothalamic levels of the catechol oestrogen, 2-hydroxyoestradiol-17β. As a result, the competition for biogenic amine binding sites between catechol oestrogens and catecholamines is disturbed. Sympathetic drive may thus be enhanced and thermo-regulatory and cardiovascular disturbances are the result. It should be noted that although pulsatile release of LH is associated with flushing episodes (Meldrum et al 1980) this relationship is not causal and LH depletion by synthetic Gn-Rh analogues does not abolish hot flushes (Lightman 1982).

End-organ atrophy

The vagina and urethra have a common embryological origin and oestrogen deficiency may result in atrophy of both. Symptomatic sequelae, which are not self-limiting, include dyspareunia, apareunia and recurrent bacterial infections. In the urethra, repeated infections may lead to fibrosis which predisposes to frequency, dysuria and urgency, the 'distal urethral syndrome' (Smith 1972).

Psychological symptoms

The controversy as to whether oestrogen deficiency *per se* gives rise to psychological symptoms has arisen for three reasons. Firstly, the various studies which have investigated the relationships between ovarian failure and psychological symptoms have been performed on different groups of women. Secondly, the results have on occasions been misinterpreted and lastly, bias has been introduced into the epidemiological investigations.

Data on the nature and incidence rates of symptoms reported to clinicians at menopause clinics (Studd et al 1977a) should be interpreted as applying only to selected groups of women and as such are valuable. These data should not be applied to unselected groups of women within the community who, for the most part, experience less severe symptoms (Jaszmann 1973). Thus, it is not surprising that comparisons between 'menopause clinic' and epidemiological data reveal inconsistencies and contradictions. Unfortunately, many of the earlier epidemiological studies were flawed and the methodological weaknesses included lack of adequate definition of menopausal status; poor sampling and the introduction of bias, the study obviously being connected with the climacteric and postmenopausal eras. These weaknesses are likely to have distorted the results and thus further fuelled the controversy surrounding oestrogen status and psychological symptomatology.

Examples of results from a recent epidemiological survey (Bungay et al 1980), which overcame most of these problems are shown in Fig. 21.2. Both sexes were studied, the men in a sense serving as controls, across a broad age band of 30–64 years. The subjects were advised that the questionnaire was investigating general health and were not aware of the true aim of the study. Peaks of prevalence of flushing and sweating were closely associated with the climacteric and interestingly, difficulty in making decisions and loss of confidence also peaked around this time. Similar responses were obtained for anxiety, forgetfulness, difficulty in concentration and feelings of unworthiness. These 'psychological' symptoms reached peak prevalence immediately prior to the mean age of menopause and the earlier observations of Jaszmann (1973) and Ballinger (1975) were thus confirmed.

These more recent data, obtained from unselected groups of women within the community without prior knowledge of the aims of the survey, provide strong evidence that psychological symptoms cluster during the climacteric.

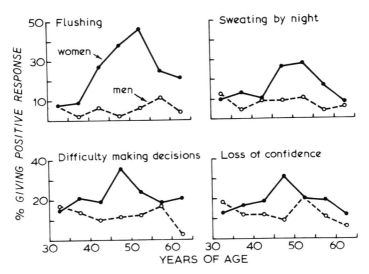

Fig. 21.2 Symptom patterns by age and sex (from Bungay et al (1980), reproduced with permission)

Possible causative factors apart from oestrogen-deficiency include concurrent, but coincidental, socio-domestic-economic crises. Importantly, analysis of data about adverse life events by Bungay et al (1980) showed little evidence of these problems clustering during the climacteric. Children tended to cause parental anxiety at this time and although there was a positive association with symptomatology, the characteristic patterns referred to previously were equally apparent in those who had no problems with their children.

Postmenopausal osteoporosis and related fractures

The relationships between ovarian failure and postmenopausal bone mass have recently been reviewed in another article in this series (Hart 1982). Since then, new data have become available on the pathogenesis and consequences of postmenopausal osteoporosis and the following comments therefore complement the previous review.

Pathophysiology

Postmenopausal bone loss apparently results from an increase in bone resorption and the relative loss of trabecular bone exceeds that of cortical bone. The pathogenesis remains to be elucidated precisely but recent studies have shed some light and should lead to a reappraisal of previous concepts. A popular belief has been that the increased bone resorption is secondary to malabsorption of calcium (Nordin 1960), with bone calcium being mobilised homoeostatically to maintain adequate plasma levels. Theoretically, two mechanisms could be responsible: a primary intestinal defect of calcium absorption or a primary defect of 1,25 dihydroxy vitamin D production by the kidney. 1, 25 dihydroxy vitamin D is the most potent of the known metabolites of vitamin D and is a powerful stimulator of calcium absorption in the intestine. If intestinal calcium malabsorption were responsible, then plasma calcium levels would tend to the lower side of normal and compensatory increases in the levels of parathyroid hormone (PTH) and 1, 25 dihydroxy vitamin D would be expected. PTH and 1, 25 dihydroxy vitamin D are the principal bone-resorbing hormones and are intimately related to maintenance of plasma calcium levels. However, it is now known that the circulating levels of PTH and 1, 25 dihydroxy vitamin D are not elevated in postmenopausal women, whether osteoporotic (Gallagher et al 1979) or non-osteoporotic (Stevenson et al 1982); indeed, they tend to be lowered. A renal defect has also been excluded by the demonstration of normal renal production of 1,25 dihydroxy vitamin D in postmenopausal osteoporotics (Riggs et al 1981).

Thus, if the postmenopausal increase in bone resorption is not primarily attributable to increases in the circulating levels of the bone-resorbing hormones or to calcium malabsorption, the concept of increased skeletal sensitivity to the *actions* of the bone-resorbing hormones becomes more tenable. A direct action of oestrogen in preventing bone resorption seems unlikely because receptors for this steroid have not been found in bone. Therefore, it is probable that oestrogen controls bone resorption indirectly. It has recently been shown that oestrogen regulates the secretion of calcitonin, a single-chain, 32 amino-acid peptide whose major function in man appears to be protection of the skeleton against excessive vitamin D-induced bone resorption (Stevenson et al 1979, 1981, Whitehead et al 1981b). There is a marked sex difference in calcitonin levels, with lower values in women (Hillyard et al 1978) and the age-related decline in secretion (Deftos et al 1980) may render the postmenopausal women particularly calcitonin-deficient. Thus, loss of ovarian function may accelerate the age-related decline in calcitonin secretion and as a result the actions of the bone-resorbing hormones are unopposed in postmenopausal women. The effects of exogenous oestrogen therapy on the circulating levels of the major calcium-regulating hormones are considered further below.

Consequences of osteoporosis

The rise in the incidence of fractures of the wrist, vertebral body and femoral neck which is associated with postmenopausal osteoporosis have been referred to previously (Hart 1982). In terms of morbidity, mortality and cost, the consequences of fracture of the femoral neck are the most important and have recently been reviewed (Stevenson & Whitehead 1982). Despite the widespread introduction of orthopaedic techniques, such as internal fixation designed to aid early mobilisation, the residual morbidity in terms of pain and loss of mobility remains 25% 12 months after fracture. By the late 1970s, fracture of the proximal femur ranked third in the list of use of non-psychiatric beds in England and Wales, and it has been calculated from the Hospital In-Patient Enquiry data that 31 618 women aged over 45 years were admitted with this diagnosis during 1977, the last year for which figures are currently available. The mortality in hospital, 16.8%, was about 20 times that expected for a population of this age and it has been calculated that the number of bed-days used by fracture of the proximal femur due to postmenopausal osteoporosis in 1977 amounted to 677, 597 at an estimated cost of £48 million (Stevenson & Whitehead 1982). If current trends continue, this drain on health resources can only increase because the incidence of femoral neck fracture has recently risen sharply and the overall increase in bed use between 1968 and 1977 was 48%. To this must be added the consequences of wrist and spinal fractures which in total are devastating both for the postmenopausal population and the resources of the National Health Service. By age 75 years, 50% of women will have sustained one or more of these three fractures.

Similar data are available from the USA. Approximately 125 000 femoral neck fractures occurred in older women in 1979 (Judd et al 1981) and the estimated costs exceed one billion dollars per year. It has been calculated that at least 15 000 women die as a result of this fracture each year in North America.

Lipids and cardiovascular disease

Although the effects of ovarian failure on plasma lipid and lipoprotein concentrations were documented many years ago (Oliver & Boyd 1959) their interpretation in terms of clinical sequelae remains controversial.

Cessation of ovarian function is followed by an increase in plasma cholesterol and triglyceride levels; a reduction in high density lipoprotein (HDL) and an increase in very low density lipoprotein (VLDL). All these changes are usually interpreted as being adverse given that an increased predisposition to ischaemic heart disease (IHD) has, at various times, been associated with hypercholesterolaemia, hypertriglyceridaemia, low levels of HDL and a reduced high density lipoprotein/low density lipoprotein (HDL/LDL) ratio (Carlson & Bottiger 1972, Yaari et al 1981). Additionally, an inverse relationship between HDL levels and the incidence of IHD has been reported (Miller & Miller 1975, Gordon et al 1977, Yaari et al 1981). Two sets of epidemiological data support this interpretation. Firstly, it is well established that premature menopause or early castration is associated with an accelerated development and increase in incidence of IHD (Vessey 1972, Gordon 1978, Rosenberg et al 1981). Secondly, the frequency of IHD is much lower in women that men under the age of 50 years but this difference is reduced with advancing age and by 80 years the death rates in the sexes are similar (Mortality Statistics 1977).

Alternative explanations of the mechanisms whereby oestrogens and the risk of IHD are linked are available. It has been suggested that this association is mediated via cigarette consumption which is known to be related to an earlier age of natural menopause and to be a risk factor for IHD. However, this concept has recently been challenged as the lowering of the mean age of menopause in tobacco users is small (Kaufmann et al 1980). It has also been proposed that the increase in incidence rates for IHD observed in older women is not real, but apparent, and result not from oestrogen deficiency but from a reduction in these rates in older men (Heller & Jacobs 1978).

DIAGNOSIS

Broadly speaking, women seeking medical advice do so either because they are already symptomatic or because, although asymptomatic, they are concerned about the long-term risks of oestrogen deficiency.

The typical nature and temporal association of acute vasomotor disturbances and the symptoms of lower genital tract atrophy with oligomenorrhoea or amenorrhoea makes their misdiagnosis unlikely. Other conditions associated with flushing and sweating, such as phaeochromocytoma, carcinoid disease and thyroid disease, cause additional symptoms which should make the diagnosis obvious. Because plasma gonadotrophin and oestrogen concentrations fluctuate widely during the climacteric (Murray & Hutton 1978), detailed biochemical investigations are often of little value in diagnosis and symptoms are always the best guide. Endocrine investigations cannot accurately predict the eventual severity and duration of symptoms nor the response to therapy. The greatest challenge to the clinician is establishing whether psychological disturbances are due to oestrogen deficiency or result from coincidental but concurrent socio-domestic-economic crises. Those 'psychological' symptoms clustering during the climacteric have been detailed above and whilst the contribution that adverse life events make to psychological retardation may be less than was previously believed (Bungay et al 1980) enquiry should always be made as to their presence. Accurate diagnosis is essential because symptoms resulting from domestic problems are best treated by psychiatrists, marriage guidance counsellors or social workers — not by drug therapy. When diagnosis proves difficult, biochemical investigations may be of value because high plasma oestrogen levels exclude ovarian failure, though the converse does not necessarily apply.

Long-term consequences

The diagnosis of severe, generalised osteoporosis and/or fractures is usually made from radiographs. Symptomatic treatment is all that can be offered, the aims being to relieve pain and to restore and then maintain mobility, however limited. This is because no therapy can restore bone mass to normal after it has been lost. Therefore, *prevention* of bone loss and osteoporotic fractures requires prophylactic therapy with an effective, bone-conserving treatment.

Loss of bone mass varies widely between postmenopausal women (Aitken 1976) but at present no simple, reliable, screening technique is available to identify the group of 'fast' bone losers most at risk of the later development of osteoporosis (Crilly et al 1978). Additionally, none of the techniques which measure bone mass accurately is suitable for screening large populations of postmenopausal women (Stevenson & Whitehead 1982). In the absence of an effective, screening programme, bone-conserving therapy has to be prescribed in an empirical fashion.

Certain groups of postmenopausal women are known to be at an increased risk of the later development of osteoporosis and these include those who have undergone premature menopause, in whom osteoporosis and related fractures develop early and tend to be severe (Johansson et al 1975); those with a strong family history of osteoporosis and those who are thin (adipose tissue converts precursors into oestrogen in postmenopausal women). Additionally, prophylactic bone-sparing therapy should also be considered in those relatively young postmenopausal women, in their late fifties or early sixties, who have already suffered an osteoporotic fracture, usually of the distal radius. The initiation of effective therapy at this stage may prevent against the later development of fractures of the vertebral body and proximal femur.

TREATMENT

Attitudes to the consequences of ovarian failure range from those who regard them as God-given events, to be endured stoically and without complaint, to those who regard the climacteric and postmenopausal years as representing a true endocrine-deficiency state with oestrogen therapy the panacea for all ills arising during this time. Informed opinion, for the most part, has remained between these two extremes with active therapy being considered when the physical/psychological well-being is adversely affected.

Non-hormonal preparations

Although widely prescribed, hypnotics, sedatives and tranquillisers have not been shown capable of relieving symptoms due to oestrogen deficiency and will not be considered further.

Clayden (1973) first observed that clonidine (Dixarit: Boehringer Ingleheim Limited) appeared to relieve hot flushes and numerous similar anecdotal reports followed. Four placebo-controlled, cross-over studies have been performed — with treatment periods ranging from only 2 to 6 weeks.

Clayden et al (1974) and Edington et al (1980) reported that both placebo and clonidine produced beneficial effects when either was given as the first course of treatment. Thus, climacteric and postmenopausal women appear to be placebo-responsive. Clonidine was better than placebo and this discrepancy was more marked in patients who started with placebo and then crossed-over to clonidine than vice-versa. In hypertensive patients, Bolli & Simpson (1975) also observed a placebo response and clonidine was more effective than placebo only when prescribed at a dosage of 150 μg daily. Ylikorkala (1975) studied younger women immediately after castration and reported beneficial clonidine effects with little placebo response.

In studies of longer duration, Lindsay & Hart (1978) reported a failure of response of vasomotor symptoms to clonidine and the two studies which have compared clonidine with oestrogen therapy (Barr 1975, Sonnendecker & Polakow 1980) both reported that oestrogen was significantly better.

Oestrogen therapy

An understanding of the effects of oestrogen administration depends upon a knowledge of the endocrinology of exogenous oestrogens. This has recently been reviewed in detail (Siddle & Whitehead 1983) and is only summarised here.

Exogenous oestrogens can be prescribed orally or parenterally, either percutaneously or trans-vaginally as creams or subcutaneously by implantation. The pharmacodynamics and biochemical effects of exogenous oestrogens can vary markedly with the route of administration.

Oral oestrogens

The oral route is most widely used, partly because of tradition and partly because of convenience. The major difference between this route and the parenteral routes is that only the oral route exposes the administered oestrogen to the gastro-intestinal tract, the portal venous system and the liver.

The gastro-intestinal tract affects oestrogen pharmacodynamics by preferentially converting oestradiol to oestrone (Ryan & Engel 1953). The portal venous system rapidly transfers the absorbed steroid, almost in the form of a 'bolus', into hepatic tissue where much of the administered oestrogen is metabolised and inactivated even before the systemic circulation is reached. This is known as the 'first pass' effect. The rapid metabolism is illustrated in Fig. 21.3 which shows the plasma levels of oestrone-3-glucuronide, an inactive metabolite, in three groups of postmenopausal women, all receiving oestradiol-preparations, at 3-hourly intervals during a 24 hour profile. Therapy had been initiated 6–8 weeks earlier. One group took oral oestradiol valerate (Progynova; Schering Chemicals), 2 mg daily; the second group administered percutaneous oestradiol cream (Oestrogel; Laboratories Besins Iscovesco), 5 g at night (containing 3 mg oestradiol), and the third group had received a subcutaneous implant of oestradiol, 50 mg. Glucuronidation of oestrogen occurs almost exclusively in the liver and percutaneous and subcutaneous oestradiol administration were not associated with an increase in plasma oestrone-3-glucuronide levels. However, the concentrations were elevated with oral therapy and surged further, following tablet ingestion at 21.00 hours, achieving a 3-fold increase above basal levels.

Delivery of the administered oestrogen into hepatic tissue has three clinical consequences. Firstly, because of the rapid inactivation, the prescribed dosage

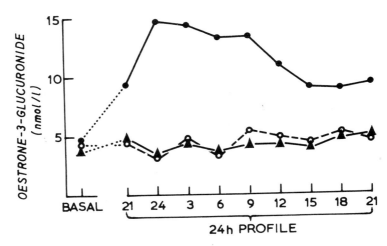

Fig. 21.3 Mean plasma oestrone-3-glucuronide levels in postmenopausal women before and then during therapy with oestradiol given orally, percutaneously or subcutaneously. For details of preparations and dosages, see text (●) oral oestradiol; (○) percutaneous oestradiol; (△) subcutaneous oestradiol (from Campbell & Whitehead (1982), reproduced with permission)

may have to be increased if effective control of symptoms which occur throughout a 24 hour period, such as daytime flushes and night sweats, is to be achieved with once daily administration. Secondly, induction of liver enzymes, particularly the glucuronidase enzymes, by other drug therapy such as hydantoin use for epilepsy, may result in such rapid oestrogen inactivation that the administered steroid is not clinically effective. Thirdly, the rates of synthesis of various hepatically-derived macromolecules are influenced by the oestrogen environment and the orally administered oestrogen may adversely or beneficially affect their production rates and thereby influence the risk of disease. For example, the liver partially or wholly synthesises renin substrate, anti-thrombin III and high and low density lipoprotein and changes in the production rates may alter the risk of hypertension (Laragh et al 1967, Eggena et al 1978), hypercoagulability and venous thrombosis (van der Meer et al 1973, Mackie et al 1978) and arterial disease (Gordon et al 1977, Yaari et al 1981), respectively. Thus, oral oestrogens should most probably not be prescribed to women predisposed to hypertension since therapy may increase renin substrate production; and should not be given to women with a history of 'clotting disorders' because anti-thrombin III activity may be depressed. In these patients, parenteral administration is to be preferred because changes in coagulation factors appear to be minimised (Elkik et al 1982). Conversely, oral oestrogens are more potent than parenterally-administered oestrogens at elevating plasma HDL-cholesterol (Fahraeus et al 1982), thereby beneficially increasing the HDL/LDL ratio. Thus, they are to be preferred in women with certain types of abnormal lipid profile who are at an increased risk of arterial disease. Such women include those with type IIa hyperlipoproteinaemia because oral natural oestrogen therapy has been shown to reduce the abnormal lipid excess, the profile becoming more normal (Tikkanen et al 1978). With other forms of abnormal lipid profile, such as hypertriglyceridaemia, the lipid excess may become gross and oestrogens are best avoided.

It should be noted that the hepatic effects of the synthetic oestrogens, such as ethinyl oestradiol and mestranol, are much more pronounced than those of the natural oestrogens, such as oestradiol valerate and piperazine oestrone sulphate (Harmogen: Abbott Laboratories). By virtue of their structure, the synthetic oestrogens have a greater affinity for the oestrogen receptor and are not substrates for the intra-cellular enzymes which normally degrade oestrogens. Because of this enhanced hepatic potency (Brenner et al 1982), the synthetic oestrogens are best avoided in postmenopausal women unless given in small dosages. The effects of 5 μg ethinyl oestradiol approximate those of 1.25 mg conjugated oestrogens (Premarin: Ayerst Laboratories) in terms of induction of renin substrate (Brenner et al 1982), but whilst there are good data showing beneficial effects of this dose of the natural oestrogen on climacteric symptomatology (Campbell & Whitehead 1977) and bone status (Meema et al 1975, Lindsay 1982), there is no evidence that such low dosages of ethinyl oestradiol are equally therapeutic.

Parenteral oestrogens

Apart from the indications stated previously, parenteral oestrogens are of value when oral therapy causes epigastric discomfort and flatulence; and when patients have a psychological aversion to taking tablets. Subcutaneous implantation produces plasma profiles of oestradiol and oestrone which most closely approximate those seen during the ovulatory cycle (Studd 1979, Campbell & Whitehead 1982); and this method of administration appears to be particularly well tolerated by women with premature menopause who may have to be on therapy for many years. When combined with subcutaneous testosterone, oestradiol implants have been shown to improve psychosexual problems, such as loss of libido and anorgasmia (Studd et al 1977b).

It should be noted that the vaginal epithelium is as effective as the gastro-intestinal tract at absorbing oestrogens because plasma oestradiol and oestrone concentrations following cream administration are in and above the ranges observed after oral ingestion of an identical oestrogen dosage (Whitehead et al 1978). Vaginal administration of oestrogens can depress gonadotrophin concentrations and lead to endometrial proliferation, eventually resulting in the development of endometrial hyperplasia (Widholm & Vartianen 1974, Whitehead et al 1978). Thus, with natural oestrogen preparations, truly 'topical or local' therapy, which only affects lower genital tract tissues and which does not stimulate distant end-organs, is not available at present because the manufacturers' minimum recommended dosages result in systemic absorption.

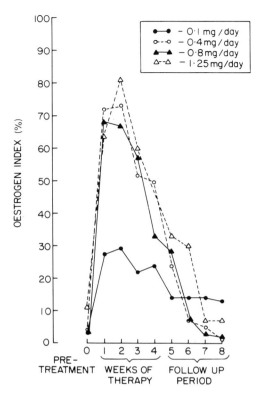

Fig. 21.4 Mean oestrogen index (vaginal Cytology) in four groups of postmenopausal women before and then during therapy with different dilutions of conjugated oestrogen cream (from Dyer et al (1982), reproduced with permission)

It has recently been shown in a dose-ranging study that much smaller oestrogen dosages can result in values for vaginal cytology which are within the pre-menopausal range (Dyer et al 1982). These data are presented in Fig. 21.4 and four different dilutions of conjugated oestrogen cream, 0.1, 0.4, 0.8 and 1.25 mg, were administered each night to postmenopausal women for 1 month. Vaginal cytology was assessed at weekly intervals during therapy and for 1 month afterwards. The lowest dose, 0.1 mg at night, induced vaginal cytology values of approximately 30% within the ovulatory cycle range. Supra-physiological responses were obtained with the higher dosages. Additionally, the lowest dose cause no appreciable increase in plasma oestrogen concentrations (data not shown) and further long-term studies are needed to determine whether this small dosage stimulates vulnerable end-organs such as the endometrium.

In summary, the manufacturers' recommended dosages of the currently available natural oestrogen preparations produce plasma oestradiol and oestrone levels within the premenopausal proliferative phase range and it is against this background that the benefits, side-effects and hazards of therapy have to be weighed.

Benefits of treatment

Symptomatic and psychological status

Lack of space prohibits a detailed review of these aspects and the interested reader is referred to recent reviews (Utian 1977, Dennerstein & Burrows 1978, Whitehead 1983). These previous reviews have emphasised the paucity of properly designed, placebo-controlled, single or double-blind (and therefore scientifically valid) studies which have evaluated the effects of oestrogens on the symptomatic and psychological status of climacteric and postmenopausal women. The importance of a cross-over and the ethical problems that placebo therapy causes the investigator have already been referred to with regard to the evaluation of clonidine in the relief of vasomotor instability. Because postmenopausal women are highly placebo-responsive, the results of uncontrolled studies are of little value.

Whilst there is good agreement between the controlled studies that oestrogens are significantly better than placebo in relieving vasomotor instability, insomnia and the symptoms of lower genital tract atrophy, the observed effects on the psychological status vary widely and these discrepancies appear due, for the most part, to differences in trial design. The duration of therapy, methods of assessment and information given to the patient have varied between the studies. An additional, and probably unforeseen problem which limited one study was the high 'drop-out' rate. Kantor et al (1973) investigated the effects of conjugated oestrogens 0.625 mg daily on prevention of deterioration in cortical function but due mainly to death, only nine of the 25 patients in the placebo group completed the trial.

The differences in response after the cross-over which were observed by Clayden et al (1974) and Edington et al (1980) during clonidine studies have also been reported in the evaluation of oestrogen therapy. Coope (1976) observed similar responses to conjugated oestrogens, 1.25 mg daily and placebo when either was given as the first course of treatment. Only after the cross-over at 3 months did Coope (1976) observe gross disparities between treatments — the group then receiving placebo experiencing a recurrence of vasomotor symptoms. For ethical reasons, patients had been informed that they were to receive an inert preparation at some stage of the trial and it is possible that with the return of hot flushes patients surmised that they were taking placebo. The objectivity of the assessments is likely to have been influenced greatly.

The two largest double-blind, placebo-controlled, cross-over studies published to date (Campbell & Whitehead 1977, Dennerstein et al 1979a, b) both reported improvements with oestrogen therapy over placebo for a variety of psychological symptoms including anxiety, agitation, depression and irritability but the authors have disagreed over the most appropriate method for assessing psychological change (Dennerstein et al 1979b). In patients with severe climacteric disturbances, Campbell & Whitehead (1977) reported that certain psychological symptoms, such as irritability, were only relieved secondary to the abolition of hot flushes and thus, a 'domino' effect appeared to be operating. However, other psychological symptoms, such as poor memory, anxiety, worry about age and worry about self were significantly improved in non-flushing patients and the authors concluded that oestrogens appear to exert a direct 'mental tonic' effect. The earlier observations of Utian (1972) were thus confirmed.

The effects of synthetic oestrogens do not appear to have been determined in placebo-controlled studies. Thus, no data are available on the physical and psychological effects of small dosages of the synthetic oestrogens.

Only one study has compared the psychological effects of oestrogen therapy with those of clonidine. Conjugated oestrogens significantly improved various measures of depression and anxiety whereas clonidine had no beneficial psychological effects (Gerdes et al 1982).

Bone Loss and Related Fractures

For once, the literature reporting the effects of oestrogens on an end-organ is in agreement and six prospective, placebo-controlled studies have established that oestrogens conserve bone mass in both non-osteoporotic (Lindsay et al 1976, 1980, Horsman et al 1977, Recker et al 1977, Nachtigall et al 1979, Christiansen et al 1980) and osteoporotic postmenopausal women (Nordin et al 1980). These studies have also clearly demonstrated that oestrogens are more effective than calcium supplementation; sodium fluoride; vitamin D; one alpha vitamin D and thiazide diuretics in this respect. Until recently, however, there was no evidence that long-term oestrogen therapy would prevent against fractures but the publication of three retrospective case-controlled studies from the United States and one prospective study from the United Kingdom now leaves little doubt that this is so (Hutchinson et al 1979, Lindsay et al 1980, Weiss et al 1980, Paganini-Hill et al 1981). The retrospective studies reported reductions in fracture rates of the distal radius and proximal femur of approximately 60%. In general, greater benefits were observed in those oestrogen-exposed women who began therapy shortly after the menopause; had received treatment for more than 5 years; were continuing to use oestrogens and those who had previously been castrated. In the prospective study which extended over 9 years, the placebo-treated group had a higher incidence of vertebral compression fractures and had experienced a significant reduction in height as compared to the oestrogen-exposed women (Lindsay et al 1980).

These bone-sparing actions are likely to weigh heavily in favour of oestrogens in any cost-benefit analysis. For reasons to be discussed below, it is now recommended that progestogens be combined with oestrogens to prevent against hyperstimulation of the endometrium. Concern has been expressed that the added progestogen might oppose the beneficial effects of oestrogen on bone status. This fear is without substantiation and combined oestrogen/progestogen regimens are now known to conserve bone mass (Nachtigall et al 1979, Christiansen et al 1981). Indeed, data are now becoming available suggesting that certain types of progestogens, such as norethisterone (Primolut; Schering Chemicals), conserve bone mass when given alone. The mechanism of action is unknown but is possibly mediated through competitive antagonism for the glucocorticoid receptor.

The response of the skeleton to termination of oestrogen therapy remains to be elucidated. Lindsay et al (1978) and Horsman et al (1979) both reported enhanced loss of bone following oestrogen withdrawal and thereby concluded that short-term therapy, of between 2 and 4 years, had no lasting beneficial effect on bone mass. These findings are at variance with those of Christiansen et al (1981) who reported that bone loss following withdrawal of therapy was not accelerated. Whereas Christiansen et al (1981) studied postmenopausal women who had undergone a natural menopause, Lindsay et al (1978) investigated castrated women in whom the rate of bone loss is known to be greater. Christiansen has suggested that the accelerated rate of bone loss observed by Lindsay's group following oestrogen withdrawal was due to the type of menopause. Further data are needed to confirm or refute this suggestion.

As stated previously, the lower calcitonin values in women and the age-related decline in calcitonin secretion may render the postmenopausal woman particularly susceptible to the actions of the principal bone-resorbing hormones, PTH and 1,25 dihydroxy vitamin D. Oral ethinyl oestradiol and percutaneous oestradiol cream significantly increase plasma calcitonin levels (Stevenson et al 1982), the data clearly showing that calcitonin secretion is oestrogen-dependent. Calcitonin opposes the bone-resorbing actions of PTH and 1,25 dihydroxyvitamin D (Stevenson et al 1979, 1981, Whitehead et al 1981b) and postmenopausal calcitonin lack would be predicted to result in a relative increase in bone resorption.

This concept explains the apparent increased sensitivity of the postmenopausal skeleton to the action of the bone-resorbing hormones (Jasani et al 1965), although the circulating levels of these hormones are not elevated (Stevenson et al 1981). It also explains the failure of vitamin D therapy to conserve bone mass. Since levels of calcitonin vary between women (Stevenson et al 1979) some may be more calcitonin deficient than others and therefore, tend to lost bone more rapidly after the menopause. Thus, they would be at greatest risk of the development of osteoporosis and calcitonin levels have been reported to be lower in osteoporotics than in controls (Milhaud et al 1978).

HAZARDS OF OESTROGENS

Thrombo-embolic disease

The risk of thrombotic disease with postmenopausal oestrogen therapy have recently been the subject of a review (Notelovitz 1982b), to which the interested reader is referred. The synthetic oestrogens appear to cause more marked changes in fibrinolytic/coagulation mechanisms and are best avoided in postmenopausal women. All but three of the epidemiological studies which have investigated the relationships between postmenopausal oestrogen use and the incidence of thrombotic disease have reported no change in risk (Boston Collaborative Drug Surveillance Program 1974, Pfeffer & van den Noort 1976, Rosenberg et al 1976, 1980, Petitti et al 1978, Pfeffer et al 1978, Bain et al 1981). Of the exceptions, Jick et al (1978), reported an increase in risk in a group of younger women in their early 40s and Gordon (1978) observed a two-fold rise in the incidence of myocardial infarction in an older population but no increase in mortality. These findings contrast sharply with those of Ross et al (1981) who reported a reduction in incidence and death rate from IHD in long-term oestrogen-exposed postmenopausal women. At present, there is no compelling evidence that postmenopausal natural oestrogen therapy is associated with adverse cardiovascular effects.

Breast

During the last decade, numerous epidemiological studies have investigated the relationship between postmenopausal oestrogen use and the incidence of breast cancer but regrettably, the majority of those published before 1976 are seriously flawed (Cramer & Schiff 1982). Failure to correct for factors known to influence the risk of breast cancer, such as type of menopause, age at menopause, parity and age at birth of first child, have greatly undermined the validity of the results. Four recent studies of a higher quality because they allow for these confounding factors (Hoover et al 1976, Jick et al 1980, Ross et al 1980, Brinton et al 1981) have suggested that there may be a small increase in the risk of breast cancer following long-term oestrogen exposure but there are major discrepancies between the results. For example, whilst Ross et al (1980) and Jick et al (1980) reported that the risk appeared to be increased most in women with a natural menopause, Brinton et al (1981) observed the converse. Overall, the epidemiological evidence that postmenopausal oestrogen therapy increases the risk of breast cancer is neither strong nor consistent but further valid studies are required before firm conclusions can be drawn. The influence of oestrogen use on the risk of breast cancer in certain sub-groups of women usually at low risk, such as multiparas and those surgically castrated, may be especially important.

Endometrium

Various authors have discussed the relationship between oestrogens and endometrial cancer (Studd & Thom 1981) and have reviewed the retrospective studies which reported that prolonged administration of oestrogens to postmenopausal women is associated with an increase in the incidence of endometrial carcinoma (Knab 1977, Cramer & Schiff 1982). Despite the methodological flaws in some of these epidemiological investigations, the data provide persuasive evidence for a causal relationship, particularly with well-differentiated, Stage I tumours. Although the results are not entirely consistent, there is a suggestion that the risk increases with higher oestrogen dose and with duration of use. The 'background' risk of one case of endometrial cancer per thousand women per annum in an untreated population is increased by a factor of approximately 0.75 per year of oestrogen use reaching 4.8 after 5 years of treatment and 8.5 after 10 years of exposure. Not surprisingly, the adverse publicity generated by these data resulted in a decline in oestrogen use which has been quickly followed by a fall in the incidence of endometrial cancer (Jick et al 1979).

Prospective histological studies in the United Kingdom which have monitored the endometrial response to exogenous oestrogens have reported a 15–30% incidence of endometrial hyperplasia with oestrogen therapy alone (Whitehead et al 1979, Studd et al 1980). Up to one-third of the hyperplasias were of the more sinister atypical pattern which in its more severe forms is a well-recognised precursor of corpus cancer (Gusberg & Kaplan 1963). Importantly, the underlying endometrial status was not reflected by the pattern of bleeding per vaginam. Abnormal breakthrough bleeding was associated with both normal and hyperplastic endometrium, and some patients with endometrial hyperplasia experienced no vaginal bleeding (Whitehead et al 1979, Studd et al 1980).

The oestrogen-related cancers are *not* associated with an increased mortality (Chu et al 1982) and possible explanations for this dichotomy include early detection of the malignancy when surgery is curative and/or the tumours being less aggressive than those arising spontaneously because they are better differentiated (Robboy & Bradley 1979). Irrespective of the reasons for the low mortality the small, but definite, increase in risk of endometrial carcinoma has led to various suggestions regarding how the treatment regimen can be modified to protect the endometrium against hyperstimulation.

Possible alternatives include reducing the oestrogen dosage, avoiding oestrone preparations, and adding a progestogen to the oestrogen therapy. These have been reviewed in detail elsewhere (Studd & Thom 1982, Whitehead et al 1983) and are only summarised here. Dosage reductions are likely to reduce the beneficial effects of oestrogens in relieving not only the physical and psychological symptoms that constitute the menopausal syndrome but also in conserving bone mass, because these are clearly dose-related (Christensen et al 1982, Lindsay 1982). The minimum effective bone-sparing dosages of oestradiol valerate and conjugated oestrogens are 2 mg (Christensen et al 1982) and 0.625 mg (Lindsay 1982), respectively, and marked endometrial proliferation has been observed with these dosages (Sturdee et al 1978, Whitehead et al 1979, 1981c, Paterson et al 1980).

It has been suggested that because almost all the retrospective, American epidemiological studies associated only conjugated oestrogens (65% of which is oestrone sulphate) with an increase in risk of endometrial carcinoma, then this preparation must possess special carcinogenic properties (Ziel & Finkle 1976) not present with other formulations such as those containing oestradiol or oestriol. The assumption, that these latter preparations can be prescribed safely without a risk of hyperstimulation, is incorrect. Conjugated oestrogens were most closely linked with endometrial carcinoma because they are the most widely prescribed oestrogen preparation in the United States. At equivalent dosages, oral oestrone sulphate and oestradiol valerate cause the same degree of endometrial stimulation as conjugated oestrogens with almost identical rates of hyperplasia (Whitehead et al 1979).

Biochemical evaluation of the degree of oestrogen stimulation applied by a particular formulation may be quantified by measurements of nuclear oestradiol and cytoplasmic progesterone receptor (King et al 1979). Oestrogens stimulate the formation of not only their own receptor proteins, but also those for progesterone. Oestradiol and progesterone receptor levels during therapy with oral conjugated oestrogens, 0.625 and 1.25 mg; oral oestradiol valerate, 2 mg; oral oestrone sulphate, 1.5 mg; subcutaneous oestradiol implant, 50 mg and percutaneous oestradiol cream, 3 mg, are well within the premenopausal, proliferative-phase range (Whitehead et al 1981c), the time of maximal oestrogenic stimulation during the ovulatory cycle. The most likely explanation for this degree of stimulation is that even in postmenopausal women, oestradiol remains the predominant intra-nuclear oestrogen within the endometrium (King et al 1980, Whitehead et al 1981a). Oestradiol is the most potent natural stimulator of cell biosynthesis (King & Mainwaring 1974). Oral oestrone-based preparations, such as conjugated oestrogens and oestrone sulphate, give rise mainly to oestrone in plasma but a percentage of this is further converted to oestradiol; and the parenteral oestradiol-based preparations, such as oestradiol implants and oestradiol creams, selectively increase plasma oestradiol levels and are, therefore, likely to be associated with marked endometrial proliferation. Thus, the high incidence of hyperplasia reported with oestradiol implants (56%) if patients did not take the prescribed progestogen (Studd et al 1980) not surprising.

At low dosages, less than 2 mg daily, oestriol appears to have little proliferative effect on the endometrium (Myrhe 1978), and has therefore been recommended as the ideal oestrogen for postmenopausal use (Follingstad 1978). However, it is doubtful whether low-dose oestriol actually imparts an oestrogenic stimulus because, unlike all other preparations studied to date, low-dose oestriol does not conserve bone mass and is no better than placebo at relieving acute vasomotor symptoms (Lindsay et al 1979). Unlike oestradiol and oestrone, oestriol is not strongly bound to plasma proteins and globulins but circulates largely as the glucuronide and this facilitates rapid renal excretion. Thus, an oral dose of oestriol is absorbed and largely excreted within 3 hours. When administered at 8-hourly intervals, oestriol has been associated with the development of endometrial hyperplasia (Englund 1979).

The third alternative, of adding a progestogen to the oestrogen therapy, has been shown to be protective to the endometrium. The duration of progestogen exposure each month appears critical because the incidence of hyperplasia, 15–30% with oestrogen therapy alone, is reduced to 3–4% with 7 days of progestogen each month (Sturdee et al 1978, Whitehead et al 1979); and is further reduced, to zero, when progestogens are administered for more than 12 days each month (Studd et al 1980, Paterson et al 1980). Importantly, epidemiological investigations have shown that the addition of a progestogen reduces the incidence of endometrial cancer to below that in an untreated population (Gambrell 1978).

PROGESTOGENS AND PROGESTERONE

To support the argument for the widespread use of progestogens with postmenopausal oestrogen therapy, it is necessary to show that the benefits outweigh the disadvantages. A comprehensive benefit/side-effect analysis is beyond the scope of this article, but appropriate reviews have recently been published (Studd & Thom 1981, Upton 1982, Whitehead et al 1982). The various side-effects associated with progestogen addition can arise either after a short period of administration or may not become apparent until much later. The immediate manifestations include the re-establishment of vaginal bleeding in some patients and, in a small percentage of women, adverse changes in the symptomatic and psychological status which may partially negate the beneficial effects of exogenous oestrogens. The longer-term effects include a putative risk of increasing the incidence of arterial thrombo-embolic disease.

The resumption of vaginal bleeding after the menopause might be regarded as a significant side-effect that would be unacceptable to the majority of women. However, only 5% of our patients refuse treatment because of the possibility of bleeding, and 5% are intolerant of it when on therapy. The most common anxiety is that resumption of bleeding indicates a return of fertility, and it is important to discuss this before commencing therapy. The pattern of uterine bleeding during combined oestrogen/progestogen therapy is much more reliable as an indicator of underlying pathology as compared to that occurring with unopposed oestrogen treatment. In our series (Whitehead et al 1979), almost half of the patients receiving unopposed oestrogens (51 of 106 patients, 48%) bled at some time during the study period; of those with breakthrough bleeding, endometrial hyperplasia was diagnosed in only 9 of 25 patients. Thus, 16 patients underwent curettage yet had a normal endometrium. With combined oestrogen/progestogen regimens, regular withdrawal bleeding occurred in 67 of 76 patients (88%) and was invariably associated with a normal endometrium. Only seven patients experienced breakthrough bleeding and two were subsequently shown to have endometrial hyperplasia. Therefore, with the combined regimens, the incidence of breakthrough bleeding that many patients find troublesome and the need for endometrial curettage were dramatically reduced.

Combined oestrogen/progestogen therapy incorporating 500 μg/dl norgestrel exerts a less beneficial effect on mood, mastalgia and breast size than oestrogen alone (Dennerstein et al 1979a, b). However, data on symptomatic and psychological changes induced by such progestogen dosages are, for reasons stated below, of limited clinical relevance. It is now known that smaller progestogen dosages are equally protective to the endometrium, and reducing the dosage is likely to lower the incidence of adverse physical and psychological effects. Identical comments may also apply to the current concern regarding the putative, major, long-term risk of progestogens, an increase in risk of thrombo-embolic disease. During oral contraceptive therapy, adverse changes in plasma HDL-cholesterol concentrations (Larsson-Cohn et al 1979) and an increase in incidence of hypertension, myocardial infarction, and cerebro-vascular accident (Kay 1980) have been linked to the progestogen component in a dose-dependent manner. It is stressed that these long-term risks are putative and require substantiation, but they may negate the benefits of oestrogens in reducing the risk of death from ischaemic heart disease (Ross et al 1981). Reducing the daily progestogen dosage is also likely to reduce the effects on carbohydrate and lipid metabolism as these are clearly dose-related (Larsson-Cohn et al 1979, Notelovitz 1982b).

For reasons stated elsewhere (Whitehead et al 1982) the currently recommended dosages of the two progestogens most widely added to oestrogen therapy, norethisterone 10 mg daily and dl norgestrel 500 μg daily, were derived more from an empirical than a scientific basis. Recent studies which included biochemical as well as histological evaluation of the postmenopausal endometrium have clearly shown that these dosages of norethisterone and dl norgestrel can be reduced to 1 mg and 150 μg daily, respectively, without loss of protective effect. Biochemically, the stimulatory actions of oestrogens upon the endometrium can be quantitated by measurements of DNA synthesis and nuclear oestradiol receptor content (King et al 1979, 1981b) and progestogen antagonism of these effects through suppression of DNA synthesis and suppression of nuclear oestradiol receptor. Additionally, progestogens induce the activities of isocitric and oestradiol dehydrogenases (Whitehead et al 1979, King et al 1981a, b) and an increase in these activities during progestogen administration indicates an end-organ response. The data are illustrated in Fig. 21.5 (Whitehead et al 1981c) and clearly show that in terms of suppression of DNA synthesis, low doses of norethisterone, 1, 2.5, and 5 mg were more effective than the 10 mg dose. All four dosages of norethisterone and both dosages of dl norgestrel, 150 and 500 μg daily, reduced nuclear oestradiol receptor levels and increased the activities of both enzymes and the magnitude of these responses equalled or exceeded those seen in the secretory phase of the ovulatory cycle. Importantly, no dose-response relationships were observed in these studies and it was concluded that even lower dosages of norethisterone and dl norgestrel warrant evaluation. The histological data showed good agreement with the biochemical results. No endometrial hyperplasia was observed during combined oestrogen/progestogen therapy and the lower dosages of norethisterone and dl norgestrel were just as effective as the higher at producing secretory changes within the endometrium (Whitehead et al 1981c).

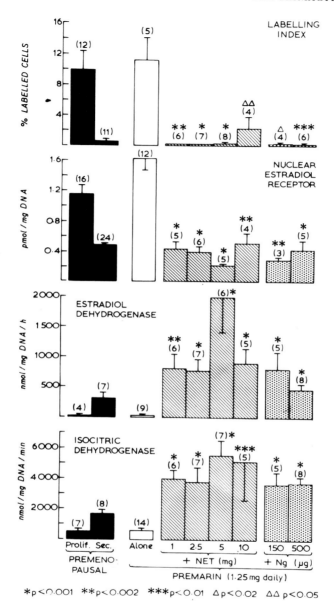

Fig. 21.5 Epithelial labelling index (DNA Synthesis), nuclear oestradiol receptor content and the activities of isocitric and oestradiol dehydrogenases in postmenopausal endometria during therapy with Premarin alone or in combination with the stated daily dose of Norethisterone (NET) or dl Norgestrel (Ng). Premenopausal proliferative (Prolif) and secretory-phase (Sec) ranges are included for comparison. Results are expressed as means ± s.e. mean. Figures in parenthesis denote numbers of observations. P values represent significant differences between treatment with Premarin alone and treatment with Premarin plus either progestogen (from Whitehead et al (1981c), reproduced with permission)

Further studies using the same methodology, the results of which are unpublished, have clearly shown that other types of progestogens also exert anti-oestrogenic effects within the endometrium and dose-response relationships have been established for oral progesterone and for dydrogesterone (Duphaston: Duphar Laboratories). Oral progesterone is well absorbed into the systemic circulation (Whitehead et al 1980) and dosages of 300 mg daily produce biochemical and histological responses similar to those observed in the secretory-phase of the ovulatory cycle. The minimum effective dosage of dydrogesterone appears to be approximately 20 mg daily. Further reductions in the dosage of norethisterone, to 0.35 mg daily, have not been associated with a loss of protective effect but a lowering of the dose of dl norgestrel, to 75 μg daily, has reduced the cellular response and approximately 20% of our patients on this low dosage have developed endometrial hyperplasia.

The development of combined oestrogen/progestogen therapies is in its infancy. It is stressed that data on adverse physical, psychological and metabolic effects induced by high daily dosages of progestogens are likely to become obsolete overnight with the introduction of the small progestogen dosage regimens. For example, in our experience, dl norgestrel 500 μg daily produces a pre-menstrual tension like syndrome with mastalgia in between 5 and 10% of patients but lowering the dosage to 150 μg daily results in a reduction in the frequency and intensity of these adverse changes. Likewise, whereas norethisterone 10 mg daily produces adverse effects on lipid and lipoprotein metabolism (Hirvonen et al 1981), norethisterone 1 mg daily does not (Christiansen et al 1983). Dosage appears all important in determining the range and severity of adverse progestogenic effects.

SUMMARY

Although the causative mechanisms remain to be determined, it is now known that hot flushes and night sweats cause profound physiological disturbances which are probably the basis of the acute physical discomfort of which so many symptomatic, climacteric and postmenopausal women complain. The importance of psychological changes is less clearly defined but the available data indicate that adverse psychological effects cluster during the climacteric. The importance of domestic-socio-economic crises as a cause of these 'mental' changes may be less than was previously believed.

In terms of morbidity, mortality and cost, the sequelae of osteoporosis must be regarded as the major consequence of oestrogen-deprivation and the primary aetiological factor in the genesis of postmenopausal bone loss is ovarian failure.

There are no scientifically valid data showing that hypnotics, sedatives and tranquillisers relieve the symptoms of the menopausal syndrome. The benefits of clonidine on vasomotor instability appear to be less than those of oestrogens, and unlike oestrogens, clonidine does not improve psychological symptoms.

Oestrogens may be prescribed orally or parenterally. The route of administration is probably of little consequence in apparently healthy women but may be important in determining the risks of oestrogen therapy in women with hypertension, abnormal coagulation/fibrinolytic mechanisms or abnormal lipid profiles. Synthetic oestrogens appear to be much more potent than their natural counterparts in altering hepato-cellular metabolism and are most probably best avoided in postmenopausal women.

In prospective and retrospective studies, oestrogens have been shown to conserve bone mass and at present, are to be regarded as the treatment of choice. They are more effective than all other therapies evaluated to date and are the only treatment which has been shown to reduce fracture rates. In the absence of a suitable screening test to identify the 'fast' bone-losers most at risk of the later development of osteoporosis, oestrogens have to be prescribed empirically. Such therapy should be mandatory following premature loss of ovarian function and should be seriously considered in high-risk patients who are thin, who have a strong family history of osteoporosis, or who have suffered an osteoporotic fracture at a relatively early age.

At the manufacturers' currently recommended dosages, all oestrone and oestradiol-based preparations cause marked endometrial proliferation and carry a risk of endometrial hyperstimulation and the later development of malignancy in predisposed individuals. Low dosages of oestriol do not appear to impart an oestrogenic stimulus because unlike all other oestrogen preparations studied to date, low dose oestriol does not conserve bone mass. At higher doses, oestriol has been associated with the development of endometrial hyperplasia.

The risk of endometrial hyperstimulation can be minimised by adding a progestogen for 12 days each calendar month. Concern has been expressed that progestogens may cause undesirable side-effects, but these risks appear to be minimised by reducing the daily progestogen dosage. Such dosage reductions are not associated with a loss of protective effect upon the endometrium. The development of combined oestrogen/progestogen therapies is in its infancy and it is probable that much research will be undertaken in the next 5 years to develop a combined regimen incorporating a progestogen devoid of adverse physical, psychological and metabolic effects.

Acknowledgements

The help of Miss H Mortimore in the preparation of this manuscript is much appreciated.

REFERENCES

Aitken J M 1976 Osteoporosis and its relation to oestrogen deficiency In: Campbell S (ed) The Management of the Menopause and Postmenopausal Years, pp 225–236. MTP Press, Lancaster

Bain C, Willett W, Hennekens C H, Rosner B, Belanger C, Speizer F E 1981 Use of postmenopausal hormones and risk of myocardial infarction. Circulation 64: 42–46

Ballinger C B 1975 Psychiatric morbidity and the menopause: screening of general population sample. British Medical Journal 3: 344–346

Barr W 1975 Problems related to postmenopausal women. South African Medical Journal 49: 437–439

Bolli P, Simpson 1975 Clonidine in menopausal flushing: a double-blind trial. New Zealand Medical Journal 82: 196–197

Boston Collaborative Drug Surveillance Program 1974 Surgically confirmed gall-bladder disease, venous thromboembolism and breast tumours in relation to postmenopausal estrogen therapy. New England Journal of Medicine 290: 15–19

Brenner P F, Mashchak C A, Lobo R A, Ryoko D-K, Eggena D, Nakamura R M, Mishell D R cited in Campbell S, Whitehead M I 1982 Potency and hepato-cellular effects of oestrogens after oral, percutaneous and subcutaneous administration. In: van Keep P A, Utian W, Vermeulen A (eds) The Controversial Climacteric, pp 103–125. MTP Press, Lancaster

Brinton L A, Hoover R N, Szklo M, Fraumeni J F 1981 Menopausal estrogen use and risk of breast cancer. Cancer 47: 2517–2522

Bungay G T, Vessey M P, McPherson C K 1980 Study of symptoms in middle life with special reference to the menopause. British Medical Journal 2: 181–183

Campbell S, Whitehead M I 1977 Oestrogen therapy and the menopausal syndrome In: Greenblatt R B, Studd J W W (eds) Clinics in Obstetrics and Gynaecology, Vol. 4. No 1, The Menopause, pp 31–47. W B Saunders, Philadelphia

Campbell S, Whitehead M I 1982 Potency and hepato-cellular effects of oestrogens after oral, percutaneous and subcutaneous administration In: van Keep P A, Utian W, Vermeulen A (eds) The Controversial Climacteric, pp 103–125. MTP Press, Lancaster

Carlson L A, Bottiger L E 1972 Ischaemic heart disease in relation to fasting values of plasma triglyceride and cholesterol. Lancet ii: 865–868

Christensen M S, Hagen C, Christiansen C, Transbol I 1982 Dose-response evaluation of cyclic estrogen/gestagen in postmenopausal women: placebo-controlled trial of its gynecologic and metabolic actions. American Journal of Obstetrics and Gynecology 144: 873–879

Christiansen C, Christensen M S, McNair P, Hagen C, Stocklund E, Transbol I 1980 Prevention of early postmenopausal bone loss; controlled 2-year study in 315 normal females. European Journal of Clinical Investigation 10: 273–279

Christiansen C, Christensen M S, Transbol I 1981 Bone mass in postmenopausal women after withdrawal of oestrogen/gestagen replacement therapy. Lancet i: 459–461

Christiansen C, Christensen M S, Grande P, Transbol I 1983 Low risk lipoprotein pattern in postmenopausal women on sequential oestrogen/gestagen treatment (submitted).

Chu J, Schweid A I, Weiss N S 1982 Survival among women with endometrial cancer. A comparison of estrogen users and non-users. American Journal of Obstetrics and Gynecology 143: 569–573

Clayden J R 1973 Effect of clonidine on menopausal flushing. Lancet ii: 1361

Clayden J R, Bell J W, Pollard P 1974 Menopausal flushing: double-blind trial of a non-hormonal medication. British Medical Journal 1: 409–412

Coope J 1976 Double-blind cross-over study of oestrogen replacement therapy In: Campbell S (ed) The Management of the Menopause and Postmenopausal Years, pp 159–168. MTP Press, Lancaster

Cramer D W, Schiff I 1982 Epidemiologic aspects of the benefits and risks of estrogen therapy. In: van Keep P A, Utian W, Vermeulen A (eds) The Controversial Climacteric, pp 137–145. MTP Press, Lancaster

Crilly R G, Horsman A, Marshall D H, Nordin B E C 1978 Postmenopausal and corticosteroid-induced osteoporosis. In: Lauritzen C, van Keep P A (eds) Frontiers in Hormone Research. Vol. 5. Estrogen Therapy, the Benefits and Risks, pp 53–70. S Karger, Basel

Deftos L J, Weisman M H, Williams G W, Karpf D B, Frumar A M, Davidson B J, Parthemore J G, Judd H L 1980 Influence of age and sex on plasma calcitonin in human beings. New England Journal of Medicine 302: 1351–1353

Dennerstein L, Burrows G D 1978 A review of studies of the psychological symptoms found at the menopause. Maturitas 1: 55–64

Dennerstein L, Burrows G D, Hyman G J, Sharpe K 1979a Some clinical effects of oestrogen-progestogen therapy in surgically castrated women. Maturitas 2: 19–28

Dennerstein L, Burrows G D, Hyman G J, Sharpe K 1979b Hormone therapy and effect. Maturitas 2: 247–259

Dyer G, Townsend P T, Jelowitz J, Young O, Whitehead M I 1982 Dose dependent effects of Premarin vaginal cream. British Medical Journal 284: 789–790

Edington R F, Chagnon J-P, Steinberg W M 1980 Clonidine (Dixarit) for menopausal flushing. Canadian Medical Association Journal 123: 1–4

Eggena P, Hidaka H, Barrett J D, Sambhi M P 1978 Multiple forms of human plasma renin substrate. Journal of Clinical Investigation 26: 367–372

Elkik F, Gompel A, Mauvais-Jarvis P cited in Campbell S, Whitehead M I 1982 Potency and hepato-cellular effects of oestrogens after oral, percutaneous and subcutaneous administration In: van Keep P A, Utian W, Vermeulen A (eds) The Controversial Climacteric, pp 103–125. MTP Press, Lancaster

Englund D E 1979 Oestrogen treatment and the menopause. Acta Universitatis Upsaliensis 335

Erlik Y, Tataryn I V, Meldrum D R, Lomax P, Bajorek J G, Judd H L 1981 Association of waking episodes with menopausal hot flushes. Journal of the American Medical Association 245: 1741–1744

Fahraeus L, Wallentin L, Larsson-Cohn U cited in Campbell S, Whitehead M I 1982 Potency and hepato-cellular effects of oestrogens after oral, percutaneous and subcutaneous administration In: van Keep P A, Utian W, Vermeulen A (eds) The Controversial Climacteric, pp 103–125. MTP Press, Lancaster

Follingstad A J 1978 Estriol: the forgotten estrogen. Journal of the American Medical Association 239: 29–30

Gallagher J C, Riggs B L, Eisman J, Hamstra A, Arnaud S B, DeLuca H F 1979 Intestinal calcium absorption and serum vitamin D metabolites in normal subjects and osteoporotic patients. Journal of Clinical Investigation 64: 729–736

Gambrell R D 1978 The prevention of endometrial cancer in post-menopausal women with progestogens. Maturitas 1: 107–112

Gerdes L C, Sonnendecker E W W, Polakow E S 1982 Psychological changes effected by oestrogen-gestagen and clonidine treatment in climacteric women. American Journal of Obstetrics and Gynecology 142: 98–104

Gordon T 1978 Coronary heart disease in young women] incidence and epidemiology In: Oliver M F (ed) Coronary Heart Disease in Young Women, pp 12–19. Churchill Livingstone, Edinburgh

Gordon T, Castelli W P, Hjortland M C, Kannel W B, Dawber T R 1977 High density lipoprotein as a protective factor against coronary heart disease. American Journal of Medicine 62: 707–714

Gusberg S B, Kaplan A L 1963 Precursors of corpus cancer. IV. Adenomatous hyperplasia as Stage O carcinoma of the endometrium. American Journal of Obstetrics and Gynecology 87: 662–678

Hart D M 1982 The prevention of osteoporosis by oestrogen therapy in postmenopausal women. In: Studd J W W (ed) Progress in Obstetrics and Gynaecology, Vol. 2, pp 241–251. Churchill Livingstone, Edinburgh

Heller R F, Jacobs H S 1978 Coronary heart disease in relation to age, sex and the menopause. British Medical Journal 1: 472–474

Hillyard C J, Stevenson J C, MacIntyre I 1978 Relative deficiency of plasma calcitonin in normal women. Lancet i: 961–962

Hirvonen E, Malkonen M, Manninen V 1981 Effects of different progestogens on lipoproteins during postmenopausal replacement therapy. New England Journal of Medicine 304: 560–563

Hoover R, Gray L A, Cole P, MacMahon B 1976 Menopausal estrogens and breast Cancer. New England Journal Of Medicine 295: 401–405

Horsman A, Gallagher J C, Simpson M, Nordin N E C 1977 Prospective trial of oestrogen and calcium in postmenopausal women. British Medical Journal 2: 789–792

Horsman A, Nordin B E C, Crilly R G 1979 Effects on bone of withdrawal of oestrogen therapy. Lancet ii: 33

Hutchinson T A, Polansky S M, Feinstein A 1979 Postmenopausal oestrogens protect against fractures of hip and distal radius. Lancet ii: 706–709

Jasani C, Nordin B E C, Smith D A, Swanson I 1965 Spinal osteoporosis and the menopause. Proceedings of the Royal Society of Medicine 58: 441–444

Jaszmann L 1973 Epidemiology of climacteric and postmenopausal complaints. In: van Keep P A, Lauritzen C (eds) Frontiers of Hormone Research, Vol. 2, Ageing and Oestrogens, pp 22–34. S Karger, Basel

Jick H, Dinan B, Rothman K J 1978 Non-contraceptive estrogens and non-fatal myocardial infarction. Journal of the American Medical Association 239: 1407–1408

Jick H, Watkins R N, Hunter J R, Dinan B J, Madsen S, Rothman K J, Walker A M 1979 Replacement estrogens and endometrial cancer. New England Journal of Medicine 300: 218–222

Jick H, Walker A M, Watkins R N, D'Ewart D C, Hunter J R, Danford A, Madsen S, Dinan B J, Rothman K J 1980 Replacement estrogens and breast cancer. American Journal of Epidemiology 112: 586–594

Judd H L, Cleary R E, Creasman W T, Figge D C, Kase N, Rosenwaks Z, Tagatz G E 1981 Estrogen replacement therapy. Obstetrics and Gynecology 58: 267–275

Johansson B W, Kaij L, Kullander S, Lenner H-C, Svanberg L, Astedt B 1975 On some late effects of bilateral oophorectomy in the age range 15–30 years. Acta Obstetrica et Gynecologica Scandinavica 54: 449–461

Kantor H I, Michael C M, Shore H 1973 Estrogen for older women. American Journal of Obstetrics and Gynecology 116: 115–118

Kaufmann D W, Slone D, Rosenburg L, Miettinen O S, Shapiro S 1980 Cigarette smoking and age at natural menopause. American Journal of Public Health 70: 420–422

Kay C R 1980 The happiness pill? Journal of the Royal College of General Practitioners 30: 8–19

King R J B, Mainwaring W I P 1974 Steroid Cell Interactions, pp 288–378. Butterworths, London

King R J B, Whitehead M I, Campbell S, Minardi J 1979 Effect of estrogen and progestin treatments on endometria from postmenopausal women. Cancer Research 39: 1094–1101

King R J B, Dyer G, Collins W P, Whitehead M I 1980 Intracellular estradiol, estrone and estrogen receptor levels in endometria from postmenopausal women receiving estrogens and progestins. Journal of Steroid Biochemistry 13: 377–382

King R J B, Townsend P T, Whitehead M I 1981a The role of estradiol dehydrogenase in mediating progestin effects on endometrium from postmenopausal women receiving estrogens and progestins. Journal of Steroid Biochemistry 14: 235–238

King R J B, Townsend P T, Whitehead M I, Young O, Taylor R W 1981b Biochemical analyses of separated epithelium and stroma from endometria of premenopausal and postmenopausal women receiving oestrogen and progestins. Journal of Steroid Biochemistry 14: 978–987

Knab D R 1977 Estrogen and endometrial carcinoma. Obstetrical and Gynecological Survey 3: 267–281

Laragh J H, Sealey J E, Ledingham J G, Newton M A 1967 Oral contraceptives; renin, aldosterone and high blood pressure. Journal of the American Medical Association 201: 918–922

Larsson-Cohn U, Wallentin L, Zador G 1979 Plasma lipids and high density lipoproteins during oral contraception with different combinations of ethinyl oestradiol and norgestrel. Hormone and Metabolic Research 11: 437–440

Lightman S L 1982 The neuroendocrinology of menopausal flushing. Journal of Maternal Health and Child Health 7: 68–76

Lindsay R, Hart D M, Aitken J M, MacDonald E B, Anderson J B, Clarke C 1976 Long-term prevention of postmenopausal osteoporosis by oestrogen. Lancet i: 1038–1041

Lindsay R, Hart D M 1978 Failure of response of menopause vasomotor symptoms to clonidine. Maturitas 1: 21–25

Lindsay R, Hart D M, Maclean A, Clarke A C, Kraszewski A, Garwood J 1978 Bone response to termination of oestrogen treatment. Lancet i: 1325–1327

Lindsay R, Hart D M, Maclean A, Garwood J, Clark A C, Kraszewski A 1979 Bone loss during oestriol therapy in postmenopausal women. Maturitas 1: 279–285

Lindsay R, Hart D M, Forrest C, Baird C 1980 Prevention of spinal osteoporosis in oophorectomised women. Lancet ii: 1151–1154

Lindsay R 1982 Dose-response studies of conjugated estrogens in conserving bone mass in postmenopausal women. Poster presented at the World Congress of Obstetrics and Gynecology. San Francisco, October 1982

Mackie M, Bennett B, Ogston D, Douglas A S 1978 Familial thrombosis: inherited deficiency of anti-thrombin III. British Medical Journal 1: 136–138

McKinlay S M, Jefferys M 1974 The menopausal syndrome. British Journal of Preventive and Social Medicine 28: 108–115

Meema S, Bunker M L, Meema H E 1975 Preventative effect of estrogen on postmenopausal bone loss. Archives of Internal Medicine 135: 1436–1440

Meldrum D R, Shamonki I M, Frumar A M, Tataryn I V, Chang R J, Judd H L 1979 Elevations of skin temperature of the finger as an objective index of postmenopausal hot flushes; Standardisation of the technique. American Journal of Obstetrics and Gynecology 135: 713–717

Meldrum D R, Tataryn I V, Frumar A M, Erlik Y, Lu K H, Judd H L 1980 Gonadotrophins, estrogens, and adrenal steroids during the menopausal hot flush. Journal of Clinical Endocrinology and Metabolism 50: 685–689

Milhaud G, Benezech-Lefevre M, Moukhtar M S 1978 Deficiency of calcitonin in age-related osteoporosis. Biomedicine 29: 272–276

Miller G J, Miller N E 1975 Plasma high density lipoprotein concentrations and the development of ischaemic heart disease. Lancet i: 16–19

Molnar G W 1975 Body temperatures during menopausal hot flushes. Journal of Applied Physiology 38: 499–503

Mortality Statistics 1974 (Causes) 1977 Office of Population Censuses and Surveys. D H 2 No 1. Her Majesty's Stationery Office, London

Murray M A F, Hutton J 1978 Plasma oestrogen levels, their significance In: Whitehead M I, Campbell S (eds) Oestrogen and the Menopause, pp 17–22. Abbott, Queenborough

Myrhe E 1978 Endometrial response to different estrogens. In: Lauritzen C, van Keep P A (eds) Frontiers of Hormone Research. Vol. 5. Estrogen Therapy, the Benefits and Risks, pp 126–143. S Karger, Basel

Nachtigall L E, Nachtigall R H, Nachtigall R D, Beckman E M 1979 Estrogen replacement therapy. I. A 10-year prospective study in relationship to osteoporosis. Obstetrics and Gynecology 53: 277–281

Nordin B E C 1960 Osteomalacia, osteoporosis and calcium deficiency. Clinical Orthopaedics 17: 235–257

Nordin B E C, Horsman A, Crilly R G, Marshall D H, Simpson M 1980 Treatment of spinal osteoporosis in post-menopausal women 280: 451–454

Notelovitz M 1982a Carbohydrate metabolism in relation to hormonal replacement therapy. Acta Obstetrica et Gynecologica Scandinavica 106 (Suppl): 51–56

Notelovitz M 1982b Coagulation risks with postmenopausal oestrogen therapy. In: Studd J W W (ed) Progress in Obstetrics and Gynaecology, Vol. 2, pp 228–240. Churchill Livingstone, Edinburgh

Oliver M F, Boyd G S 1959 Effect of bilateral ovariectomy on coronary artery disease and serum lipid levels. Lancet ii: 690–694

Paganini-Hill A, Ross R K, Gerkins V R, Henderson B E, Arthur M, Mack T M 1981 A case-control study of menopausal estrogen therapy and hip fractures. Annals of Internal Medicine 95: 28–31

Paterson M E L, Wade-Evans T, Sturdee D W, Thom M H, Studd J W W 1980 Endometrial disease after treatment with oestrogens and progestogens in the climacteric. British Medical Journal 1: 822–924

Pettiti D B, Wingerd J, Pellegrin F, Ramcharan S 1978 Oral contraceptives, smoking and other factors in relation to risk of venous thromboembolic disease. American Journal of Epidemiology 180: 480–485

Pfeffer R, van den Noort S 1976 Estrogen therapy and stroke risk in postmenopausal women. American Journal of Epidemiology 103: 445–456

Pfeffer R J, Whipple G H, Kurosaki T T, Chapman J 1978 Coronary risk and estrogen use in postmenopausal women. American Journal of Epidemiology 107: 467–487

Recker R R, Saville R D, Heaney R P 1977 Effects of estrogens and calcium carbonate on bone loss in postmenopausal women. Annals of Internal Medicine 87: 649–655

Riggs B L, Hamstra A, DeLuca H F 1981 Assessment of 25-hydroxyvitamin D 1-alpha-hydroxylase reserve in postmenopausal osteoporosis by administration of parathyroid extract. Journal of Clinical Endocrinology and Metabolism 53: 833–835

Robboy S J, Bradley R 1979 Changing trends and prognostic features in endometrial cancer associated with exogenous estrogen therapy. Obstetrics and Gynecology 54: 269–277

Rosenburg L, Armstrong B, Jick H 1976 Myocardial infarction and estrogen therapy in postmenopausal women. New England Journal of Medicine 294: 1256–1259

Rosenberg L, Slone D, Shapiro S, Kaufmann D, Stolley P D, Miettinen O S 1980 Non-contraceptive estrogens and myocardial infarction in young women. Journal of the American Medical Association 244: 339–342

Rosenberg L, Hennekens C H, Rosner B, Berlanger C, Rothman K J, Speizer F E 1981 Early menopause and the risk of myocardial infarction. American Journal of Obstetrics and Gynecology 139: 47–51

Ross R K, Paganini-Hill A, Gerkins V R, Mack T M, Pfeffer R, Arthur M, Henderson B E 1980 A case-control study of menopausal estrogen therapy and breast cancer. Journal of the American Medical Association 243: 1635–1639

Ross R K, Paganini-Hill A, Mack T M, Arthur M, Henderson B E 1981 Menopausal oestrogen therapy and protection from ischaemic heart disease. Lancet i: 858–860

Ryan K J, Engel L L 1953 The interconversion of estrone and estradiol by human tissue slices. Endocrinology 52: 287–291

Siddle N C, Whitehead M I 1983 Pharmacodynamic and biochemical effects of estrogens after different routes of administration. Contemporary Obstetrics and Gynecology (In Press).

Smith P 1972 Age changes in the female urethra. British Journal of Urology 44: 667–676

Sonnendecker E W W, Polakow E S 1980 A comparison of oestrogen/progestogen with clonidine in the climacteric syndrome. South African Medical Journal 58: 753–756

Stevenson J C, Whitehead M I 1982 Postmenopausal osteoporosis. British Medical Journal 285: 585–588

Stevenson J C, Hillyard C J, MacIntyre I, Cooper H, Whitehead M I 1979 A physiological role for calcitonin: protection of the maternal skeleton. Lancet ii: 769–770

Stevenson J C, Hillyard C J, Abeyasejera G, Phang K G, MacIntyre I, Campbell S, Townsend P T, Young O, Whitehead M I 1981 Calcitonin and the calcium-regulating hormones in postmenopausal women: effect of oestrogens. Lancet i: 693–695

Studd J W W, Chakravarti S, Oram D 1977l The climacteric. In: Greenblatt R B, Studd J W W (eds) Clinics in Obstetrics and Gynecology, Vol. 4, No 1, The Menopause, pp 3–29. W B Saunders, Philadelphia

Studd J W W, Collins W P, Chakravati S, Newton J R, Oram D H, Parsons A 1977b Oestradiol and testosterone implants in the treatment of psycho-sexual problems in the postmenopausal woman. British Journal of Obstetrics and Gynaecology 84: 314–315

Studd J W W, Dubiel M, Kakkar V V, Thom M, White P J 1978 The effect of hormone replacement therapy on glucose tolerance, clotting factors, fibronolysis and platelet behaviour in postmenopausal women. In: Cooke I D (ed) The Role of Oestrogen/Progestogen in the Management of the Menopause, pp 41–59. MTP Press, Lancaster

Studd J W W 1979 The Climacteric syndrome. In: van Keep P A, Serr D M, Greenblatt R B (eds) Female and Male Climacteric, pp 23–33. MTP Press, Lancaster

Studd J W W, Thom M H, Paterson M E L, Wade-Evans T 1980 The prevention and treatment of endometrial pathology in postmenopausal women receiving exogenous oestrogens. In: Pasetto N, Paoletti R, Ambrus J L (eds) The Menopause and Postmenopause, pp 127–139. MTP Press, Lancaster

Studd J W W, Thom M H 1981 Oestrogens and endometrial cancer. In: Studd J W W (ed) Progress in Obstetrics and Gynaecology. Vol. 1, pp 182–198. Churchill Livingstone, Edinburgh

Sturdee D W, Wade-Evans T, Paterson M E L, Thom M H, Studd J W W 1978a Relations between bleeding pattern, endometrial histology and oestrogen treatment in menopausal women. British Medical Journal 1: 1575–1577

Sturdee D W, Wilson K A, Pipili E, Crocker A D 1978b Physiological aspects of menopausal hot flush. British Medical Journal 2: 79–80

Tikkanen M J, Nikkila E A, Vartianen E 1978 Natural oestrogen as an effective treatment for Type II hyperlipoproteinaemia in postmenopausal women. Lancet 3: 490–491

Thompson B, Hart S A, Durno D 1973 Menopausal age and symptomatology in a general practice. Journal of Biosocial Science 5: 71–82

Upton G V 1982 The perimenopause: Physiologic correlates and clinical management. Journal of Reproductive Medicine 1: 1–27

Utian W H 1972 The true clinical features of postmenopause and oophorectomy and their response to oestrogen therapy. South African Medical Journal 46: 732–737

Utian W H 1977 Current status of menopause and postmenopausal estrogen therapy. Obstetrical and Gynaecological Survey 32: 193–204

van der Meer J, Stoepman van Dalen E A, Jensen J M S 1973 Anti-thrombin III deficiency in a dutch family. Journal of Clinical Pathology 26: 532–538

Voda A M 1981 Climacteric hot flush. Maturitas 3: 73–90

Vessey M P 1972 Gender differences in the epidemiology of non-neurological disease. In: Ounsted C, Taylor D C (eds) Gender Differences — their Ontogeny and Significance, pp 203–213. Churchill Livingstone, Edinburgh

Weiss N S, Ure C L, Ballard J H, Williams A R, Daling J R 1980 Decreased risk of fractures of the hip and lower forearm with postmenopausal use of estrogen. New England Journal of Medicine 303: 1195–1198

Whitehead M I 1983 Hormone 'replacement' therapy: the controversies. In: Dennerstein L, Burrows G D (eds) Handbook of Psychosomatic Obstetrics and Gynaecology pp 445–481. Elsevier Biomedical Press, Amsterdam

Whitehead M I, Minardi J, Kitchin Y, Sharples M J 1978 Systemic absorption of estrogen from Premarin vaginal cream In: Cooke I (ed) The Role of Estrogen/Progestogen in the Management of the Menopause, pp 63–71. MTP Press, Lancaster

Whitehead M I, King R J B, McQueen J, Campbell S 1979 Endometrial histology and biochemistry in climacteric women during oestrogen and oestrogen/progestin therapy. Journal of the Royal Society of Medicine 72: 322–327

Whitehead M I, Townsend P T, Gill D K, Collins W P, Campbell S 1980 Absorption and metabolism of oral progesterone. British Medical Journal 289: 825–827

Whitehead M I, Lane G, Dyer G, Townsend P T, Collins W P, King R J B 1981a Oestradiol: the predominant intra-nuclear oestrogen in the endometrium of oestrogen-treated postmenopausal women. British Journal of Obstetrics and Gynaecology 88: 914–918

Whitehead M I, Lane G, Young O, Campbell S, Abeyasekera G, Hillyard C J, MacIntyre I, Phang K G, Stevenson J C 1981b Interrelations of the calcium regulating hormones during normal pregnancy. British Medical Journal 1: 10–12

Whitehead M I, Townsend P T, Pryse-Davies J, Ryder T A, King R J B 1981c Effects of estrogens and progestins on the biochemistry and morphology of the postmenopausal endometrium. New England Journal of Medicine 305: 1599–1605

Whitehead M I, Siddle N C, Townsend P T, Lane G, King R J B 1982 The use of progestins and progesterone in the treatment of climacteric and postmenopausal symptoms In: Bardin C W, Milgrom E, Mauvais-Jarvis P (eds) Progesterone and Progestins, pp 277–294. Raven Press, New York

Whitehead M I, Lane G, Siddle N C, Townsend P T, King R J B 1983 Avoidance of endometrial hyperstimulation in estrogen-treated postmenopausal women. In: Speroff L (ed) Seminars in Reproductive Endocrinology, pp 41–53. Thieme-Stratton, New York

Widholm O, Vartianen E 1974 The absorption of conjugated estrogen and sodium estrone sulphate from the vagina. Annales Chirurgiae et Gynecologiae Fenniae 63: 186–190

Yaari S, Goldbourt U, Even-Zohar S, Neufeld H N 1981 Associations of serum high density lipoprotein and total cholesterol with cardiovascular and cancer mortality in a 7 year prospective study of 10,000 men. Lancet i: 1011–1015

Ylikorkala O 1975 Clonidine in the treatment of menopausal symptoms. Annales Chirurgiae et Gynaecologica Fenniae 64: 242–245

Ziel H K, Finkle W D 1976 Association of estrone and the development of endometrial cancer. American Journal of Obstetrics and Gynecology 124: 735–740

Urinary tract injuries during gynaecological surgery

Injury to the urinary tract is a rare complication of gynaecological surgery, despite the fact that the ureters lie concealed in extraperitoneal tissue immediately adjacent to the ovarian and uterine vessels and the cervix, and the bladder and urethra are closely applied to the anterior wall of the vagina. The incidence of such injuries varies with the experience of the surgeon, but in the hands of a competent gynaecologist, and with modern techniques, they probably occur in only 0.5/1.0% of all pelvic operations (Mattingly & Borkowf 1978), possibly rising to nearer 2% with radical hysterectomy (Macasaet et al 1976). These injuries would undoubtedly be more common, were it not for the gynaecologist's constant awareness of this hazard, and the great care that is taken to identify and preserve these structures. Nevertheless, injury does occasionally occur, and when it does, it may lead to difficult convalescence, with prolonged hospitalisation and additional complicated surgical procedures.

In this chapter, the conditions that predispose to injury to the ureters and bladder are outlined, and principles underlying the management of suspected or definite urinary tract damage are described, first when recognised at operation, and secondly, when evidence of injury only becomes evident during convalescence. Experience gained from dealing with 33 urinary fistulas and 12 obstructed ureters associated with, or following gynaecological surgery during the past 12 years will be used to illustrate the principles involved, and the overall results will be summarised at the end.

PREDISPOSING FACTORS

Congenital anomalies pose a constant challenge to the gynaecologist, as they inevitably increase the possibility of damage as a result of capricious and unpredictable variations in the normal anatomy. Duplex ureters occur in about 1 in 125 of the normal population, most commonly in females, and 1 in 6 of them are bilateral. A kidney may be absent in 1 in 1100, ectopic in 1 in 900, situated in the pelvis in 1 in 2100, and both solitary and ectopic in 1 in 22 000. Crossed ectopia, taking the ureter in a grossly abnormal path across the pelvis, occurs in 1 in 2000 (Perlmutter et al 1979). Fused lump or disc kidneys, usually situated in the pelvis, may present to the gynaecologist and should of course be left alone as they generally comprise all the functioning renal tissue that the patient has. Congenital reproductive organ abnormalities often co-exist with urinary anomalies, especially in females: for example, they can be expected in 25 to 50% of cases with unilateral renal agenesis.

The ureters are usually injured either at a relatively high level near the pelvic brim, where they lie adjacent to the ovarian vessels, or low down beside the cervix, where they are crossed by the uterine vessels. The ureters may be included in ligatures which are used to control these vessels; they may be crushed in clamps and subsequently undergo necrosis; or they may simply be partially or completely divided. These complications are most likely to occur in the presence of dense adhesions — as may be produced by pelvic inflammatory disease or endometriosis — or when the normal anatomy of the pelvis is distorted, for example by fibroids or ovarian tumours growing into the broad ligament, which may displace the ureter from its normal position. Occasionally, the ureter may become devitalised and slough after extensive pelvic dissection, as in a Wertheim's hysterectomy, due to interference with its blood supply, particularly after previous pelvic irradiation. Very rarely, the extreme lower end of the ureter may be caught in the high stitches inserted beside the cervix in pelvic floor repair or vaginal hysterectomy.

The bladder may be perforated during abdominal or vaginal hysterectomy, during its separation from the cervix and lower uterine segment, or during anterior colporrhaphy. This danger is greatly increased if there have been previous attempts at repair, or if there has been long standing prolapse, with dense adhesions between the bladder, uterus and cervix.

A preoperative intravenous urogram may alert the gynaecologist to possible future trouble (Fig. 22.1) and thus allow arrangements to be made for more detailed urological assessment (Fig. 22.2) and if necessary, a collaborative approach in the operating theatre.

INJURIES RECOGNISED OR SUSPECTED AT OPERATION

If the ureter is injured during operation, or if there are grounds for suspecting that it may have been crushed, divided or included in a ligature, the entire length of the pelvic ureter is exposed, and the nature and extent of the injury is defined. This may frequently be facilitated by stripping the peritoneum from the side-wall of the pelvis on that side, identifying the ureter, and following it down to the bladder. If injury to the extreme lower end of the ureter is suspected, the bladder should be opened without hesitation, by an anterior cystotomy, and the appropriate ureteric orifice is catheterised. If the catheter ascends easily and no injury is found, the bladder is simply closed with two layers of chromic catgut, and a small Malecot suprapubic tube or urethral catheter is left in for 10/14 days. The bladder usually heals well and nothing is lost. If, on the other hand, ureteric injury is found, reconstruction or reimplantation can proceed without delay, using tissues that are fresh and easily identified.

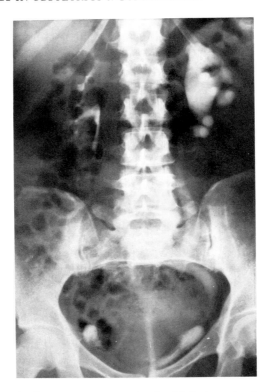

Fig. 22.1 Preoperative intravenous urogram showing left hydronephrosis and hydroureter, cause unknown

If a high ureteric injury is found, direct end-to-end anastomosis is performed (Fig. 22.3). The circumference of the cut ends of the ureters is increased by a 1 cm vertical incision, and they are then joined using fine chromic catgut sutures (*not* silk). This anastomosis is best performed over a ureteric splint. A No. 8 F.G. infant's oesophageal feeding tube (Portex) passed up from the bladder is ideal for this purpose, as it has a Luer connection at its distal end for joining up to the bedside apparatus. Some surgeons prefer a T tube, but this necessarily involves a second hole in the ureter. A corrugated drain is laid down to the anastomosis extraperitoneally, and removed after 4/5 days. The ureteric splint is usually removed after about 10 days (Fig. 22.4).

If a low ureteric injury is found, it is usually possible to reimplant the ureter into the bladder. The lower end of the ureter is dissected out, and may be reimplanted directly into the nearest part of the bladder; or, preferably, the bladder may be opened, and the ureter is then reimplanted with a reflux-preventing procedure into the posterior or lateral wall.

The most important technical point is to ensure that the ureteric reimplantation is performed without tension. This is best achieved by suturing the apex of the bladder to the psoas muscle on that side (the 'bladder hitch')

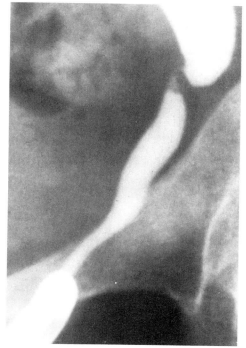

Fig. 22.2 Ascending ureterogram clarifies the situation: endometriosis involving the left ureter

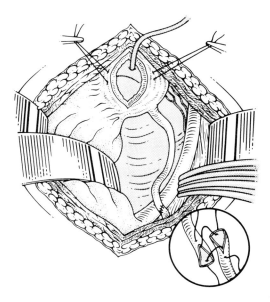

Fig. 22.3 High ureteric injuries are best repaired by end-to-end anastomosis over a splint. An extraperitoneal drain is advisable

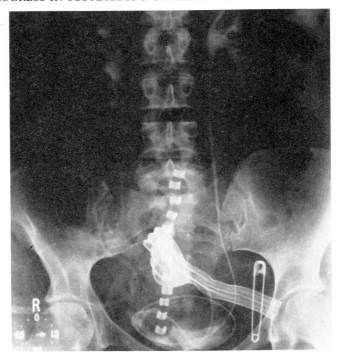

Fig. 22.4 Injury to left ureter (involved with endometriosis) recognised immediately and repaired

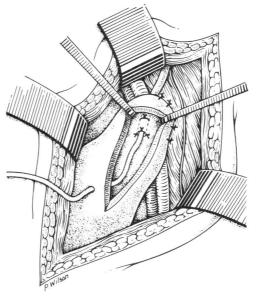

Fig. 22.5 Reimplantation of ureter with reflux preventing submucosal tunnel: note psoas hitch to prevent tension on the anastomosis

(Fig. 22.5). The ureter is brought through a hole in the posterior wall of the bladder, and led down a submucosal tunnel about 2 cm in length, in order to prevent vesico-ureteric reflux. The anastomosis may be splinted as previously described, and the bladder is drained by suprapubic or urethral catheter for 2 weeks.

After radiotherapy or in the presence of dense adhesions, it may not be possible to elevate the peritoneum sufficiently well to perform the ureteric reconstruction extraperitoneally. Under these circumstances, a transperitoneal Boari flap procedure may be preferable (Fig. 22.6): the bladder flap is rolled into a tube and joined to the lower end of the ureter over a splint. This

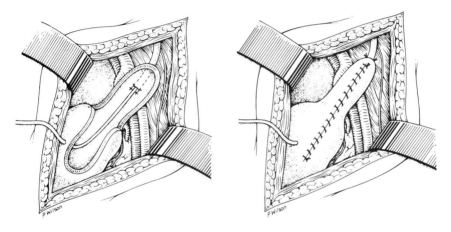

Fig. 22.6 Boari flap: this technique is particularly useful after pelvic irradiation

procedure has the advantage of using well vascularised bladder wall to bridge the gap to the lower end of the ureter, and this is particularly important after previous deep X-ray treatment. However, it is more difficult to prevent reflux with this technique (Figs 22.7 and 22.8) than with the direct reimplant with submucosal tunnel.

During dissection of the cervix and upper vagina, the bladder may be punctured. The opening should be brought into view and its margins defined; the opening is surrounded by a purse-string suture of chromic catgut, and closed. A series of further purse-string sutures may then be inserted, to invaginate the repair. A urethral catheter is then left in for 10/14 days. Occasionally, more extensive opening of the supratrigonal part of the bladder may be necessary — for example, during local excision of a small vault recurrence; under these circumstances, formal two layer closure with omental interposition should be done as in closure of a vesico-vaginal fistula, especially if the patient has previously been irradiated. Specialist urological help should be sought without hesitation in such a case if required.

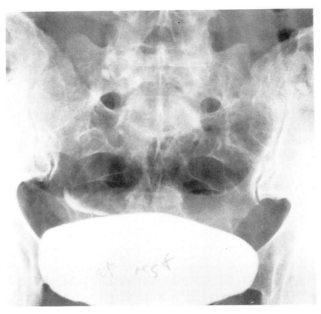

Fig. 22.7 Cystogram at rest showing successful Boari flap reconstruction of lower end of right ureter

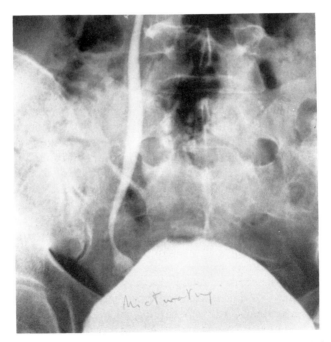

Fig. 22.8 On micturition, gross reflux is seen. This lady had recurrent urinary infection post-operatively

INJURIES RECOGNISED DURING CONVALESCENCE

Ureteric injuries may present after operation in an urgent or non-urgent manner. If the damaged ureter continues to drain urine into the extraperitoneal tissues, pelvic cellulitis may follow; if it drains into the peritoneal cavity, urinary peritonitis will be produced; or if both ureters are injured, anuria may result. On the other hand, ligation of one ureter may produce little more than transient loin pain. Probably the most common delayed presentation is by the development of a urinary fistula, presenting usually per vaginam, or occasionally through the wound.

Where evidence of ureteric damage becomes evident after operation, the precise nature of the injury should be defined before deciding on the best approach to repair. In urgent cases, investigations may be performed as an emergency; in other cases careful evaluation of the lesion may proceed more slowly. A midstream or catheter specimen of urine is sent for bacteriological culture and sensitivities as soon as the possibility of urinary complications is suspected, and repeated specimens should be sent twice a week thereafter. Urological reconstruction is always safer with a sterile urine, but if the urine is infected, sensitivity studies will allow surgery to be performed under appropriate antibiotic cover, and will also provide invaluable guidance on the correct management of septicaemia, should this potentially fatal complication occur.

Blood urea and electrolytes should be checked routinely prior to surgery, and dehydration or electrolyte imbalance may require correction.

A high-dose intravenous urogram is essential, and if correctly performed, will nearly always demonstrate the nature of the complication, although great care must be taken to confirm its exact location, especially since a complex fistula may involve both bladder and ureter. If the site of the injury is not clearly seen on the intravenous urogram, cystoscopy and ascending ureterogram will show in more exactly (Figs 22.9 and 22.10).

Once the nature of the lesion has been defined, a decision on the best form of management can be reached. In some early cases, simple ureteric drainage with a whistle tip or flute-ended catheter may allow a small fistula to heal (Hulse et al 1968). It is always worth waiting for a few days with ureteric or even urethral catheter drainage to see whether the leak will subside. If it does not dry up quickly, however, some form of operative intervention is necessary and there is little point in further delay (Beland 1977). If a ureter is completely obstructed, reconstruction or reimplantation should be undertaken within 3 weeks if worthwhile kidney function is to be preserved.

The operative approach to the repair of ureteric injuries proceeds along similar lines to those outlined in the preceding section: the ureter is generally approached extraperitoneally, and either repaired or reimplanted, with or without a bladder hitch or Boari flap. If a considerable defect has to be bridged, it may occasionally be necessary to do a high transuretero-ureterostomy (Fig. 22.11), or even interpose an isolated loop of ileum between the ureter or ureters

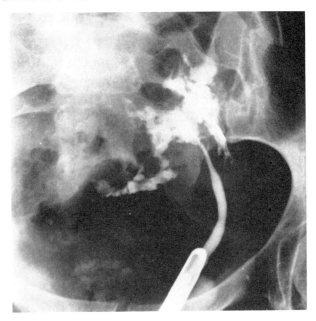

Fig. 22.9 Ascending ureterogram showing urinary extravasation at a high (ovarian renal) level

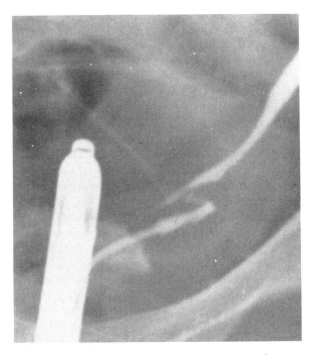

Fig. 22.10 Typical appearance of low uretero-vaginal fistula

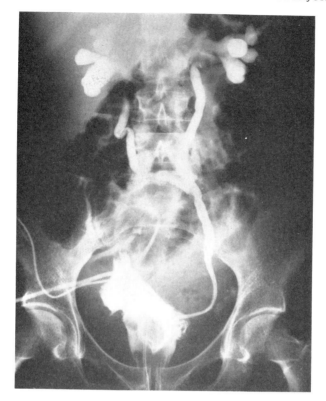

Fig. 22.11 Extensive radionecrotic fistula of right side of bladder and lower right ureter: trans-uretero-ureterostomy and failed primary repair of bladder; *subsequent* ileal loop diversion

and the bladder as uretero-ileo-neocystostomy (Kontturi & Larni 1972, Boxer et al 1979). The latter alternative is particularly useful with bilateral ureteric damage after heavy irradiation and surgery, for example, post-radiotherapy Wertheim's hysterectomy (Figs 22.12–22.14). Rarely, ileal conduit diversion may be the only safe solution to the problems posed by a massive post radiation fistula.

When a vaginal leak occurs after gynaecological surgery, it may not be clear whether it is coming from the bladder or the ureter or both. Under these circumstances, the investigations outlined above — including the intravenous urogram — should be completed in every case, since complicated or double fistulas are by no means uncommon. The 3-swab test may be helpful, but cystoscopy and examination under anaesthetic is essential to confirm the diagnosis, and in planning the repair (Fig. 22.15).

At least 2 months should elapse before considering operative treatment for vesico-vaginal fistula. A few smaller fistulas may heal spontaneously, and in the remainder this time allows infection and oedema to subside, and tissue planes to

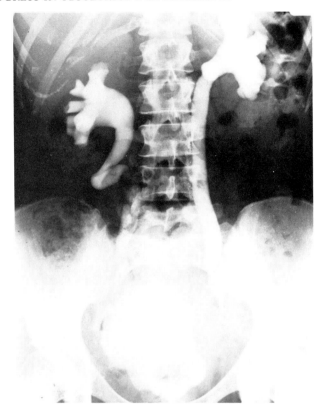

Fig. 22.12 Urinary incontinence 3 months after radiotherapy and Weitheim's hysterectomy — IVP shows bilateral hydroureter and hydronephrosis

be re-established. Closure of vesico-vaginal fistula may be performed vaginally for low lesions (Lawson 1972), transvesically for high lesions, or by a combined approach for large or complex lesions. The author's preference (Fig. 22.16) is for transperitoneal, vesical bivalve repair (Javadpour et al 1973) with omental interposition (Turner-Warwick 1972, Kiricuta & Goldstein 1972). After the repair the bladder is drained by both suprapubic Malecot and urethral Foley catheters for 14 days to ensure adequate drainage.

ANALYSIS OF 45 CASES (1972–1983)

The sites of 33 gynaecological fistulas seen over a 12 year period are shown in Table 22.1. Four ureteric fistulas dried up before they could be operated on — one within a few hours of scheduled reimplantation, much to the surprise of all concerned. A common feature in these cases was clearly visible efflux from the affected ureteric orifice at cystoscopy, even though a ureteric catheter would not go up the ureter. Ureteric reimplantation over an 8Ch splint with psoas

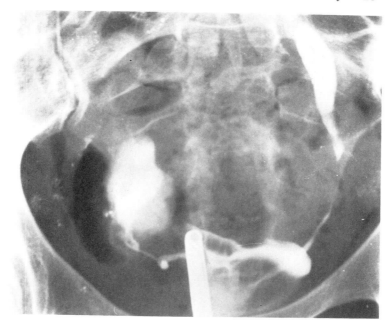

Fig. 22.13 Ureterograms show fistula on right side, stenosis on left

hitch has worked uniformly well, and Boari flap has not been used. Experience of the difficulties associated with a large complex post-irradiation fistula has led to primary use of ileum to by-pass the affected pelvic portions of ureter (Figs 22.12–22.14), either directly reconnected to the bladder if it is intact or diverted to the skin surface if the bladder is hopelessly damaged. Awareness of the possibility of combined bladder and ureteric fistulas has led to routine cystoscopy and bilateral ureterograms prior to definitive repair — a policy also recommended by Murphy et al (1982). The transperitoneal approach to vesico-vaginal fistula with routine omental interposition has given very satisfactory results (three had had previous failed vaginal attempts at repair), but failed once in a bladder with massive post-radiation and post-surgical tissue deficit; primary instead of secondary ileal loop urinary diversion would have been wiser in that case. Overall, the success rate compares favourably with that reported in 47 patients by Goodwin & Scardino (1980).

Twelve patients developed unilateral or bilateral ureteric obstruction associated with or following their gynaecological treatment (Table 22.2). Perry et al (1975) have made the point that uraemia following surgery or radiotherapy for carcinoma of cervix does not necessarily indicate tumour recurrence, and described six long-term survivors with uretero-ileo-neo-cystostomy — we have two such patients, plus another with an ileal conduit. One lady recently required bilateral ureterolysis (with reimplantation on one side) for retroperitoneal fibrosis following apparently successful chemotherapy for

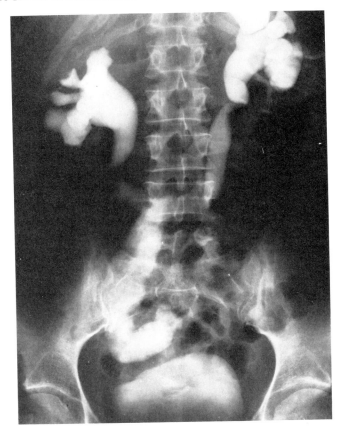

Fig. 22.14 Four years later, after uretero-ileo-neocystostomy, patient well and symptom free

ovarian cancer. Sudden obstructive anuria developed during radiotherapy for advanced carcinoma of cervix in one case, and was relieved by percutaneous nephrostomies (Lang et al 1979) which were removed 3 months later once the tumour had regressed. Urinary diversion has not been favoured in the presence of inoperable recurrent pelvic malignancy, since the prognosis is often so poor (Brin et al 1975), unless fistula formation and uncontrollable wetting has demanded attention (Henry 1978). However, the recently introduced 'double-J' splints which can be inserted cytoscopically can often prolong life comfortably in patients with advanced malignancy.

CONCLUSIONS

Occasional injury to the urinary tract appears to be inevitable, during or after gynaecological surgery due either to congenital anomalies, distortion or

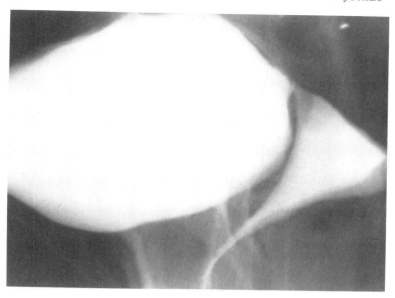

Fig. 22.15 Cystogram showing supratrigonal vesico-vaginal fistula, following hysterectomy

Table 22.1 Management techniques and outcome in 33 gynaecological patients with urinary fistulas (1972–83)

Site of Fistula	Management	Successful outcome/ number of patients
Uretero-vaginal	Conservative	4/4
	Ureteric re-implant	9/9
	Uretero-ileo-neocystostomy	1/1
Vesico-vaginal	Abdominal repair with omentum	14/14
Combined uretero- and vesico-vaginal	Primary repair with reimplant	1/1
	Primary repair (failed) with trans-uretero-ureterostomy; later converted to ileal conduit	0/1
Uretero rectal with bilateral reflux	Ileal conduit	1/1
Vesico-rectal	Primary repair with omentum	1/1
	Pelvic exenteration with ileal conduit	1/1
Total		32/33 (97%)

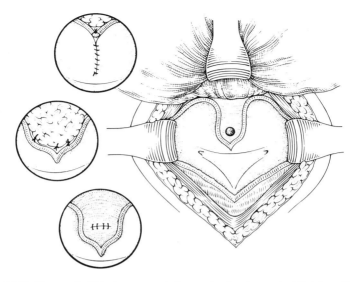

Fig. 22.16 Transvesical bivalve approach for repair of vesico-vaginal fistula, with omental interposition

Table 22.2 Causes of acquired ureteric obstruction and management techniques in 12 patients with gynaecological disease

Cause of obstruction	Number of cases	Management
Post radiation/	1	Ureteric reimplant
chemotherapy/	1	Ureterolysis
surgical fibrosis	2	Uretero-ileo-neo- cystostomy
(patient with		
malignant disease)	1	Ileal conduit
Active carcinoma of cervix	1	Bilateral nephrostomies and radiotherapy
	1	Uretero-ileo-neo- cystostomy
Endometriosis	1	Excision and end-to-end ureteric anastomosis
Surgical ligature	1	Ureterolysis
	1	Ureteric reimplant
	1	Nephrectomy
Pelvic haematoma	1	Conservative

involvement of the tissues by disease, or technical difficulty. If the injury is recognised at the time, primary repair will give the best results. If the damage only becomes evident post-operatively, extreme care must be exercised to locate the injury or injuries accurately, and then to choose the optimum timing and the surest technique for its repair, since failure of the first attempt at repair is profoundly depressing for all concerned.

The gynaecologist must not hesitate to ask for skilled assistance as soon as urinary tract injury is encountered — the urologist has access to diagnostic techniques, and is familiar with reconstructive methods, which should ensure that the problem is dealt with as safely and effectively as possible, with a minimum of delay.

ACKNOWLEDGEMENT

I wish to thank my father, Mr D. W. Hendry, MD, FRCOG, for helpful advice and criticism. Also I would like to thank Mr Philip Wilson for the drawings.

REFERENCES

Beland G 1977 Early treatment of ureteral injuries found after gynecological surgery. Journal of Urology 118: 25–27

Boxer R J et al 1979 Replacement of the ureter by small intestine: clinical application and results of the ileal ureter in 89 patients. Journal of Urology 121: 728–731

Brin E N, Schiff M, Weiss R M 1975 Palliative urinary diversion for pelvic malignancy. Journal of Urology 113: 619–622

Goodwin W E, Scardino P T 1980 Vesicovaginal and ureterovaginal fistulas: a summary of 25 years of experience. Journal of Urology 123: 370–373

Hendry W F 1978 Management of urinary complications of recurrent pelvic malignancy in gynaecological practice. Journal of the Royal Society of Medicine 71: 516–519

Hulse C A, Sawtelle W W, Nadig P W, Wolff H L 1968 Conservative management of ureterovaginal fistula. Journal of Urology 99: 42–49

Javadpour N, John T, Wilson M R, Bush I M 1973 Transperitoneal vesical bivalve in repair of recurrent vesico-vaginal fistula. Obstetrics and Gynecology 41: 469–473

Kiricuta I, Goldstein A M B 1972 The repair of extensive vesico-vaginal fistulas with pedicled omentum: a review of 27 cases. Journal of Urology 108: 724–727

Kontturi M, Larni T K I 1972 Utilisation of the intestine in surgery for major urological complications following gynaecological cancer. Annales Chirurgiae et Gynaecologiae (fenniae) 61: 306–311

Lang E K, Lanasa J A, Garrett J, Stripling J, Palomar J 1979 The management of urinary fistulas and structures with percutaneous ureteral stent catheters. Journal of Urology 122: 736–740

Lawson J 1972 Vesical fistulae into the vaginal vault. British Journal of Urology 44: 623–631

Macasaet M A, Lu T, Nelson J H 1976 Uretero-vaginal fistula as a complication of radical pelvic surgery. American Journal of Obstetrics and Gynecology 124: 757–760

Mattingly R F, Borkowf H I 1978 Acute operative injury to the lower urinary tract. Clinics in Obstetrics and Gynaecology 5: 123–149

Murphy D M, Grave P A, O'Flynn J D 1982 Ureterovaginal fistula: a report of 12 cases and review of the literature. Journal of Urology 128: 924–925

Perlmutter A D, Retik A B, Bauer S R 1979 Anomalies of the upper urinary tract. In: Harrison J H et al (ed) Campbell's Urology, 4th edn, pp 1309–1398. W B Saunders, Philadelphia

Perry C P, Massey F M, Moore J N, Erickson C A 1975 Treatment of irradiation injury to the ureter by ileal substitution. Obstetrics and Gynecology 46: 517–522

Turner-Warwick R 1972 The use of pedicle grafts in the repair of urinary tract fistulae. British Journal of Urology 44: 644–656

Cancer of the cervix in young women

Both the incidence of and the mortality from cancer of the cervix uteri in young women are increasing. In the two South Thames Regions, the *incidence* of carcinoma *in situ* and of cancer of the cervix have increased considerably in women aged under 40; between 1970 and 1980 the incidence of carcinoma *in situ* has more than doubled in the 30–34 year old age group and the incidence of cancer of the cervix has more than doubled in the 35–39 year old age group (Table 23.1). The *mortality* from cancer of the cervix in England and Wales in the 25–34 year old age group has almost trebled (Table 23.2).

The results of treatment of early cancer of the cervix with radiotherapy or with radical surgery or with a combination of the two are very good (Table 23.2). However, the aim should be to give the young patient with cancer of the cervix a normal life span with minimal morbidity. In the author's view this is best achieved with radical surgery used alone.

AETIOLOGY

There is now abundant evidence that squamous cell cancer of the cervix is a sexually transmitted disease. It is more common if coitus begins at an early age, if there have been several sexual partners, if the socio-economic group is low and if parity is high. Jewish women have a low incidence, especially if they are orthodox. Nuns have a low incidence while prostitutes have a high incidence (Rotkin 1973).

If the husband has an occupation which involves frequent absence from home, the wife has a high risk of contracting cancer of the cervix. (Beral 1974, Skegg et al 1982). In Beral's study wives of 'clerks of work' had a standardised mortality ratio of 40, whereas wives of 'deck and engineroom ratings, barge and boatmen' had a standardised mortality ratio of 263. Presumably these marked differences occur because extramarital coitus is more common in the latter group. Barrier techniques of contraception seem to protect against cancer of the cervix (Wright et al 1978). In the study of Wright et al (1978) diaphragm users had a low incidence (0.17 per 1000 women–years) compared with users of oral contraceptives (0.95 per 1000 women–years) or intra-uterine devices (0.87 per 1000 women–years). Even after adjusting for age at first coitus and number of
378

Table 23.1 Incidence per 100 000 women of carcinoma-in-situ and carcinoma of the cervix in the two South Thames Regions (from The South Thames Cancer Registry)

Age	Carcinoma *in situ* 1970	1980	Cancer 1970	1980
20–24	6.3	14.5	0	1.4
25–29	19.8	38.8	3.2	8.1
30–34	26.3	56.1	6.1	11.7
35–39	21.7	39.1	7.8	16.4
40–44	30.6	22.0	17.8	14.9
45–49	21.1	14.2	24.1	18.0
50–54	11.4	6.7	31.7	17.0
55–59	6.3	2.3	28.2	20.1

Table 23.2 Deaths per million population from cancer of the cervix (from the Office of Population Censuses and Surveys)

Age	1970	1975	1980
25–34	11	20	30
35–44	59	49	56
45–54	184	135	110
55–64	203	207	190
Over 65	239	216	209
All ages	94	85	82

sexual partners, diaphragm users still had only about one-quarter of the risk of those using the other two methods of contraception.

What is the sexually transmitted factor which causes squamous cancer of the cervix? The herpes simplex type 2 virus and the genital wart virus seem to be likely contenders (Meisels 1981).

In a recent four year study of the 114 patients with mild dysplasia, 23% (7 of 31) with herpes simplex type 2 antibodies developed severe dysplasia whereas only 9% (6 of 66) of those with herpes simplex type 1 antibodies only had lesions which progressed (Coleman 1983). It has also been shown that in a high proportion of cervical cancers, herpes simplex type 2 virus RNA is present (Eglin et al 1982).

A theory linking the herpes simplex type 2 virus and the genital wart virus has been described recently (Zur Hansen 1982). The genital wart virus can produce flat lesions on the cervix which are difficult to distinguish colposcopically or cytologically from dysplasia, the virus being demonstrable by electron microscopy and producing the characteristic histological changes of koilocytosis, double nucleation and dyskeratosis (Kirkup et al 1982).

A viral cause would be particularly interesting because vaccination might substantially reduce the incidence of cancer of the cervix.

Table 23.3 Five year percentage survivals of patients with Stage I cancer of the cervix after radiotherapy and after radical surgery (after Peel, 1978)

Radiotherapy		
Newton	(1975)	74
Masabuchi	(1969)	88
Joslin	(1976)	94

Radical surgery (+ postoperative radiotherapy if nodes involved)		
Newton	(1975)	81
Masabuchi	(1969)	90
Hoskins	(1976)	87
Stallworthy	(1976)	82 ⎫
Kolstad	(1973)	88 ⎬ +preoperative intra-cavitary radiotherapy
Currie	(1971)	86 ⎭

CERVICAL INTRA-EPITHELIAL NEOPLASIA

In theory the detection and treatment of cervical intra-epithelial neoplasia should reduce the incidence of frank cancer. Cervical smears should begin to be taken when coitus begins, since cervical pre-malignancy and malignancy are sexually transmitted conditions; and women at particular risk, such as those who begin sexual activity at an early age, or who have had a genital viral infection, should have a cervical smear test every year. In the author's view other women should have cervical smear tests at least every 2 years but this may strain local cytology services.

In British Columbia an intensive cervical cytology campaign has reduced the incidence of cervical cancer from 28.4 per 100 000 in 1955 to 8.6 per 100 000 in 1974 while the mortality has fallen from 11.4 per 100 000 in 1958 to 4.8 per 100 000 in 1974.

The subject of cervical intra-epithelial neoplasia has been dealt with in a previous article (Jordan 1982). However, the principles of management are as follows.

Before puberty there is a linear junction between the squamous epithelium overlying the ectocervix and the columnar epithelium lining the endocervix. Oestrogen makes the cervix pout so that columnar epithelium comes onto the ectocervix. This happens particularly at puberty, with oestrogen containing oral contraceptives and during pregnancy. This columnar epithelium, exposed to acidic conditions within the vagina, undergoes physiological squamous metaplasia gradually turning into squamous epithelium. It is in this zone that cervical intra-epithelial neoplasia may develop. Abnormal cervical smears can be investigated by colposcopy after application of 3% acetic acid to the cervix which makes areas of CIN go white or show a mosaic pattern or punctation pattern of abnormal capillaries. Biopsies can be taken from these abnormal areas with a punch biopsy forceps and, if invasion is excluded histologically, the whole transformation zone can be destroyed with diathermy, laser, cryocoagulation or the 'cold' coagulator. Laser is probably the most satisfactory because the depth of destruction can be accurately controlled; it is important to destroy to a depth of 7 mm to ensure destruction of any abnormal epithelium in gland crypts. Furthermore general anaesthesia is not necessary for laser treatment.

If the whole transformation zone cannot be seen because the upper limit lies in the cervical canal or if there are colposcopic features suggestive of malignancy, such as an irregular surface contour or abnormal capillaries, a traditional cone biopsy must be taken. The aim of a cone biopsy is to excise the whole transformation zone. Cone biopsy is best avoided in young women because of its adverse affect on subsequent pregnancy, midtrimester miscarriage, pre-term labour and prolonged labour due to cervical stenosis necessitating delivery by Caesarean section all being more common (Jones et al 1979).

Conveniently most young women have a transformation zone clear of the external os making conservative management easy. It remains to be seen if young women treated with local destructive techniques perform better in a subsequent pregnancy than those treated with traditional cone biopsy.

MICROINVASION

Microinvasive squamous cell cancer of the cervix is an important entity because it can be treated effectively without radical surgery or radiotherapy. It is symptomless and usually diagnosed by histological examination of a cervical biopsy.

There is considerable dispute about where to draw the line between microinvasion and macroinvasion. A reasonable view seems to be that microinvasion means that the tumour has not gone more than 4 mm below the basement membrane with no involvement of lymphatic vessels (Ullery et al 1965). However, some authors draw the line at invasion for 1 mm (Friedell & Graham 1959) and others at as much at 9 mm (Morton 1964). Recently there have been attempts to define microinvasion as meaning a volume of invasive tumour of 500 mm^3 or less (Burghardt 1977, 1979).

Another problem is that different histologists may have different views about whether invasion of any kind is present or not. Involvement of a gland crypt may look very like invasion beyond the basement membrane.

Treatment of microinvasive cancer is also controversial. Most gynaecologists would advise hysterectomy but there is no need to remove the ovaries, parametrium or pelvic lymph nodes. If the transformation zone extends onto the vagina a cuff of vagina should be removed this being most conveniently achieved during vaginal hysterectomy. The vaginal vault is treated with Lugol's iodine which stains normal squamous epithelium mahogany brown. If the incisions are placed in this normal epithelium, no dysplastic epithelium should be left.

Some authors advise an even more conservative approach to microinvasive cancer of the cervix regarding cone biopsy as adequate treatment since spread to the uterine fundus from a microinvasive cervical cancer has never been reported (Burghardt 1977). This view may well be appropriate to a young woman who wants a pregnancy but close cytological and colposcopic follow-up is indicated. It may be wise to ask for a second opinion on the microscopic appearance in such cases. If the pathologists are uncertain about whether the diagnosis is of carcinoma *in situ* or of microinvasion, a conservative approach is reasonable. If the difficulty is in deciding between microinvasion and macroinvasion, then hysterectomy is the minimum appropriate treatment.

EARLY INVASIVE CANCER OF THE CERVIX

Clinical features

A very early cancer of the cervix may be symptomless and diagnosed from microscopical examination of a biopsy taken as part of the investigation of an abnormal cervical smear. There may be post coital bleeding, intermenstrual bleeding or vaginal discharge and the cervix should always be inspected and a smear taken for cytology in any patient with one of these symptoms. Any suspicious lesion must be biopsied especially as cervical cytology may be normal in the presence of a frank cancer; the necrotic tissue overlying the cancer may be all that is scraped off. The lesion may be a polyp or an ulcer; however with an infiltrating lesion the cervix may be simply bulky and friable. An early adenocarcinoma of the endocervix may be particularly difficult to diagnose as the cervix may look completely normal.

Advanced cancer of the cervix may cause pain from involvement of pelvic nerves or lethargy from renal failure secondary to bilateral ureteric obstruction.

Staging

Staging is based on clinical features and patients with suspected cancer of the cervix need thorough examination under general anaesthesia performed by or at least supervised by an experienced gynaecologist. Firstly, cystoscopy should be done to ensure that there is no invasion of the bladder. Secondly, a vaginal examination should be performed with biopsy of the lesion on the cervix and curettage of the uterine cavity. Thirdly, a rectal examination should be made to assess rectal or parametrial involvement and also to see if there are any pelvic side wall masses. 'Parametrial induration' may in fact be adnexal induration from chronic salpingitis or endometriosis.

Clearly radical surgery will be curative only if the cancer is limited to the cervix or involving a small amount of the upper vagina or involving the uterine cavity. If there is any parametrial involvement the resection line may cross malignant tissue and if there is involvement of the bladder or rectum, these structures will have to be removed as well making radical surgery much more dangerous. An intravenous pyelogram should always be done. Obstruction of the ureters may be due to malignant involvement and since the ureters are

Table 23.4 The spectrum of cervical intraepithelial neoplasia (CIN) and cervical malignancy

CIN 1:	mild dysplasia
CIN 2:	moderate dysplasia
CIN 3:	severe dysplasia or carcinoma *in situ*
Stage IA cancer:	microinvasion
Stage IB cancer:	macroinvasion
Stage IIA cancer:	spread to upper two-thirds of the vagina
Stage IIB cancer:	spread to parametrium
Stage IIIA cancer:	spread to lower third of the vagina
Stage IIIB cancer:	spread to pelvic side wall
Stage IV cancer:	spread into bladder, into rectum or beyond pelvis

pelvic wall structures, involvement of them precludes surgery. It should be remembered that there are other causes of abnormal intravenous pyelography. There may be a long standing ureteric calculus or stricture or one kidney may be congenitally absent. Chest X-ray and an ultrasound scan of the liver rarely show evidence of metastases and computerised axial tomography of the pelvis does not yet have any obvious advantage over clinical examination in staging.

Staging is of fundamental importance to the individual patient ensuring that she has appropriate treatment. It is also important to the assessment of the results of treatment and to comparison of results from different oncological centres.

Treatment, surgery or radiotherapy

If the patient is young and fit and if the tumour is at Stage I or very early stage IIA, then in the author's opinion radical surgery has overwhelming advantages over radiotherapy used alone or radiotherapy followed by radical surgery. Cure rates are similar (Table 23.3) but there is much less morbidity with radical surgery.

What is meant by the words 'young and fit'? Women aged under 50 are clearly young and require treatment which will conserve vaginal function and if possible ovarian function as well. Women aged over 50 are also 'young' if they are in other respects fit and if they do not have problems which would make surgery or general anaesthesia unduly hazardous such as obesity, cardiac disease or respiratory disease.

Radiotherapy has several disadvantages in the young woman. It is in itself *carcinogenic*; the radium menopause has fallen into disfavour mainly for this reason. The latent period is long so that this is less of a problem in older women.

Radiotherapy may cause *radiation cystitis* with frequency and haematuria. Although a Wertheim hysterectomy partially denervates the bladder and bladder sensation may be reduced, this is not usually an incapacitating symptom.

Radiotherapy may cause *radiation proctitis* with diarrhoea and rectal bleeding or even a rectal stricture, the latter usually associated with the placement of an isotope in the vagina rather than with external radiotherapy.

Radiotherapy may cause *radiation vaginitis* with narrowing, discharge and dyspareunia. This problem is aggravated by oestrogen deficiency caused by destruction of ovarian function during radical pelvic radiotherapy, unless oestrogen replacement therapy is given.

In a study of 75 patients, 78% of those treated with radiotherapy alone had sexual dysfunction compared with 6.2% of those treated with surgery alone and 33% of those treated with surgery and radiotherapy together (Abitbol & Davenport 1974).

Of the 28 radiotherapy patients in this study, 12 had lack of libido and disappearance of sexual climax, 11 had dyspareunia, 15 had the feeling during coitus that the vagina was narrow or short, four were afraid of recurrent cancer and three stated that their husbands had stopped coitus because of 'lack of satisfaction'. The lubrication of the vagina and the ballooning of its upper two-thirds, both of which normally precede orgasms are impaired by the lack of vascularity and elasticity of the vagina after radiotherapy. Similar views on the adverse effect of radiotherapy on sexual function have been reached in other studies (Seibel et al 1980).

Oestrogen deficiency is inevitable after radiotherapy to the pelvis. With a Wertheim hysterectomy it is permissible to leave one or both ovaries with a stage I well differentiated tumour. However whether the ovaries have been removed or irradiated, oestrogen tablets or implants can be given to correct oestrogen deficiency.

The main disadvantages of radical surgery are that there is an operative mortality, a risk of pulmonary embolism and a risk of ureteric fistula. The *operative mortality* should be low and most studies report mortalities of about 1% or less.

The risk of *pulmonary embolism* should be substantially reduced by covering every Wertheim hysterectomy with subcutaneous heparin injections (Kakkar 1972).

The risk of *ureteric fistula* formation is low in most recent series (Mascasaet et al 1976) and in any event a ureteric fistula due to a Wertheim hysterectomy can be cured and is not life threatening although it can be a considerable nuisance to the patient and an embarrassment to the surgeon.

Technique of Wertheim's hysterectomy

Wertheim performed the first radical hysterectomy in 1898 and reported a series of 270 cases in 1905 (Wertheim 1905). The operation was first extensively performed in this country by Victor Bonney. There are numerous detailed accounts of operative technique in the textbooks of operative gynaecology.

The object of the operation is to remove the uterus, tubes, ovaries (usually), parametrium, upper third of the vagina (at least) and the pelvic lymph nodes. Most surgeons remove the external iliac nodes, internal iliac nodes, obturator nodes and common iliac nodes but some remove the para-aortic nodes as well, this addition increasing the morbidity of the operation and the time taken to perform it. The ureters have to be identified and dissected from the pelvic brim to their entrance into the bladder but the dissection should not be so tidy and meticulous as to render them avascular so causing avascular necrosis with a ureteric fistula. The uterine vessels should be ligated lateral to the ureters so that a reasonable amount of parametrium can be removed. The operation can be performed perfectly adequately through a long Pfannenstiel incision, but this does not allow access to the para-aortic lymph nodes.

Post-operative management

Although the pelvic drain, wound drain and intravenous infusion can be removed usually after 48 hours, a Foley catheter should be left in the bladder for 10 days. The urine should be kept sterile by the administration of prophylactic antibiotic (e.g. amoxycillin) and by culturing catheter specimens of urine, promptly treating any infection. Heparin 5000 units with the premedication and twice daily for 7 days reduces the risk of venous thrombo-embolism. Shock or post-operative anaemia should be corrected by transfusion. The patient should be mobilised early and given chest and lower limb physiotherapy. If a watery vaginal discharge occurs there may be a *urinary fistula*. Pyridium should be given orally; this makes the urine bright orange and this test will confirm that the watery fluid emerging from the vagina is in fact urine. A uretero vaginal fistula can be distinguished from a vesico vaginal fistula by instilling methylene blue into the bladder; a swab placed in the vagina will be stained blue if the fistula is vesico vaginal in which case leaving a Foley catheter in the bladder for 2–3 weeks should result in healing of the fistula which may otherwise be closed surgically by a vaginal or trans-vesical approach. If the fistula is ureterovaginal, the ureters should be catheterised if possible via a cystoscope. If this splinting is achieved, the fistula may heal without further treatment. Otherwise formal re-implantation of the ureter into the bladder six months later may be necessary unless the fistula heals spontaneously during this period which 50% do (Macasaet et al 1976).

A *rectovaginal fistula* may occur. This may heal spontaneously especially if the stools are made firm with a bulk laxative such as Normacol. Otherwise formal repair vaginally or abdominally with a temporary defunctioning transverse colostomy may be necessary.

If *venous thrombosis* or *pulmonary embolism* are suspected, the diagnosis should be confirmed with phlebography or an isotopic lung scan and full anti coagulation instituted. This complication should be uncommon if subcutaneous heparin has been given prophylactically. If histological examination shows *pelvic lymph node metastases* the five year survival rate for stage I cases is almost half that for such cases without lymph node metastases (Masubuchi et al 1969, Currie 1971). For this reason postoperative external radiotherapy is usually advised although there is no clear evidence that survival rates are increased.

Young women who have had both ovaries removed should be prescribed *oestrogen therapy*.

ADVANCED INVASIVE CANCER

Radiotherapy is indicated if the cervical cancer has advanced beyond a very early stage IIA. Radium was the first agent to be used in various techniques. The Stockholm method was established in 1914, the Paris method in 1919 and the Manchester method in 1938. An intrauterine tube and two vaginal ovoids of radium deliver a high dose of radiation to the cervix with rapid diminution of dose with distance. The parametrium and pelvic side walls can then be treated with external radiotherapy. The disadvantage of intracavitary treatment with radium is that the operator has to insert the radium with some exposure therefore to the radiation. Furthermore the patient has to be nursed on a ward usually for about 24 hours; care is necessary to ensure that other patients are not unduly close to her and that the radium when removed is placed immediately in a lead-lined box and returned to the isotope curator. Losing a radium source is clearly a serious matter.

For these reasons *after loading techniques* are now popular. Applicators are placed in the uterus and vagina and their position adjusted without hurry. The applicators are then connected to a remote radiation safe through a system of flexible tubes and the radioactive sources are then moved mechanically into the patient. The patient stays in a shielded room while the treatment personnel leave, observing the patient through a closed circuit television system. Using the Cathetron with radioactive cobalt, as at St Thomas's Hospital, London, each treatment takes a few minutes only.

SPECIAL PROBLEMS

Adenocarcinoma of the cervix

These constitute 5–10% of cervical cancers. The aetiology is not clear cut but there is a link between clear-cell adenocarcinomata of the cervix and diethyl stilboestral exposure in utero (Herbst et al 1971). They are said to be less radiosensitive than squamous cell cancers and the arguments in favour of radical surgery for cases occurring in young women are even stronger therefore.

Cervical cancer in pregnancy

A cervical smear test suggestive of cervical intra-epithelial neoplasia or cervical cancer in pregnancy should be investigated by colposcopy and if there are no features suggestive of invasion the colposcopy can be repeated every two months and the lesion dealt with in the normal way after delivery. Cervical biopsy in pregnancy may cause heavy vaginal bleeding and a formal cone biopsy may cause miscarriage or premature labour.

Cervical cancer presents with vaginal bleeding in pregnancy and the diagnosis may be confused with threatened miscarriage or antepartum haemorrhage. The cervix should always be inspected in such patients and any lesion suspected of being invasive should be biopsied.

In early pregnancy a Wertheim hysterectomy can be performed and although no gynaecological oncologist can claim a large experience of this problem, anecdotes indicate that the operation is not unduly difficult.

In late pregnancy steroids can be administered to accelerate fetal lung maturation, an amniocentesis can be performed to ensure that the lecithin sphingomyelin ratio is satisfactory, and the baby can be delivered by Caesarean section, a Wertheim hysterectomy being performed at the same time.

Recurrence

If cervical cancer recurs after a Wertheim hysterectomy, radiotherapy may be used. Recurrence after radiotherapy may be treated with a Wertheim hysterectomy only if the recurrence is limited to the cervix. Because the tissues are devascularised, fistulae and pelvic fibrosis are more common in these circumstances. Treatment of recurrence despite these treatments is difficult but a recent report suggests that bromocriptine may be worth trying (Guthrie 1982).

Terminal cases

A young woman dying of cervical cancer despite treatment will often have many domestic problems and the sympathetic help of a social worker may be needed especially to ensure that any children are properly looked after. Pain can be relieved with opiates in full dosage and sometimes epidural injections of phenol may help. Nausea and anxiety can be relieved with phenothiazines, given rectally if necessary, and depression can be relieved with tricyclic antidepressants. The patient should remain at home for as long as possible preferably with visits from a special Support Team of nurses experienced in the care of the dying. When the patient comes into hospital to die, every effort should be made to ensure that her death is as dignified as possible with medical investigation or intervention only if designed to make her more comfortable.

SUMMARY

Cervical cancer is becoming commoner in young women probably because of the changes in attitudes to sex and in contraceptive technique which occurred in the 1960s. There are strong arguments in favour of primary treatment with radical surgery rather than with radiotherapy. If it is found that cervical cancer is caused by a virus, then vaccination may reduce the risk. Women at particular risk of cervical cancer because of their sexual behaviour should have annual cervical smear tests.

ACKNOWLEDGMENTS

The author thanks Mr R. G. Skeet of The South Thames Cancer Registry for providing statistics showing the incidence of carcinoma *in situ* and cancer of the cervix.

REFERENCES

Abitbol M M, Davenport J H 1974 Sexual dysfunction after therapy for cervical carcinoma. American Journal of Obstetrics and Gynecology 119 2: 189

Beral V 1974 Cancer of the cervix: a sexually transmitted infection? Lancet i: 1037

Burghardt E, Holzer E 1977 Diagnosis and treatment of microinvasive carcinoma of the cervix uteri. Obstetrics and Gynecology 49: 641

Burghardt E 1979 Microinvasive carcinoma. Obstetrical and Gynaecological Survey 34: 836

Coleman D V 1983 Herpes simplex virus and cervical cancer. Personal communication

Currie D W 1971 Operative treatment of carcinoma of the cervix. Journal of Obstetrics and Gynaecology of the British Commonwealth 78: 385

Eglin R P, Sharp F, Maclean A B, Cordiner J W, Kitchener H C, Macnab J C M, Clements J B, Wilkie N M 1982 Herpes Simplex virus — type 2 coded material in cervical neoplasia In: Jordon J A, Sharp F, Singer A (eds) Preclinical Neoplasia of the cervix, p. 31. Royal College of Obstetricians and Gynaecologists, London

Friedell G H, Graham J B 1959 Regional lymph node involvement in small carcinoma of the cervix. Surgery, Gynaecology and Obstetrics 108: 513

Guthrie D 1982 Treatment of carcinoma of the cervix with bromocriptine. British Journal of Obstetrics and Gynaecology 89: 853

Herbst A L, Ulfelder H, Poskanzer D C 1971 Adenocarcinoma of the vagina: association of maternal stilboestral therapy with tumor appearance in young women. New England Journal of Medicine 284: 878

Hoskins W J, Ford J H, Lutz M H, Averette H E 1976 Radical hysterectomy and pelvic lymphadenectomy for the management of early invasive cancer of the cervix. Gynaecologic Oncology 4: 278

Jones J M, Sweetnam P, Hibbard B M 1979 The outcome of pregnancy after cone biopsy of the cervix: a case control study. British Journal of Obstetrics and Gynaecology 86: 913

Jordan J A 1982 The management of pre-malignant conditions of the cervix. In: Studd J (ed) Progress in Obstetrics and Gynaecology, Vol. 2, p. 151. Churchill Livingstone, Edinburgh

Joslin C A 1976 Management of cervical malignant disease — radiotherapy. In: Jordan J, Singer A (eds) The Cervix, p. 494. W B Saunders, London

Kakkar V V, Corrigan T P, Spindler J, Fossard D P, Flute P T, Crellin R Q, Wessler S, Yin E T 1972 Efficacy of low doses of heparin in prevention of deep vein thrombosis after major surgery. Lancet ii: 101

Kirkup W, Evans A S, Brough A K, Davis J A, O'Loughlin T, Wilkinson G, Monaghan J M 1982 Cervical intraepithelial neoplasia and 'warty' atypia: a study of colposcopic, histological and cytological characteristics. British Journal of Obstetrics and Gynaecology 89: 571

Kolstad P 1973 Gynaecologic Oncology: present status and future aspects. American Journal of Obstetrics and Gynaecology 115: 597

Macasaet M A, Lu T, Nelson J H 1976 Uterovaginal fistula as a complication of radical pelvic surgery. American Journal of Obstetrics and Gynecology 124: 757

Masubuchi K, Tenjin Y, Kubo H, Kimura M 1969 Five year cure rate for carcinoma of the cervix uteri. American Journal of Obstetrics and Gynecology 103: 566

Meisels A, Roy M, Fortier M, Morin C, Casas-Cordero M, Shah K V, Turgeon H 1981 Human papillomavirus infection of the cervix: the atypical condyloma. Acta Cytologica 25: 7

Morton D G 1964 Incipient carcinoma of the cervix. American Journal of Obstetrics and Gynecology 90: 64

Newton M 1975 Radical hysterectomy or radiotherapy for stage I cervical cancer. American Journal of Obstetrics and Gynecology 123: 535

Peel K R 1978 Surgery of Cervical Carcinoma In: Lees D H, Singer A (eds) Clinics in Obstetrics and Gynaecology, Vol. 5, p. 659. W B Saunders, London

Rotkin I D 1973 A comparison review of key epidemiological studies in cervical cancer related to current searches for transmissible agents. Cancer Research 33: 1353

Seibel M M, Freeman M G, Graves W L 1980 Carcinoma of the cervix and sexual function. Obstetrics and Gynaecology 55: 484

Skegg D C G, Corwin P A, Paul C 1982 Importance of the male factor in cancer of the cervix. Lancet ii: 581

Stallworthy J, Wiernik G 1976 Management of cervical malignant disease — combined radiotherapy and surgical techniques. In: Jordan J A, Singer A (eds) The Cervix, p. 474. W B Saunders, London

Ullery J C, Boutselis J G, Botschner A C 1965 Microinvasive carcinoma of the cervix. Obstetrics and Gynaecology 26: 866

Wertheim E 1905 A discussion on the diagnosis and treatment of cancer of the uterus. British Medical Journal 2: 689

Wright N H, Vessey M P, Kenward B, McPherson K, Doll R 1978 Neoplasia and dysplasia of the cervix uteri and contraception: a possible protective effect of the diaphragm. British Journal of Cancer 38: 273

Zur Hausen H 1982 Human genital cancer: synergism between two virus infections or synergism between a virus infection and initiating events. Lancet ii: 1370

Carcinoma of the vulva — which operation when?

For approximately 30 years it was accepted that carcinoma of the vulva should be treated by radical vulvectomy together with groin and pelvic node dissection. This belief was founded on the work of Taussig (1935) and Way (1954), both of whom demonstrated the very much improved survival statistics when patients were treated in this manner. In spite of these figures, critics have been unhappy, especially when these radical procedures were carried out on old women, resulting in death or prolonged stay in hospital awaiting the healing of large groin wounds. Little, if any, evidence was available to show that this standard approach could be modified or tailored to the individual patient until the early '70s. At this time it was suggested (Rutledge et al 1970) that those patients with small tumours (T1,NO,MO), with a depth of invasion of less than 5 mm may not require a groin node dissection, as there was little evidence of metastases in this group of patients. Wharton et al 1974, reported on a series of 25 patients who met these criteria, 15 of whom were treated with radical vulvectomy alone and 10 of whom had additional pelvic node dissection. They reported a 100% 5 year survival rate.

These reports stimulated a considerable amount of study and comment; it rapidly became clear sadly that the parallel with microinvasive carcinoma of the cervix was an over simplification and far from the truth. Many authorities subsequently reported cases and series showing nodal metastases and deaths in patients with T1,NO,MO, tumours with less than 5 mm of invasion (Nakao 1974, Parker et al 1975, Diapola et al 1975, Jafari & Cartnick 1976, Yasigi et al 1978).

INDIVIDUALISATION OF TREATMENT

A number of factors must be considered before _individualisation_ of treatment can become a reality in carcinoma of the vulva. These factors and other determinants of metastatic potential will be discussed.

General medical condition of the patient

Carcinoma of the vulva is most commonly seen in women in the seventh decade of life, consequently these patients often have significant medical problems including hypertension, obesity, diabetes and heart and lung disease. It is important that these complicating factors are assessed prior to any decision about the type of operative procedure to be performed. This assessment must be made by the surgeon and his anaesthetist, not arbitrarily by a physician who will not be involved in the surgery, anaesthesia or after care of the patient. The judgement must be made in the light of the experience of the surgeon and anaesthetist; if they work closely together in a department dealing with a large number of such cases then the operability rate will inevitably rise, increasing further with the use of spinal and epidural anaesthesia. Reports from major centres commonly quote operability rates of the order of 96% (Monaghan & Hammond 1984, Podratz et al 1982).

Stage of tumour

The staging of carcinoma of the vulva has always been unsatisfactory, it clearly requires an operative staging system but over the years has been bedevilled by using the TNM non-operative method of staging. This system was adopted by FIGO in 1970 but has severe limitations which include:

1. Size of tumour is only recorded at 2 cm and does not allow for larger lesions (see later data).
2. No account is taken of the position of the tumour.
3. No account is taken of the histology of the tumour.
4. Inaccuracy of palpation of groin nodes (see later data).

Errors in clinical staging of vulval squamous carcinoma can be unacceptably high, reaching 25% (Podratz et al 1980), and in a series of malignant melanomas from the same institution, 31% inaccurate assessments were noted (Podratz et al 1983). The TNM system has more serious staging limitations in malignant melanoma in that many tumours are less than 2 cm in diameter but conversely are extremely aggressive and tend to have wide spread metastatic patterns (Podratz et al 1983, Monaghan & Hammond 1984).

Histology and differentiation of tumour

Most carcinomas of the vulva are squamous in type (85%). Approximately 9% are melanomas and the remaining 6% are made up of carcinomas of the Bartholin's gland, sarcomas and other rare cancers. Among the squamous carcinomas are included basal cell carcinomas and verrucous carcinomas, both of which are relatively benign and can be adequately dealt with by simple surgery, usually in the form of wide local excision (see Table 24.1).

Thus it is important that an adequate biopsy is taken prior to any decision about the extent of surgery. Both basal cell and verrucous carcinomas have a very low propensity for lymphatic metastases (Japaze et al 1981), therefore anything more than a vulvectomy or a wide local excision is quite unnecessary. Conversely although many melanomas are very small when diagnosed, their

Table 24.1 Relative aggression of carcinoma of the vulva

Tumour		Treatment
Basal cell carcinoma	Least aggressive	Local excision or vulvectomy
Verrucous carcinoma	Least aggressive	Local excision or vulvectomy
Squamous carcinoma	More aggressive	Radical vulvectomy + groin node dissection
Melanoma	Most aggressive	Radical vulvectomy +/− pelvic & groin node dissection
Carcinoma of Bartholin's gland	Most aggressive	Radical vulvectomy +/− pelvic & groin node dissection
Sarcomas	Most aggressive	Radical vulvectomy +/− pelvic & groin node dissection

high node metastasis rate indicates that an en bloc dissection of at least the groin nodes is essential. In those patients affected by squamous cell carcinomas the degree of differentiation is closely related to the metastatic potential. In 1960 Way showed almost a two fold increase in metastases when anaplastic squamous carcinomas were compared with well differentiated tumours. Iversen et al (1981) found no difference in the two groups. Andreasson et al (1981) found a lower metastatic rate in better differentiated tumours only in those cases less than 4 cm in diameter, but the author has found a statistically significant difference when squamous carcinoma differentiation was related to nodal metastases (Table 24.2).

Penetration

A further sophistication of assessment has been advocated for malignant melanoma by Clark et al (1969) assessing depth of penetration of the tumour (Clark's levels), and by Breslow (1970) measuring the depth of penetration. A progressive decrease in survival is seen as the melanoma reaches the lower levels

Table 24.2 Vulval carcinoma histology and nodal metastasis

Tumour		Groin nodes		Pelvic nodes	
		n	+ve	n	+ve
Squamous cell	Well differentiated	97	19(19.5%)	53	2(3.7%)
	Moderately differentiated	29	15(52%)	16	1(6%)
	Poorly differentiated	37	17(46%)	17	2(12%)
	$\chi^2 = 15.51$ $P<0.001$				
Melanoma		7	3(43%)	2	0
TOTAL		170		88	

of the epithelium (level II-V), so that when the disease reaches the subcutaneous levels (level V), then the survival drops rapidly and the recurrence rates reaches 78% (Podratz et al 1983). It also appears that only those patients with disease in levels IV and V exhibit nodal metastases. There is considerable evidence that an en bloc dissection of the inguinal and/or pelvic lymph nodes with radical vulvectomy is the optimum management for lesions reaching these deeper levels. In the author's series although groin node metastases occurred in 43% of patients none had involvement of the pelvic nodes.

Primary carcinoma of the Bartholins gland is rare, representing approximately 1–3% of all vulval tumours. This disease is characterised by a high node metastasis rate (37.3%, Leuchter et al 1982), in this quoted series there was an 18% pelvic node involvement. Even those patients with negative groin nodes have a poor 5 year survival of 52% (Leuchter et al 1982). This compares very badly with squamous carcinoma of the vulva where similar node negative patients can expect to have a 94% chance of surviving 5 years (Monaghan et al 1984). Pelvic node dissection as part of the basic management may not be necessary unless more than four groin nodes are involved, (Curry et al 1980), and when pelvic nodes are involved the prospects for salvage are extremely poor. It is commonly written that carcinoma of the Bartholins gland has a capacity for direct spread to the pelvic lymph nodes, however the only case reported is that of Barclay et al (1964).

Size of tumour

Podratz et al (1982) showed that the larger the tumour the greater the chance of metastases. In the author's present series of over 160 groin and/or groin and pelvic node dissections it has been observed that there is a clear cut-off point at 4 cm diameter between those with pelvic node metastases (> 4 cm), and those without (< 4 cm) (Table 24.3). A similar observation was noted by Andreasson et al (1980). Thus by reserving pelvic node dissection only for those patients with tumours greater than 4 cm a small but significant salvage would be achieved without subjecting all patients to the procedure.

Table 24.3 Size of tumour related to nodal metastases

Size of tumour	Groin nodes		Pelvic nodes	
	n	+ve	n	+ve
<4 cm diameter	84	19 (22.6%)	40	0
>4 cm diameter	80	32 (40.0%)	47	5 (10.6%)
		$\chi^2 = 4.99\ P < 0.05$	Fishers exact test $P < 0.0415$	

Site of tumour

Most carcinomas of the vulva affect the labia, the left slightly more often than the right; the second commonest site is the clitoris. It has been thought that carcinomas affecting the clitoris required more aggressive management. The lymphatics of the clitoris were thought to communicate directly with the pelvic lymphatics, (Parry-Jones 1963). This direct communication has never been satisfactorily demonstrated and recent work by Iversen & Aas (1983) did not find any evidence of such a communication. They also demonstrated the frequent bilateral flow of the clitoral lymphatics and evidence of contralateral flow alone from laterally placed injection of radionucleide in the labia (28/42, 67%). They did not demonstrate higher lymph flow rates from any particular part of the vulva. However care must be used in interpreting this study as they used patients with *carcinoma of the cervix* and no allowance was made or could be made for any disturbance of lymphatic drainage in the presence of *vulvar carcinoma*.

There is no evidence that the pelvic nodes should be routinely dissected simply because the clitoris is involved, unless the groin nodes are heavily infiltrated and in these circumstances the salvage is low.

In the author's series the clitoris was involved in 54 out of 200 cases, 47 of which had nodal dissections. Twenty five (53%) had metastases to the groin nodes but only two (4.2%) had metastases to the pelvic nodes, thus giving little support for the routine dissection of pelvic nodes. Piver & Xynos (1977), in a similar sized series, came to the same conclusion.

Laterality

It has been proposed that when a vulvar carcinoma affects the labia alone and does not impinge on the clitoris, urethra, vagina, fourchette or perianal region, that it may be practicable to carry out a local excision or vulvectomy plus an ipsilateral groin node dissection, the contralateral nodes being preserved. This proposal is based on the belief that contralateral spread alone and bilateral spread from a laterally placed tumour is extremely rare. Hacker et al (1984) stated that they had never seen positive contralateral nodes with negative ipsilateral nodes, they developed their argument further by stating that if ipsilateral nodes are found to be negative then a contralateral dissection is unnecessary. This has not been the author's experience (Table 24.4), a small but significant number of patients with very small tumours have contralateral

Table 24.4 Site of tumour (200 cases, 199 had site recorded)

Left side tumours n = 44			Right side tumours n = 41		
		NODE METASTASES			
Ipsilateral	Contralateral	Bilateral	Ipsilateral	Contralateral	Bilateral
7	2	0	6	1	1

n = node dissections

alone or bilateral spread. It is impossible at the moment to accurately determine which tumours will spread to the contralateral nodes and to date preoperative assessments by palpation, fine needle aspiration and lymphography have proved of little value.

Groin node status

Palpation of groin nodes has been notoriously inaccurate in the author's experience (Table 24.5). Benedet et al (1979) quoted error rates of between 13% and 39%. *Lymphography* has also been disappointing in spite of the relative accessibility of the groin nodes, giving false positive results for fatty nodes and false negative for nodes totally replaced by tumour. This technique demands great skill and interest and unfortunately varies in reliability from one centre to another. *Fine needle aspiration* may be able to assist in confirming significant metastases, but is limited where there are small metastases and peripheral sinus emboli.

Intra-operative sampling has been used to determine whether to proceed to pelvic node dissection. Curry et al (1980) stated that where four or more nodes were involved pelvic node dissection should be carried out.

Monoclonal radionucleide labelling may have a role to play in the assessment of involvement of nodes by metastatic disease.

Table 24.5 Palpation of groin nodes v metastases

	Number cases	Groin nodes	
	n	–ve	+ve
Not palpable	118	89 (75%)	29 (25%)
Palpable — mobile	48	27 (56%)	21 (44%)
Palpable — fixed	4	1 (25%)	3 (75%)

'Microinvasion'

After the initial enthusiasm of Rutledge (1970) and Wharton et al (1974) it was shown in some studies that lymph node metastases could occur with depths of invasion below 3 mm (Yasigi et al 1978, Andreasson 1981, Hacker et al 1983). It is not uncommon to see node metastasis rates of between 8 and 20% quoted for tumours invading less than 5 mm. It is clear that it is not only depth of invasion which determines the tumour's capacity for metastasis. These other factors will include vascular space involvement, plasma cell/lymphocyte infiltration, and confluence of tumour.

Vascular space involvement. Parker et al (1975) and Iversen et al (1981) both commented that vascular space involvement by tumour was the most important prognostic factor in determining metastases in tumours invading less than 5 mm.

Plasma cell/lymphocytic infiltration. Andreasson et al (1981) found improved survivals with severe or moderate local immune cellular reaction.

Confluence. Depth of invasion and confluence and nodal metastases were found to be strongly related by Hoffman et al (1983). Their series showed 17 out of 47 cases (36%) which exhibited confluence had nodal metastases, whereas none out of 31 cases without confluence had any nodal spread.

Conclusion.

It is now becoming clear that it is not justifiable to dispense with groin node dissection unless the depth of invasion is less than 1 mm (Hacker et al 1984). The groin node dissection must include all nodes, no attempt should be made to distinguish between the superficial and the deep inguinal node systems.

SPREAD OF VULVAR CARCINOMA — EMBOLISATION OR PERMEATION?

When surgery for carcinoma of the vulva is limited to vulvectomy alone the results are very poor. The very good long-term results following radical surgery and groin node dissection speak for themselves (Table 24.6). The extremely high survival rates in patients with negative nodes frequently tempts less experienced operators and some who should know better, to adopt a more conservative technique, dispensing with the groin node dissection. The usual

Table 24.6 Life tables for vulval carcinoma (January, 1984)

	Cases (n)	Five year survivals
All cases	200	68.3%
RV + GND negative nodes	46	94.7%
RV, GND + PND negative nodes	107	89.6%
RV + PND	61	88.2%
RV, GND + PND positive nodes	50	27.9%

RV — radical vulvectomy; GND — groin node dissection;
PND — pelvic node dissection.

end result is disaster. It is clear that the groin node dissection is not only capable of dealing with gross metastases in the nodes, but also effectively removes micrometastases which are not histologically visible. These are removed when the groin nodes are removed en bloc, in direct continuity with the vulvar dissection. Would the same result occur if the groin nodes were dissected as a separate bloc from the vulvar operation?

There are no large series comparing the results of dissection in continuity with those of separate incisions. The separate incisions will depend for their success on the hypothesis that squamous carcinoma of the vulva spreads by embolisation and not by permeation (Willis 1973). The author believes that small tumours spread by embolisation primarily and then later will fill the lymphatic channels and spread by permeation. It is also frequently seen that in large tumours the groin lymphatics become obstructed and then retrograde lymphatic permeation occurs especially down the lymph channels running alongside the saphenous vein. The author feels that it is important that the relative merits of separate groin incisions versus the traditional dissection in continuity with the vulva should be fully evaluated, but feels that success will only be achieved where the tumour has spread by embolisation and therefore the separate incision procedure should probably be reserved for very small early tumours.

METASTATIC VULVAR CARCINOMA.

Unfortunately vulvar carcinoma is a disease characterised by delay both on the part of the patient and of the attending medical practitioner; it is not uncommon to see delays of a number of years being reported. The consequence of this is that frequently the patient presents with widespread disease. It is important to realise that, even with diseases involving the pelvic organs or fungating groin nodes, it may still be possible to cure the patient or at worst improve her state to such an extent that she can live (and die) with a degree of dignity.

Distant metastases are not a contraindication to carrying out a radical vulvectomy and groin node dissection. It is frequently possible to completely remove all local disease and leave the patient with a clean vulva and groin, and although the patient will die from the distant metastases, the mode of death will be much improved.

Fungating groin nodes should be removed in continuity with the vulva, and ideally combined with a pelvic node dissection. Occasionally it is found that the pelvic nodes are clear of tumour and the prospects for the patient are very much improved (Table 24.6).

Pelvic organ involvement including the bladder, anus and rectum and vagina demands a more aggressive approach. If the patient is fit she should be considered for an exenterative procedure using the techniques of total, anterior or posterior exenteration to achieve clearance of all tumour. Lesions which extend into the anus but do not invade further than the pectinate line may be treated by radical ano-vulvectomy rather than posterior exenteration. Lesions extending further into the anus and rectum must be treated by exenterative techniques because of the different lymphatic drainage. If the tumour invades bone, the bones of the pubic arch being most commonly affected, then it may be effectively removed by resecting a segment of bone in with the specimen. A patient so treated is able to walk without difficulty in spite of the loss of a segment of her bony pelvis.

Recurrent disease

Following radical vulvectomy and groin node dissection most recurrences occur on the vulva with very few in the groin. One of the reasons for this to occur is because although most surgeons will produce adequate lateral margins for the resection it is very common to see structures such as the end of the urethra being preserved at all costs, whereas by removing the end 1–1.5 cm the risk of recurrence can be markedly reduced. Most recurrences should be managed by surgery using the standard principles of adequate margins and wide local excision. Occasionally surgery may be combined with radiotherapy or chemotherapy to deal with a recurrence in a difficult position.

Groin recurrences are very difficult to deal with and unless they are small may need local radiotherapy to attempt to treat them. One must therefore be very cautious before dispensing with groin node dissection as an integral part of the basic management of this disease.

There can be nothing worse than to have had an inadequate primary procedure and then to have a recurrence of the carcinoma presenting multiple management problems.

As with all cancers the first chance of treatment is the best chance.

SUMMARY

Except where the patient's medical condition does not allow the radical vulvar operation and groin node dissection, this procedure should be regarded as the optimum minimal surgery for carcinoma of the vulva.

Only when the tumour invades less than 1 mm can groin node dissection be dispensed with.

Conversely, pelvic node dissection should only be added to the basic procedure when there is a significant risk of metastases, i.e. when the tumour is greater than 4 cm in diameter or when the tumour is poorly differentiated, or a melanoma.

REFERENCES

Andreasson B, Bock J E, Weberg E 1980 Invasive cancer in the vulva region. *Ugeskr.Laeg.* 1942: 1067–1071

Andreasson B, Bock J E, Visfeldt J 1981 Prognostic role of histology in squamous carcinoma in the vulvar region. Gynecologic Oncology 24: 373–381

Barclay D L, Collins C R, Macey A B 1964 Cancer of the Bartholin gland: A review and report of 8 cases. Obstetrics and Gynecology 24: 329

Benedet J L, Turko M, Fairey R N, Boyes D A 1979 Squamous carcinoma of the vulva: results of treatment, 1938 to 1976. American Journal of Obstetrics and Gynecology 134: 201–207

Breslow A 1970 Thickness, cross sectional areas and depth of invasion in the prognosis of cutaneous melanoma. Annals of Surgery 172: 902–908

Clark W H, From L, Bernadino E A, Mihm M C 1969 The histogenesis and biologic behavior of primary human malignant melanomas of the skin. Cancer Research 29: 705–726

Curry S L, Wharton J T, Rutledge F N 1980 Positive lymph nodes in vulvar squamous carcinoma. Gynecologic Oncology 9: 63–67

Diapola G R, Gomez-Rueda N, Arrighi L 1975 Relevance of microinvasion in carcinoma of the vulva. Obstetrics and Gynecology 45: 647–649

Hacker N H, Berek J S, Lagasse L D, Nieberg R K 1983 Microinvasive carcinoma of the vulva. Obstetrics and Gynecology 62: 134–135

Hacker N F, Berek J S, Lagasse L D, Nieberg R K, Leuchter R S 1984 Individualisation of treatment for Stage I squamous cell vulvar carcinoma. Obstetrics and Gynecology 63: 155–162

Hoffman J S, Kumar N B, Morley G W 1983 Microinvasive squamous carcinoma of the vulva: search for a definition. Obstetrics and Gynecology 61: 615–618

Iversen T, Abeler V, Aalders J 1981 Individualised treatment of stage I carcinoma of the vulva. Obstetrics and Gynecology 57: 85–89

Iversen T, Aas M 1983 Lymph drainage of the vulva. Gynecologic Oncology 16: 179–189

Jafari K, Cartnick E N 1976 Microinvasive squamous cell carcinoma of the vulva. Gynecologic Oncology 4: 158–166

Japaze H, Van Dinh T, Woodruff J D 1981 Verrucous carcinoma of the vulva: study of 24 cases. Obstetrics and Gynecology 60: 462–466

Leuchter R S, Hacker N F, Voet R L, Berek J S, Townsend D E, Lagasse L D 1982 Primary carcinoma of the Bartholin gland: a report of 14 cases and review of the literature. Obstetrics and Gynecology 60: 361–368

Monaghan J M, Hammond I G 1984 Pelvic node dissection in the treatment of vulval carcinoma — is it necessary? British Journal of Obstetrics and Gynaecology 91: 270–274

Nakao C Y, Nolan J F, Disaia P J, Futoran R 1974 'Microinvasive' epidermoid carcinoma of the vulva with an unexpected natural history. American Journal of Obstetrics and Gynecology 120: 1122–1123

Parker R T, Duncan I, Rampone J, Creasman W 1975 Operative management of early invasive epidermoid carcinoma of the vulva. American Journal of Obstetrics and Gynecology 123: 349–355

Parry-Jones E 1963 Lymphatics of the vulva. British Journal of Obstetrics and Gynaecology 70: 751–765

Piver M S, Xynos F P 1977 Pelvic lymphadenectomy in women with carcinoma of the clitoris. Obstetrics and Gynecology 49: 592–595

Podratz K C, Symmonds R E, Taylor W F, Williams T J 1980 Treatment of invasive squamous cell carcinoma of the vulva at the Mayo clinic 1955–1975. (Abstract) Gynecologic Oncology 10: 362

Podratz K C, Symmonds R E, Taylor W F 1982 Carcinoma of the vulva: analysis of treatment failures. American Journal of Obstetrics and Gynecology 143: 340–351

Podratz K C, Gaffey T A, Symmonds R E, Johansen K L, O'Brien P C 1983 Melanoma of the vulva: an update. Gynecologic Oncology 16: 153–168

Rutledge F N, Smith J P, Franklin E W 1970 Carcinoma of the vulva. American Journal of Obstetrics and Gynecology 106: 1117–1130

Taussig F J 1935 Primary cancer of the vulva, vagina and female urethra: five year results Surgery Gynecology and Obstetrics 60: 477

Way S 1954 Results of a planned attack on carcinoma of the vulva. British Medical Journal 2: 780

Way S 1960 Carcinoma of the vulva. American Journal of Obstetrics and Gynecology 79: 692–698

Wharton J T, Gallagher S, Rutledge F N 1974 Microinvasive carcinoma of the vulva. American Journal of Obstetrics and Gynecology 118: 159–162

Willis R A 1973 The Spread of Tumours in the Human Body, 3rd edn, pp 19–30. Butterworth, London

Yasigi R, Piver M, Tsukada Y 1978 Microinvasive carcinoma of the vulva. Obstetrics and Gynecology 51: 368–370

Index

400

PROGRESS IN OBSTETRICS AND GYNAECOLOGY

Contents of Volume 3